HEALTHY INSPIRATION

REFLEXOLOGY

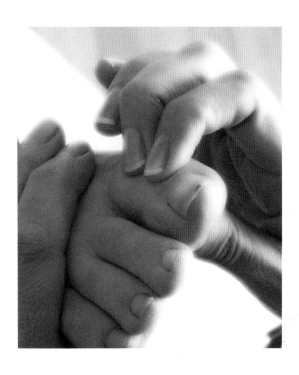

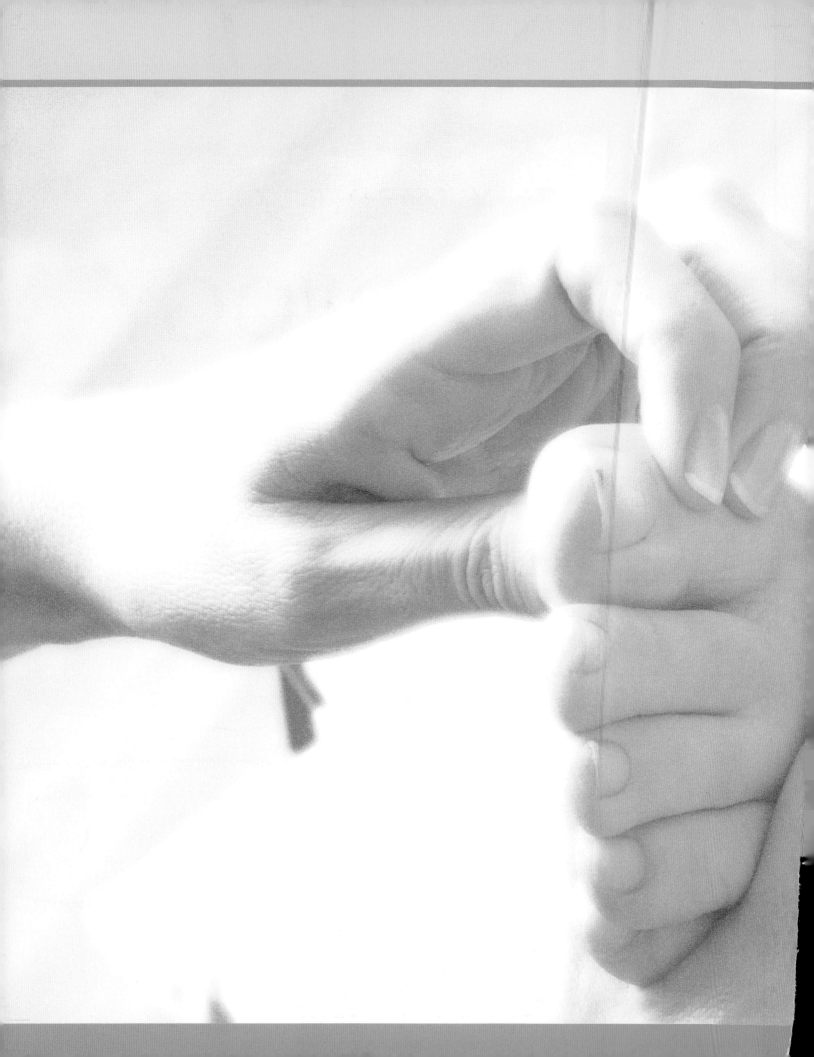

HEALTHY INSPIRATION

REFLEXOLOGY

Denise Whichello Brown

Published by SILVERDALE BOOKS
An imprint of Bookmart Ltd
Registered number 2372865
Trading as Bookmart Ltd
Blaby Road
Wigston
Leicester LE18 4SE

© 2006 D&S Books Ltd

D&S Books Ltd
Kerswell,
Parkham Ash, Bideford
Devon, England
EX39 5PR

e-mail us at:- enquiries@d-sbooks.co.uk

This edition printed 2005

ISBN 1-84509-274-0

DS0139. Healthy inspirations Reflexology

Creative Director: Sarah King
Editor: Clare Haworth-Maden
Project editor: Nicky Barber
Designer: Debbie Fisher & Co.
Photographer: Paul Forrester

Fonts: Rotis Sans Serif and Vag Rounded

Printed in China

1 3 5 7 9 10 8 6 4 2

Contents

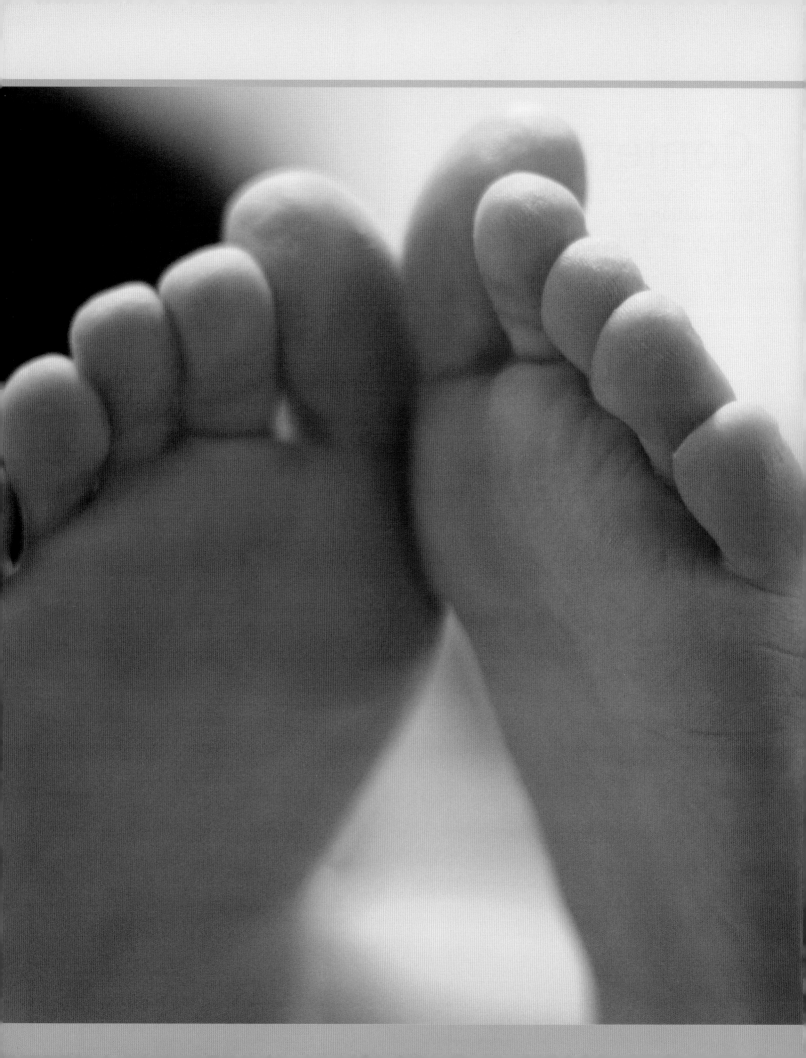

Introduction –
reflexology is for everyone!

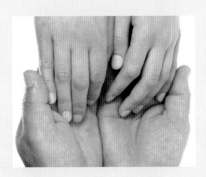 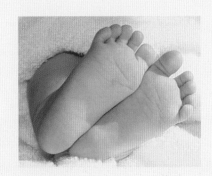 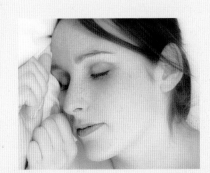

The ancient healing art of reflexology can be practised and enjoyed by everyone!

It is an invaluable tool, both for helping yourself and for improving the health of your

friends and family.

This simple, straightforward, yet comprehensive, guide is fully illustrated and very easy to follow. It is suitable for the absolute beginner, as well as for the student reflexologist who is embarking upon professional training. There are many guides to foot reflexology, but very few books have been written about hand reflexology, making this book a must because it covers both hand and foot reflexology. It is your choice whether to work on the hands or the feet, and you may even decide to use a combination of foot and hand reflexology.

Whether you treat the feet or the hands, or both, reflexology is so simple, yet you can achieve the most amazing results with it. So if you are looking for a way of relieving the stress of everyday life, or are seeking a therapy with which to alleviate common ailments, let this book be your guide and your inspiration.

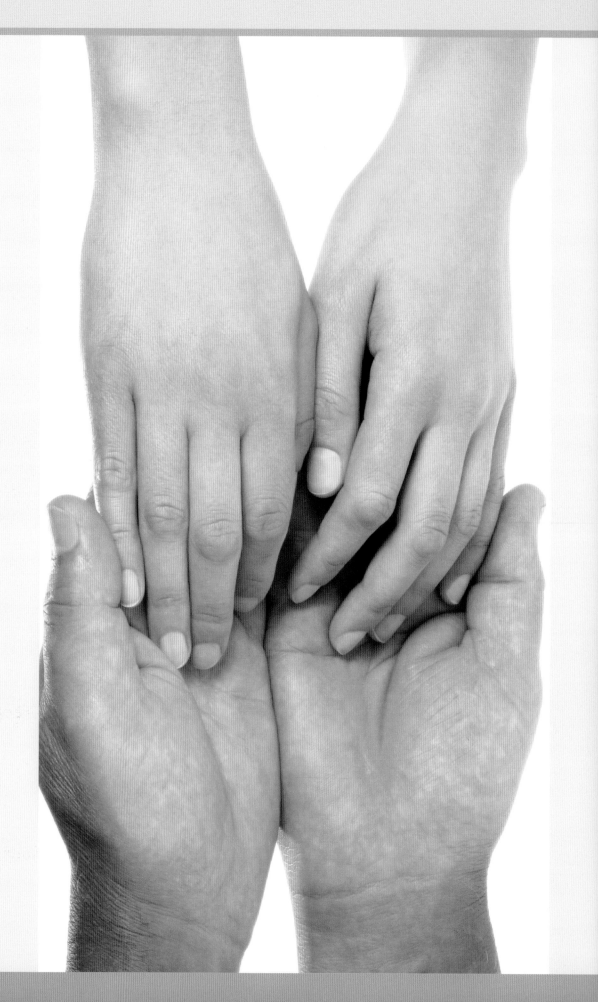

What is reflexology?

Reflexology is a simple, natural and non-invasive touch therapy that has many health benefits. To touch and to be touched is a fundamental, instinctive need in all of us. Indeed, the first sense that the human embryo develops is that of touch, and the close bond that develops between mother and baby is the basis of our human need for touch. We all instinctively have the power in our hands to touch and to heal, and to enable others to enjoy the benefits of reflexology.

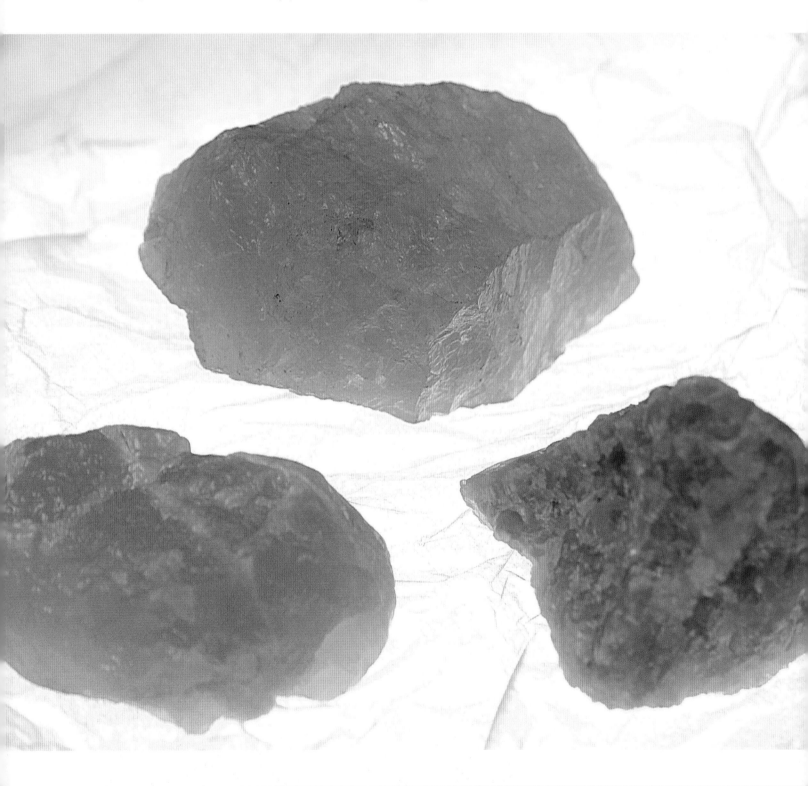

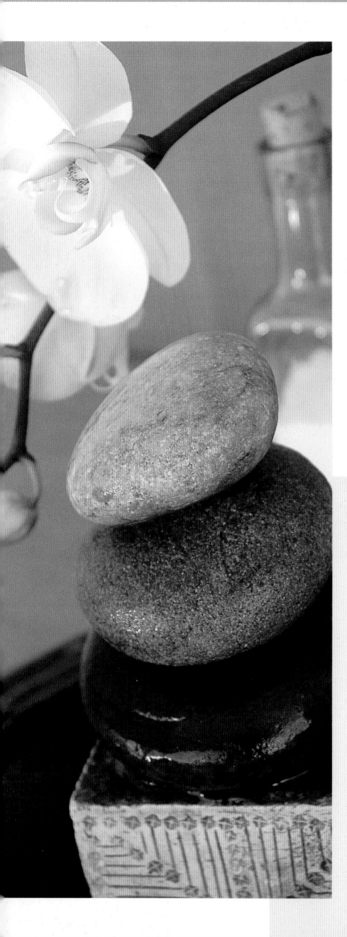

Reflexology is a treatment that involves the application of gentle pressure to reflex points located on all of the surfaces of the feet and hands. According to reflexology, these points relate to all of the organs, glands and bodily parts, which, remarkably, are represented in the same arrangement as in the physical body. The feet and hands can thus be seen as a mirror, or a mini-map, of the body, and the reflex points accurately and clearly reflect the physical, mental, emotional and even the spiritual health of each individual. Your entire life's history can be revealed through your hands and feet! As these reflex points are massaged, the body's natural recuperative abilities are stimulated, so that any ailments, whether minor or major, and no matter how longstanding, can be alleviated. Vital energy is encouraged to flow freely, energy blockages may be dissipated, physical toxins are gently flushed away, together with any emotional blockages, and optimum health and inner peace can be restored.

As well as combating disease and distress, reflexology is an effective therapy for maintaining health and wellbeing, and for preventing problems from occurring. Through the ancient art of reflexology, you can thus regain and maintain your health, and become healthy and whole.

Reflexology is a natural way to promote health and wellbeing. ▶

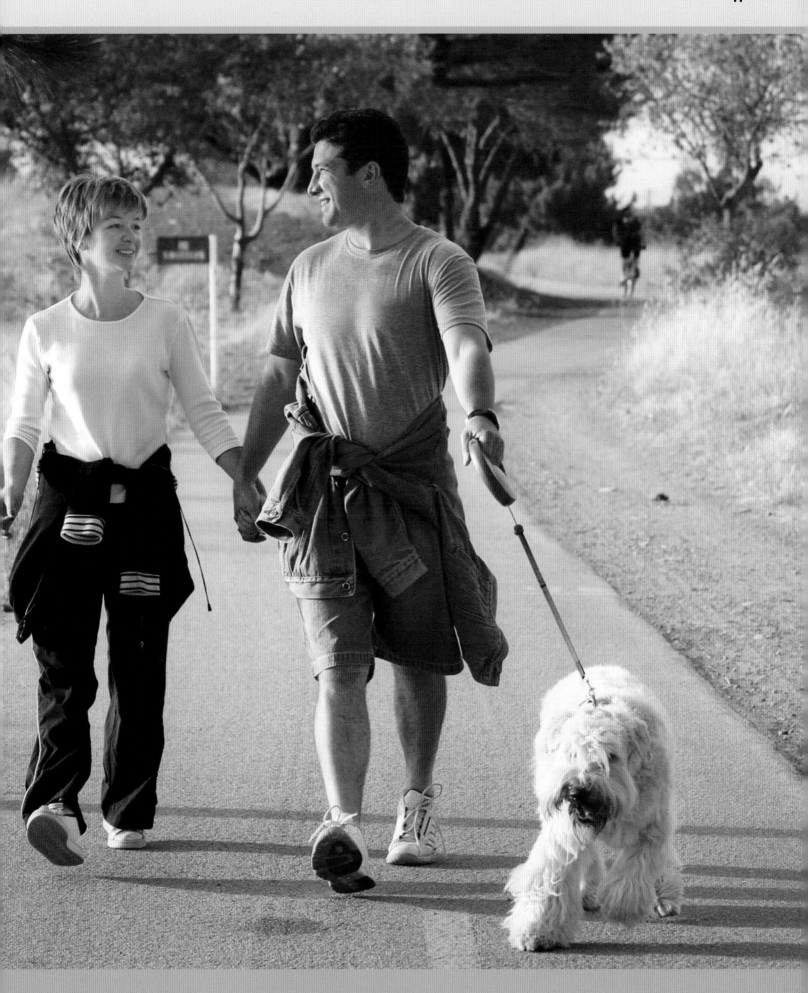

Foot versus hand reflexology

Traditionally, foot reflexology is employed more frequently by the professional reflexologist than hand reflexology because some consider the feet to be the most sensitive to treatment. However, both can achieve equally good results.

There are occasions when working on the hands becomes a necessity because foot reflexology is impossible. For instance, if a foot is fractured or sprained, then hand reflexology is the natural option. If part of a foot is infected with, for example, athlete's foot, or if a verruca is present, then these areas should be avoided and the relevant areas on the hands should be treated instead. Similarly, if there are problems with the hands, then foot reflexology is advantageous. Some individuals also love to have their feet worked on (I am certainly one of them!), whereas others may be ticklish or may be embarrassed to expose their feet, in which case hand reflexology is ideal.

Whether you decide to work on the hands or the feet, or both, your treatments will be equally effective.

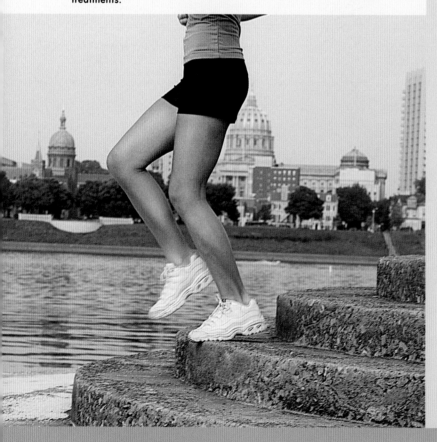

▼ **Joints will become more flexible and mobile with regular reflexology treatments.**

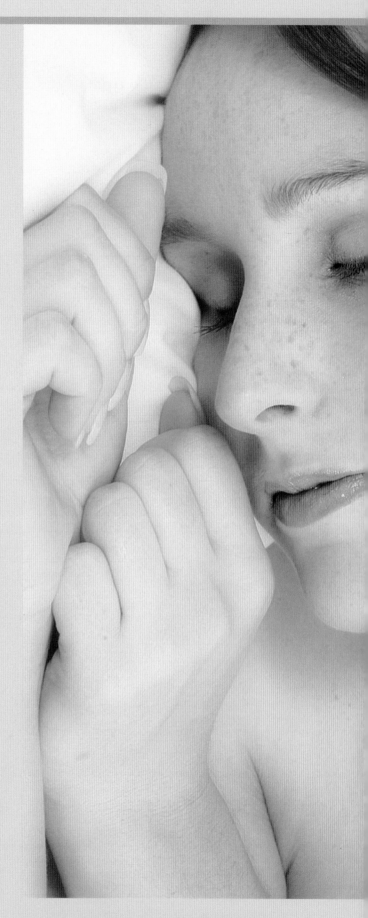

▲ **Enjoy a deep, relaxing sleep after a reflexology session.**

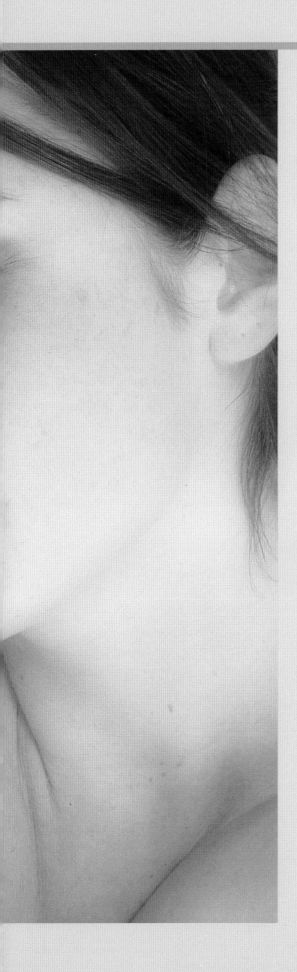

The benefits of reflexology

The benefits of reflexology are so numerous and wide-ranging that it is impossible to convey all that it has to offer. It is highly effective for treating and enhancing the body, mind and spirit, and everyone can derive benefits from this ancient therapeutic art.

The physical benefits

The following physical benefits result from reflexology.

- Reflexology improves the circulation of blood to every single part of the body. Blood carries oxygen and vital nutrients to all of the body's cells.
- Reflexology balances blood pressure and relieves strain on the heart.
- Reflexology cleanses the body of impurities and encourages harmful waste products to be eliminated more efficiently.
- Reflexology boosts the immune system. As a result, illnesses are less likely to occur and recovery from them is swifter and more complete. Chronic fatigue syndrome, which is becoming increasingly common in today's stressful society, can also be alleviated.
- Reflexology aids digestion and elimination. It keeps the digestive system in excellent working order, combating such problems as indigestion, constipation, irritable bowel syndrome, food allergies and flatulence.
- Reflexology relieves aches and pains. No matter how persistent they are, and wherever they are, muscular problems can be alleviated.
- Reflexology improves the mobility of the joints. Stiff and painful backs, knees, necks, hips, shoulders, wrists and hands, and ankles and feet can become more flexible and mobile following treatment.
- Reflexology alleviates problems associated with the reproductive system. Menstrual problems, such as premenstrual syndrome (PMS), painful, scanty, heavy or irregular periods, endometriosis, polycystic ovarian syndrome and the menopause, can all be treated. Problems with conception, male and female infertility and loss of libido also respond positively to reflexology.
- Reflexology relieves urinary problems such as cystitis.
- Reflexology counteracts fluid retention.
- Reflexology encourages deep sleep and alleviates insomnia.
- Reflexology eliminates mucus and catarrh and restores deep breathing. All respiratory problems, including asthma, chest infections, coughs and colds, ear, nose and throat problems, can be eased with reflexology.
- Reflexology alleviates such skin problems as acne, eczema, psoriasis and rashes, and reduces itching, irritation and allergic reactions. The condition, tone and texture of the skin improve enormously after reflexology treatments.
- Reflexology slows down such progressive illnesses as Parkinson's disease and multiple sclerosis.
- Reflexology is an essential treatment for terminal illnesses such as cancer, and hospices often employ reflexology practitioners.

The mental benefits

The mental benefits of reflexology include the following.

- Reflexology restores mental alertness.
- Reflexology improves focus and concentration.
- Reflexology enhances and stimulates creativity and productivity.
- Reflexology calms an overactive mind.
- Reflexology boosts confidence.
- Reflexology reduces, or eliminates, the need for such harmful substances as drugs, tobacco and alcohol.

▼ **Reflexology enhances creativity.**

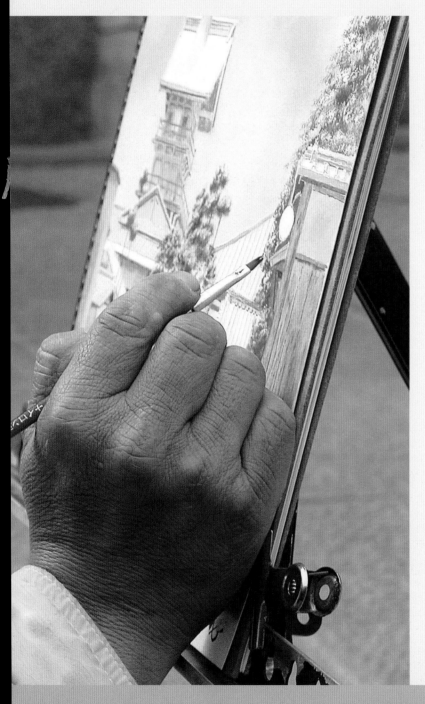

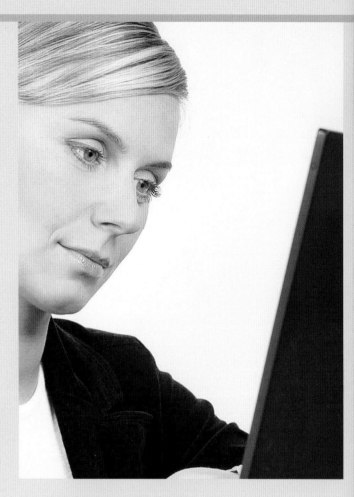

▲ **Reflexology improves concentration**

The emotional benefits

The following number among the emotional benefits of reflexology.

- Reflexology relieves stress, inducing a deep sense of relaxation.
- Reflexology reduces emotional turmoil.
- Reflexology soothes fears and anxieties.
- Reflexology releases the memory of, and heals, past traumas.
- Reflexology calms anger, frustration and impatience and reduces the tendency to overreact to minor issues.
- Reflexology induces courage and strength, helping the receiver to cope with difficult situations and problems.
- Reflexology lifts depression.
- Reflexology increases such positive emotions as happiness, joy, enthusiasm and satisfaction with life.
- Reflexology assists in resolving emotional conflicts.

Reflexology promotes happiness ▶

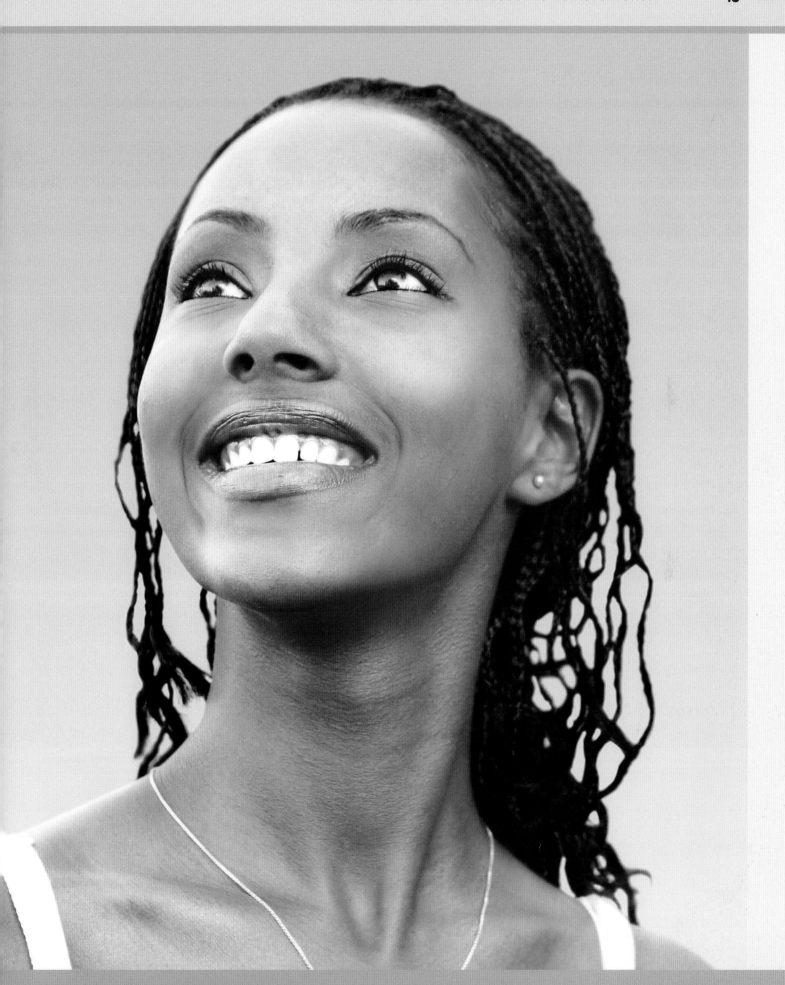

The spiritual benefits

The spiritual benefits of reflexology include the following.

- Reflexology encourages spiritual growth and development and helps to break down any obstacles in your path.
- Reflexology enables you to fulfil your spiritual truth.

Overall, reflexology revitalises and harmonises the body, mind and spirit, enabling you to lead a more fulfilling and rewarding life. Make reflexology part of your life, and you'll be jumping out of bed in the morning raring to go!

Can reflexology and orthodox medicine work together?

Reflexology and orthodox medicine can indeed work remarkably well together. In fact, they are an ideal combination, and the medical profession is now recognising reflexology as the powerful tool that it is. Reflexologists are even employed by some hospitals in maternity, oncology and rheumatology departments, as well as in many others.

Caution

Reflexology should not be used instead of orthodox medicine. A reflexologist should never diagnose an illness or condition (this is the prerogative of a doctor), promise a cure or otherwise give false hope.

▼ Orthodox and complementary practitioners can work together to improve health and well-being.

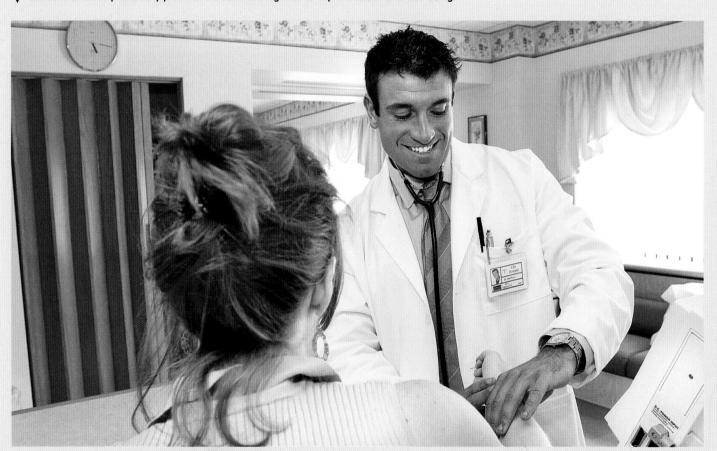

Acceleration of ▶
spiritual growth is
one of the benefits
of reflexology.

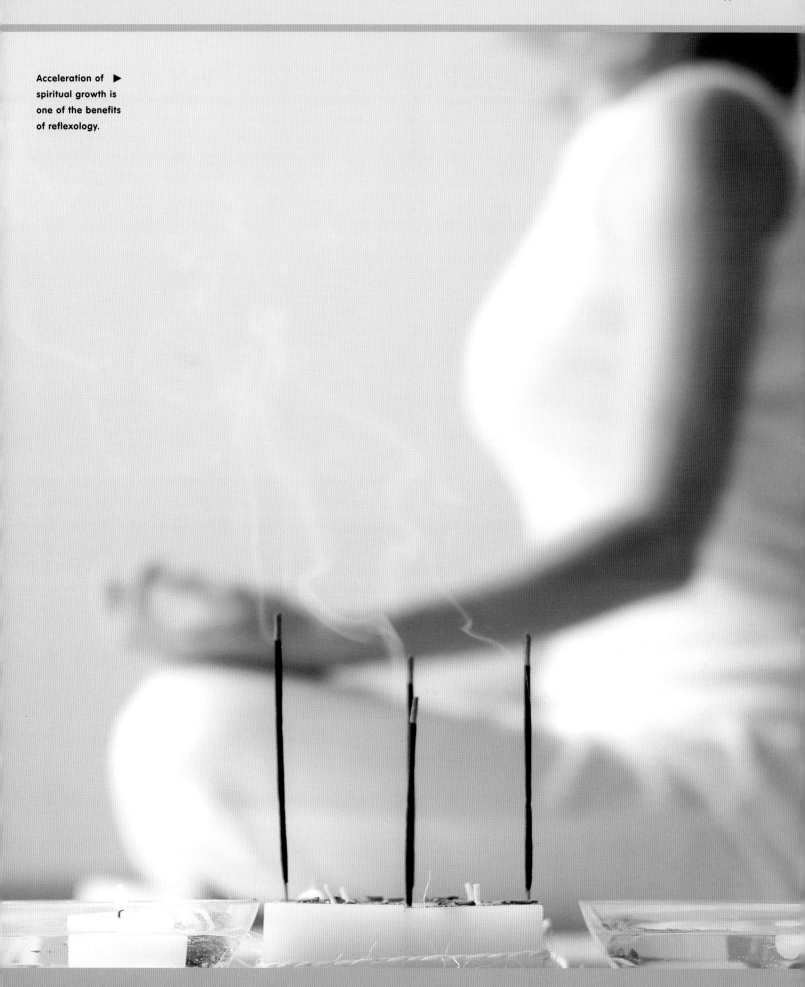

The roots of reflexology

Although the origin of reflexology is unclear, it is certain that it is a very ancient art that has been practised by many diverse cultures in various forms for thousands of years. The Egyptians and Chinese, in particular, appear to have played a major part in its development. In Egypt, evidence can be seen in Saqqara, in the tomb of the Egyptian physician Ankmahor. On the wall is a drawing dating back to about 2330 BC that depicts a reflexology treatment taking place. Four people are shown; one person is working on a foot and another is treating a hand. The hieroglyphics read as follows:

'Do not let it be painful' (patient); 'I shall act so you praise me' (practitioner).

Reflexology is thought by some to have been employed by the Chinese five thousand years ago, and it is believed that it preceded acupuncture, which was developed by the Chinese in around 2500 BC. Others have speculated that the Incas invented this ancient art in around 12,000 BC. Reflexology has been used for thousands of years by the Native Americans, who still practise a form of reflexology today.

As far as Europe is concerned, Dr Adamus and Dr A'tatis, two eminent physicians from Leipzig, Germany, published a book on 'zone therapy' in 1582. There are also historical references to the Italian sculptor Benvenuto Cellini (1500–71) applying pressure to his fingers and toes in order to administer pain relief, and also to US president James Garfield (1831–81) using reflex zone therapy on himself after an assassination attempt.

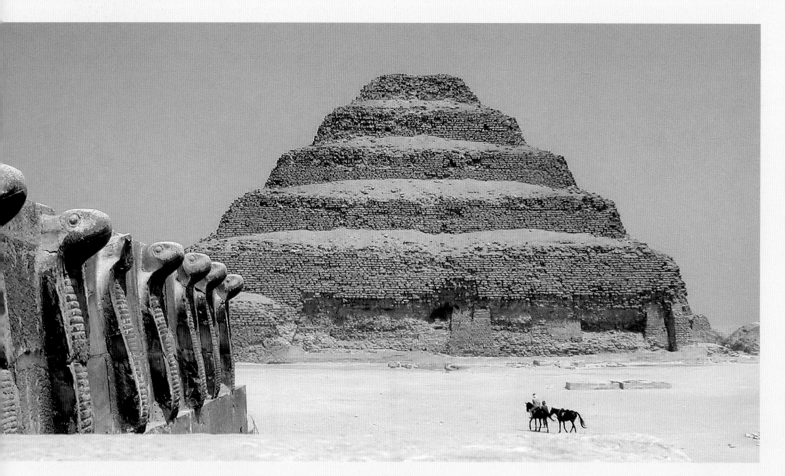

▲ A reflexology treatment is depicted on the wall of Ankmahor's tomb in Saqqara, Egypt.

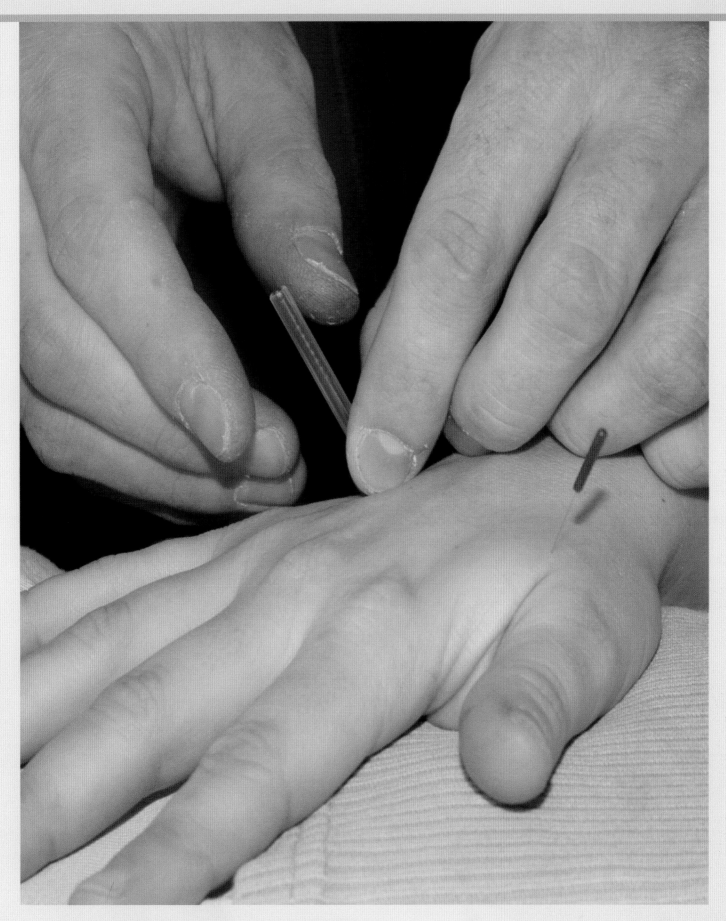

▲ Some believe that acupuncture was developed from the practice of reflexology.

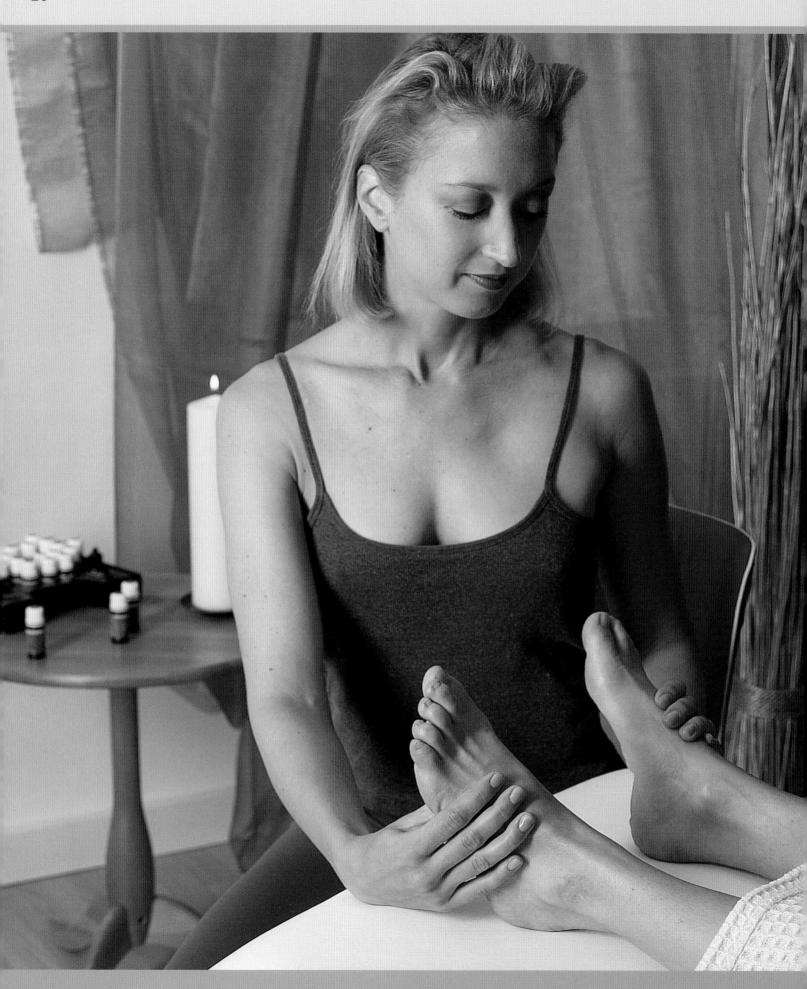

The US physician Dr William Fitzgerald (1872–1942) can be regarded as the father of reflexology, however. After graduating from the University of Vermont in 1895, he practised at Boston City Hospital, at the Central London Ear, Nose and Throat Hospital in England, and at an ear, nose and throat (ENT) hospital in Vienna, Austria, before becoming the senior ENT surgeon at St Francis Hospital, Hartford, Connecticut. While working there, Dr Fitzgerald developed his concept of 'zone therapy', and in 1917 published a book with his colleague Dr Edwin Bowers entitled *Zone Therapy*. In this book, he described how he could relieve pain and induce an anaesthetic effect by applying pressure to specific areas of the hands and feet, as well as to other parts of the body.

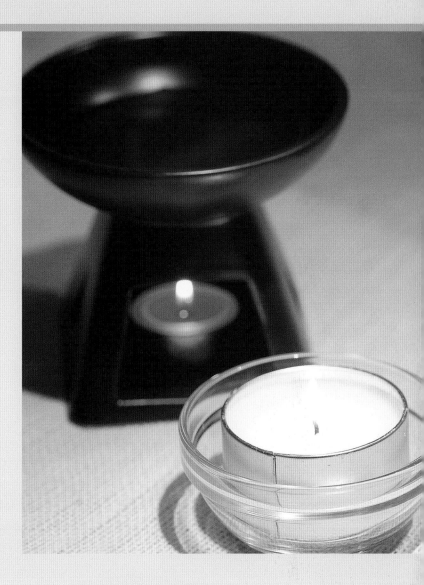

Dr Fitzgerald taught many courses, and one colleague in particular, Dr Joseph Shelby-Riley, took his theories on board, later publishing several books on zone therapy himself. Dr Shelby-Riley's most famous pupil was Eunice Ingham (1879–1974), now acknowledged as the 'mother' of reflexology and the author of two classic reflexology texts that I use even today while lecturing at my college: *Stories the Feet Can Tell* was published in 1938, followed by *Stories the Feet Have Told*. Eunice Ingham mapped out the reflex points for the whole body on the feet and hands, and dedicated her life to the teaching and practising of reflexology. And it was one of Eunice Ingham's students, Doreen Bayley, who brought reflexology to the UK during the 1960s.

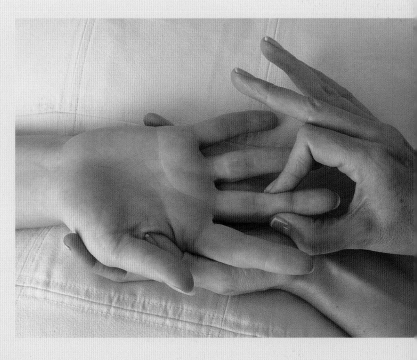

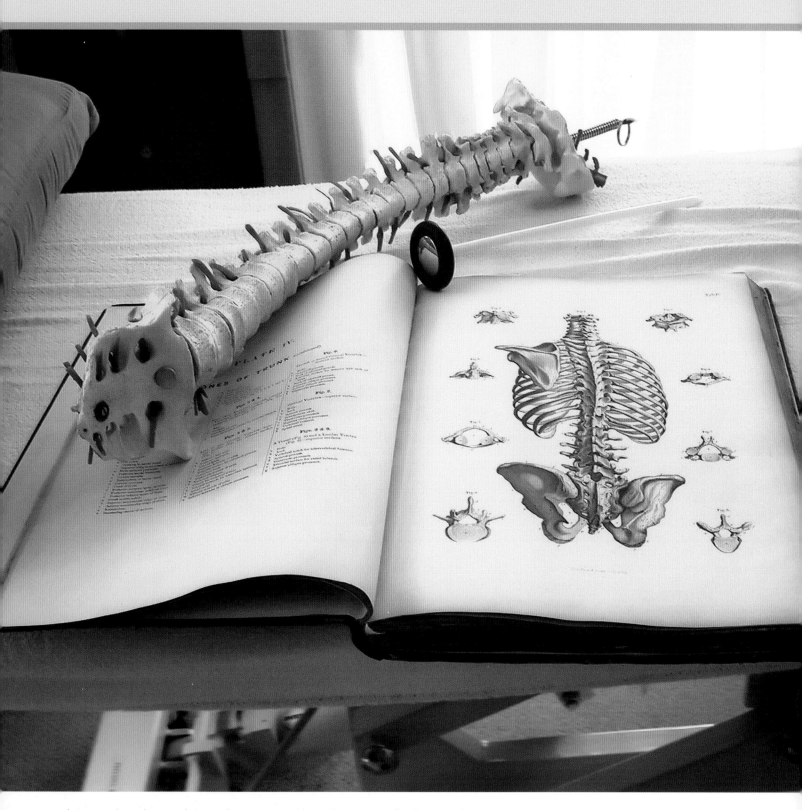

▲ Osteopaths and many other complementary practitioners incorporate reflexology into their practice.

Reflexology is an extremely fast-growing therapy, and it now has many thousands of practitioners all over the world. During my career, I have carried out in excess of fifty thousand treatments, and there are many more to come! I am delighted that the art of reflexology is gaining increasing recognition within the medical profession. Not only are reflexology practitioners today to be found in many hospital departments, but it is encouraging that many doctors, nurses, osteopaths, physiotherapists, chiropractors, chiropodists, acupuncturists and homoeopaths are increasingly incorporating reflexology into their work.

The basic principles of reflexology

According to reflexology, the body is divided into longitudinal (vertical) and transverse (horizontal) zones, enabling us to pinpoint the different reflexes with precision.

The ten longitudinal zones

There are ten invisible, longitudinal (vertical) energy zones. These zones run from the tips of the toes to the top of the head and out to the fingertips and vice versa. If an imaginary line were to be drawn through the centre of the body, there would be five zones located to the right of this midline and five to the left.

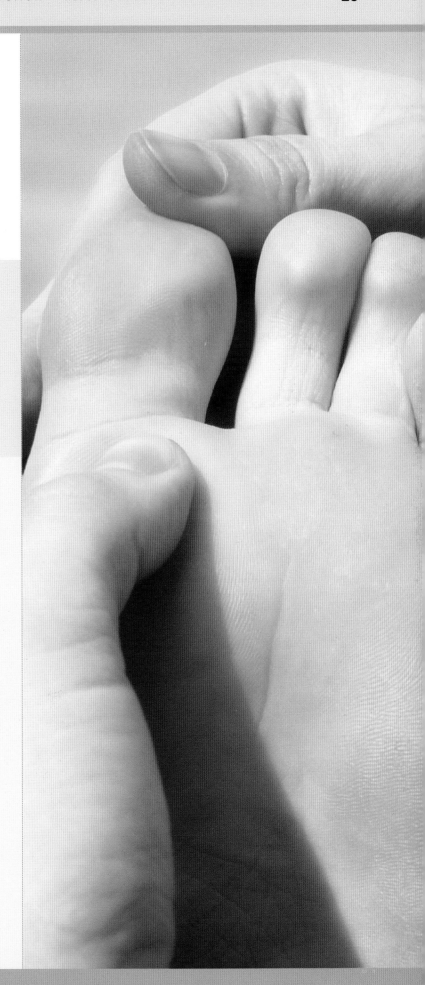

Try tracing these zones on each side of your body.

- **Zone 1:** go from your big toe up your leg, up the centre of your body to your head, and then down to your thumb.

- **Zone 2:** go from your second toe up to your head, and then down to your index finger.

- **Zone 3:** go from your third toe up to your head, and then down to your third finger.

- **Zone 4:** go from your fourth toe up to your head, and then down to your fourth finger.

- **Zone 5:** go from your little toe up to your head, and then down to your little finger.

All of the organs, glands and bodily parts are located in one or more of these zones. And all points within a zone are related to each other, so that if, for instance, a reflex point is worked on in zone 1, all of the reflex points in zone 1 will be treated.

Ten longtitudinal zones of the hands

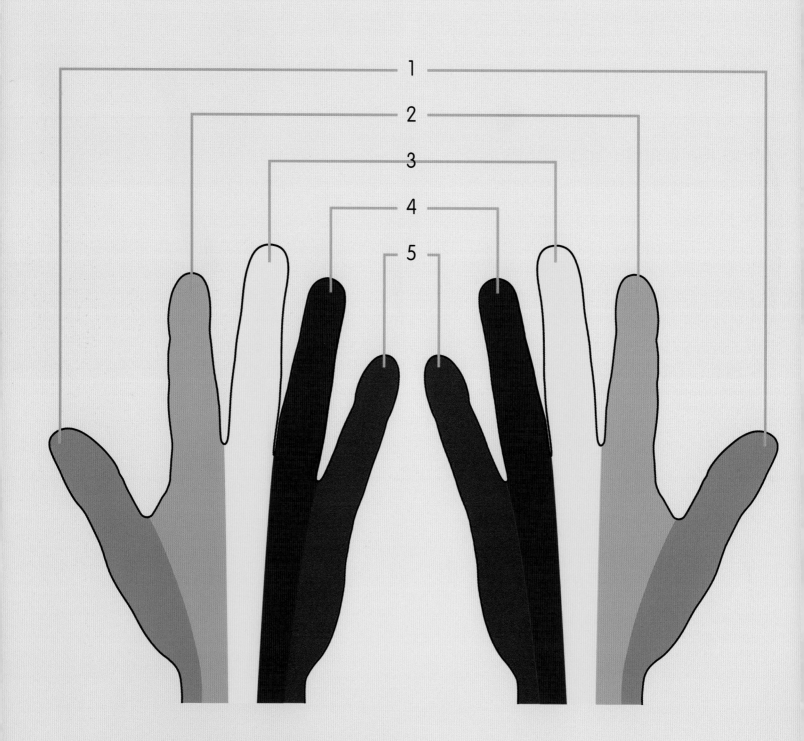

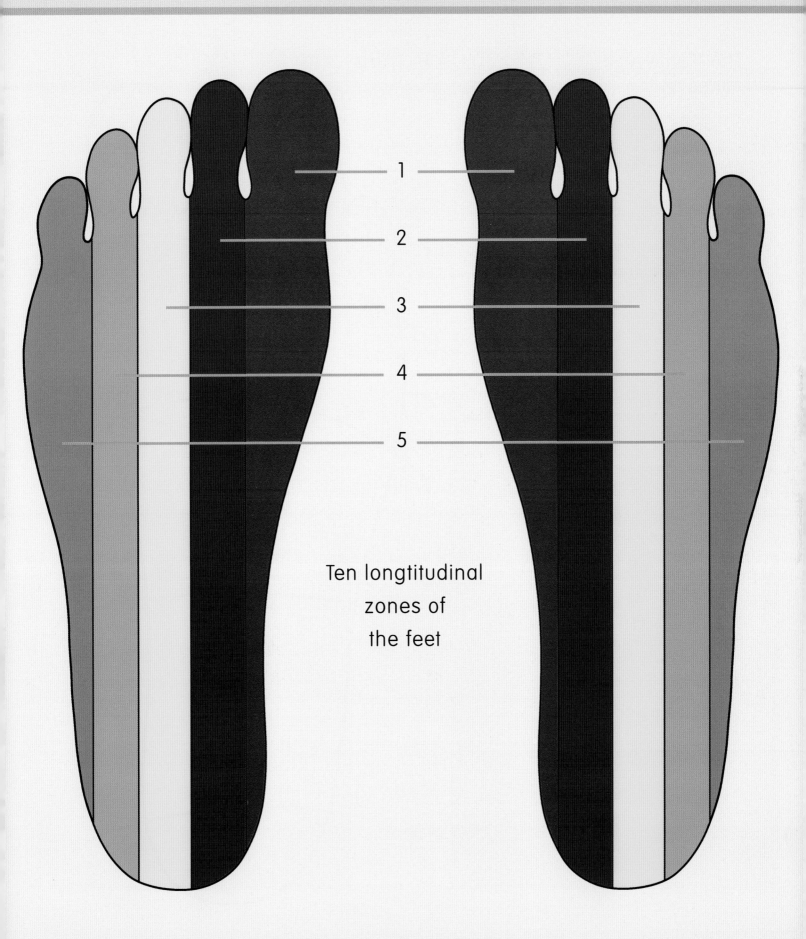

1

2

3

4

5

Ten longtitudinal
zones of
the feet

The transverse zones

The feet and hands can be mapped out even more accurately by drawing imaginary transverse (horizontal) lines across the hands or feet.

The transverse zones of the feet

First of all, let us look at the transverse lines of the feet.

1. The shoulder girdle line: this is located just below the base of the toes. Anatomically, the shoulder girdle line relates to the region where the toes (phalanges) meet the bones of the foot (metatarsals). The reflexes of all areas found above the shoulder girdle, such as those of the head and brain, neck, face, sinuses, ears, eyes and teeth, are located here.

2. The diaphragm line: this is located just under the ball of the foot. Reflexes of the thorax, such as those of the lungs and the heart, are found between the shoulder girdle line and the diaphragm line.

The four transverse zones of the feet

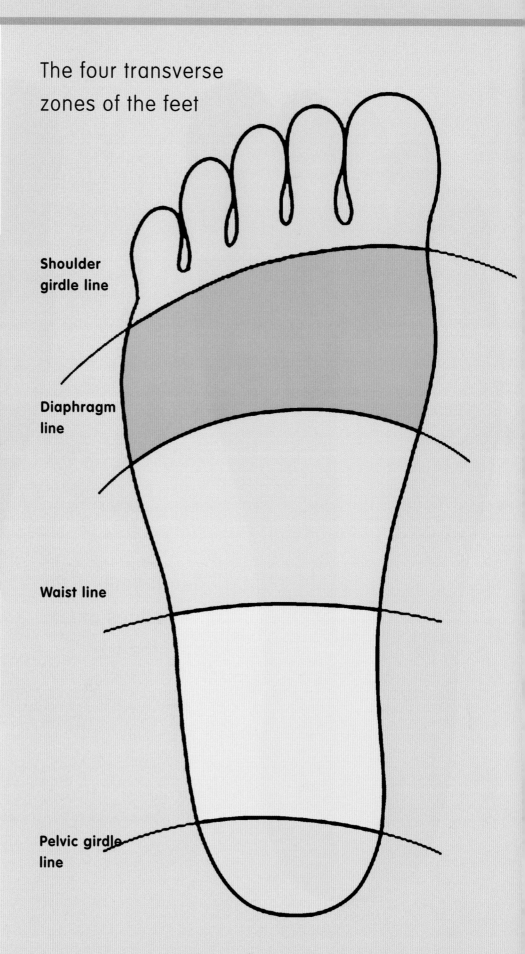

Shoulder girdle line

Diaphragm line

Waist line

Pelvic girdle line

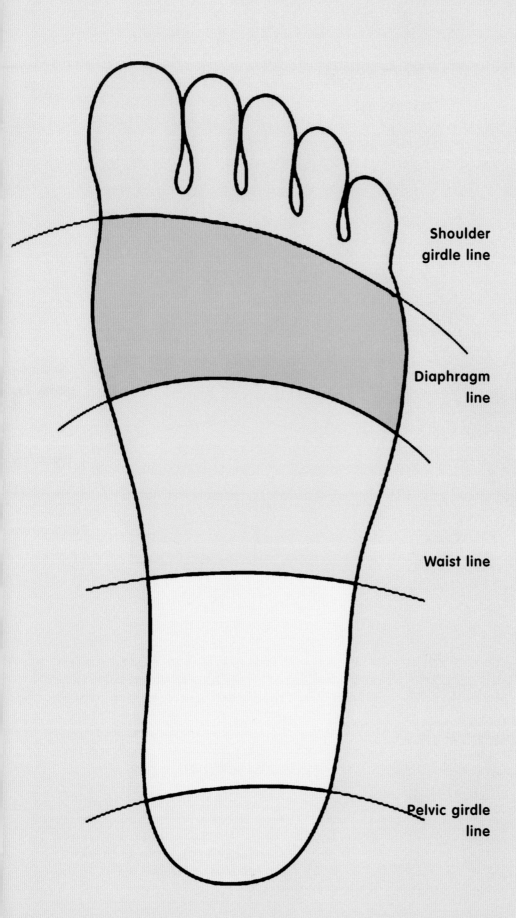

Shoulder girdle line

Diaphragm line

Waist line

Pelvic girdle line

3. The waist line:
this is located approximately in the middle of the foot. Anatomically, the waist line relates to the region where the foot bones (metatarsals) meet the anklebones. The bulge on the outside edge of your foot is the fifth metatarsal. The reflexes of organs of the upper abdomen, such as those of the liver, gallbladder, stomach, pancreas and spleen, are found between the diaphragm line and the waist line.

4. The pelvic girdle line:
place one of your index fingers on your outer anklebone and one on your inner anklebone and imagine a line running between them – this is the pelvic girdle line. The reflexes of organs of the lower abdomen, such as those of the intestines, are found between the waist line and the pelvic girdle line.

The transverse zones of the hands

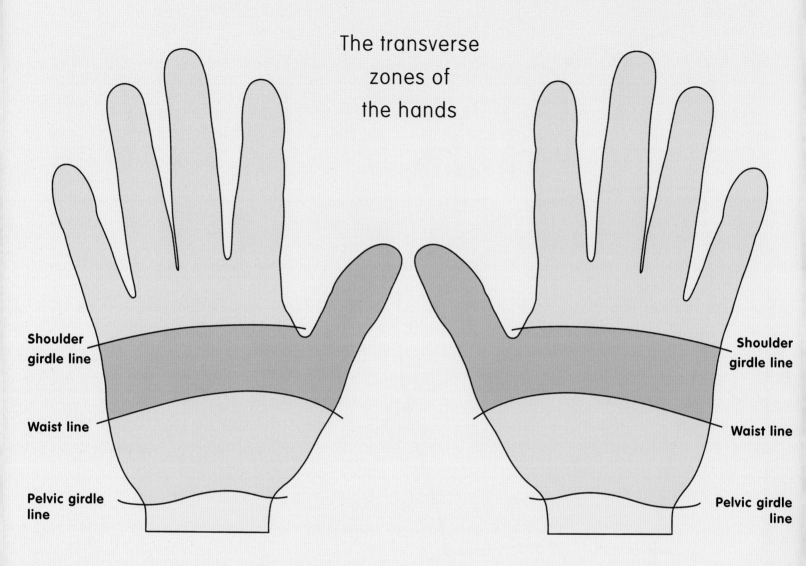

Shoulder girdle line

Waist line

Pelvic girdle line

Shoulder girdle line

Waist line

Pelvic girdle line

The transverse zones of the hands

Now let us explore the transverse lines of the hands.

1. **The diaphragm line:** this is located just below the padded area of the fingers, about 2.5cm (1in) below where the index finger joins the hand. Such reflexes as those of the head and brain, neck, throat, face, sinuses, eyes, ears and teeth are located here.

2. **The waist line:** this line runs from where the bottom of the thumb joins the hand across to the other side of the hand.

3. **The pelvic line:** the pelvic line circles the wrist.

Because the hands and feet mirror the body, the reflexes of any organs and structures found on the right side of the body are located in the right hand or the right foot. The left side of the body is reflected in the left hand or the left foot. The reflexes of paired organs and structures, such as the lungs, kidneys and knees, will be found in both hands and feet. Where there is only one organ, such as the liver or gallbladder, its reflex will usually be located in only one hand or foot, in these instances, the right one. Where a structure or an organ is central and lies along the midline of the body (for example, the spine or the bladder), its reflex can be found in both hands and feet. However, there are exceptions to this rule, which will be made clear in the step-by-step sequences.

Contraindications and cautions

Reflexology is a very safe therapy, but there are a small number of cases where treatments are not advisable, or where extra care needs to be taken. If you are in any doubt, seek a doctor's permission to give treatments or ask a professional reflexologist for advice.

▼ If there is a danger of miscarriage reflexology should not be given.

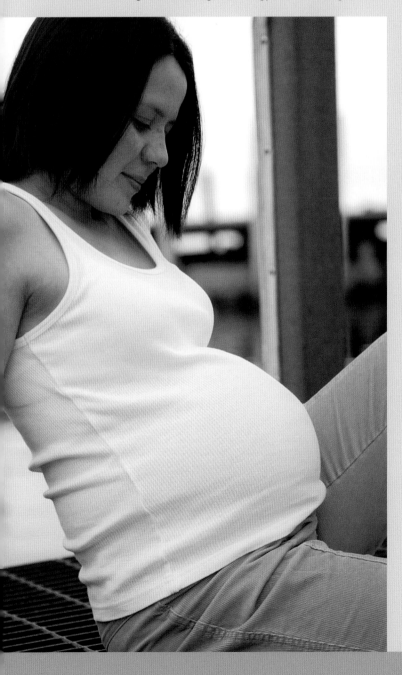

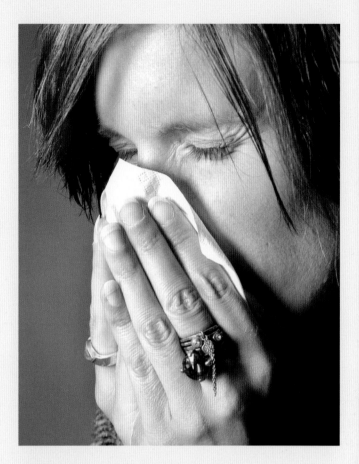

▲ Reflexology is not advisable in cases of contagious conditions such as 'flu.

Do not give reflexology

If a prospective receiver is undergoing medical treatment for a serious condition, check with a doctor that reflexology is acceptable before providing therapy. Do not give a reflexology treatment in the following instances.

- If the receiver has a contagious skin disease, such as scabies, ringworm, impetigo or chickenpox (you neither want to catch it yourself nor to spread it to others).

- If the receiver has a fever (the treatment may release more toxins, when the body already has enough to contend with).

- If the receiver has deep-vein thrombosis (you could dislodge the clot).

- If the receiver has just undergone surgery (there is the risk of thrombosis).

- If the receiver is under the influence of drugs or alcohol.

- If the receiver is pregnant and has a history of miscarriage.

► Any sore or tender areas should not be
treated during a reflexology session.

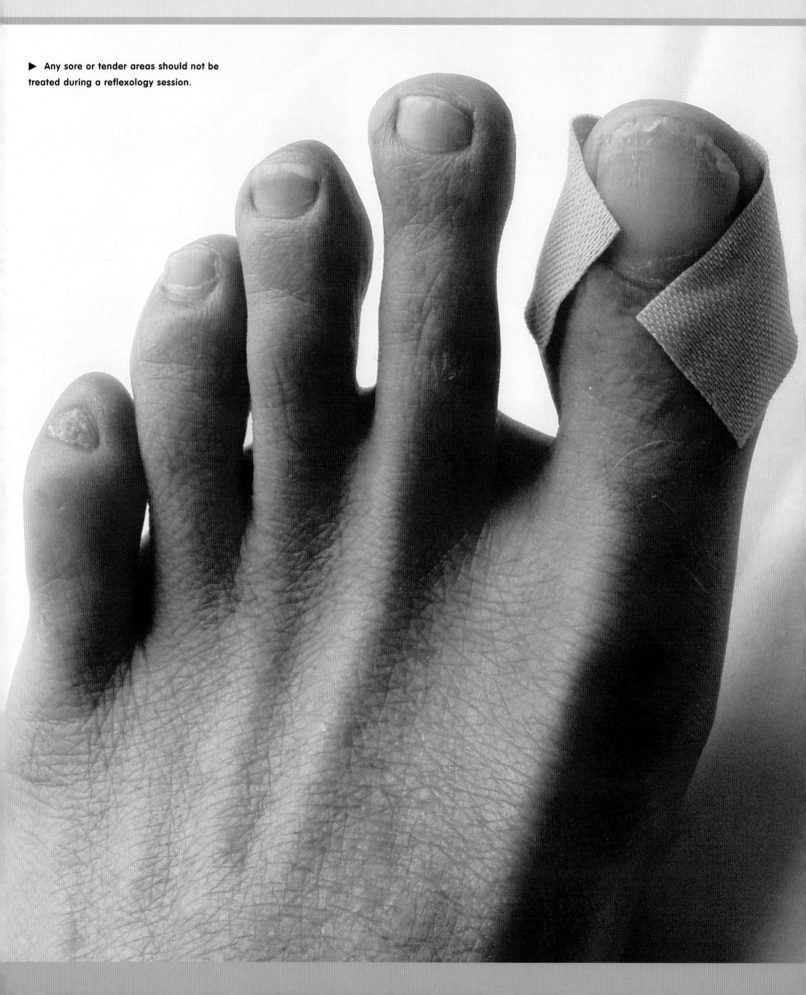

Exercise caution

When giving a reflexology treatment, exercise caution in the following instances.

- Over any parts of the hands or feet that are injured.
- Over cuts, bruises, recent scars, varicose veins and any other areas that may be tender to the touch.
- Over any painful corns, calluses or bruises (use a more gentle pressure).
- Over verrucae and warts (which should be covered up with a plaster or avoided during the treatment).
- Over areas of inflammation, such as an inflamed, arthritic joint.
- If there is puffiness, for instance, around the ankles.
- If the menstrual flow is heavy (then exert only gentle pressure over the reproductive organs).
- Over the uterus area if there is an intrauterine device (IUD) fitted.
- If the receiver has osteoporosis (use only light pressure on his or her fragile bones).
- If the receiver has epilepsy (take care over the head and brain reflex zones).

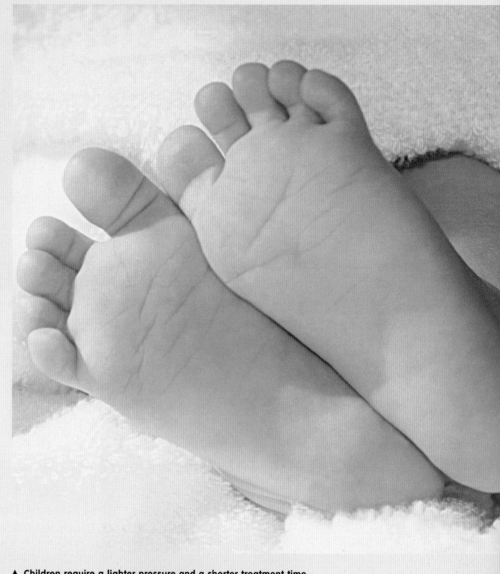

▲ **Children require a lighter pressure and a shorter treatment time.**

- If the receiver has diabetes (use only gentle pressure, particularly over the reflex area of the pancreas). Remember that diabetics may have thinner skin, bruise more easily, have less sensitivity and a slower healing rate and may be more prone to ulceration of the legs and feet than non-diabetics.
- If the receiver has cancer (use only light pressure), but be heartened that reflexology encourages relaxation, elimination and provides pain relief.
- If the receiver is elderly (use only gentle pressure and, if necessary, reduce the treatment time in accordance with the fitness of the receiver).
- If the receiver is terminally ill (use a lighter pressure than usual and shorten the duration of the treatment to suit the receiver).
- If the receiver is a baby or child. (In the case of babies, simply stroke the feet or hands very gently and use your index finger to touch any problem area gently. In the case of children, use gentle pressure and reduce the treatment time depending on the age of the child. For young children, the treatment should consist mostly of stroking movements.)

Possible reactions

There are many reactions that may occur as a result of a reflexology treatment, both during the treatment and particularly between treatments, but it is impossible to predict if, and how, a person is likely to react. Reactions should be seen as a positive indication that treatment is working, however, being perfectly natural and part of the healing process that is taking place.

If receivers are nervous about suffering reactions, reassure them that they will certainly not experience all of them! In most cases, only one or two reactions will occur, and these will be short-lived, usually disappearing within 24 hours.

▼ **If a sensitive area is palpated the receiver may frown.**

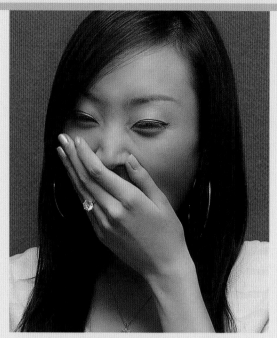

▲ **Expect to feel relaxed and sleepy during the treatment.**

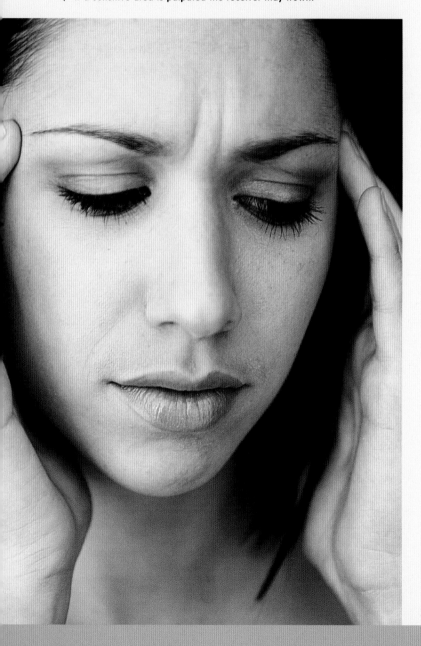

Possible reactions during a reflexology treatment

The following reactions may occur during a reflexology treatment.

- A state of deep relaxation.
- Feelings of peace and tranquillity.
- Feelings of euphoria.
- Sleepiness.
- Changes in expression, such as smiling or, perhaps, frowning if a sensitive area is palpated. (Note that if a sharp, pin-prick-like sensation is experienced, this usually indicates an acute problem, whereas a dull ache normally indicates a chronic problem that has existed for a while.)
- Tingling sensations and rushes of energy and warmth.
- Twitching or jerking.
- Muscular contraction, for example, the receiver may move his or her neck as the reflex area is treated.
- Audible noises, such as deep sighs, laughing or crying.
- A runny nose.
- Coughing and clearing the throat.
- Noises emanating from the abdomen.
- Itchy or watery eyes.
- The receiver may see beautiful colours as healing takes place.

You may see the most beautiful colours during your reflexology session. ▶

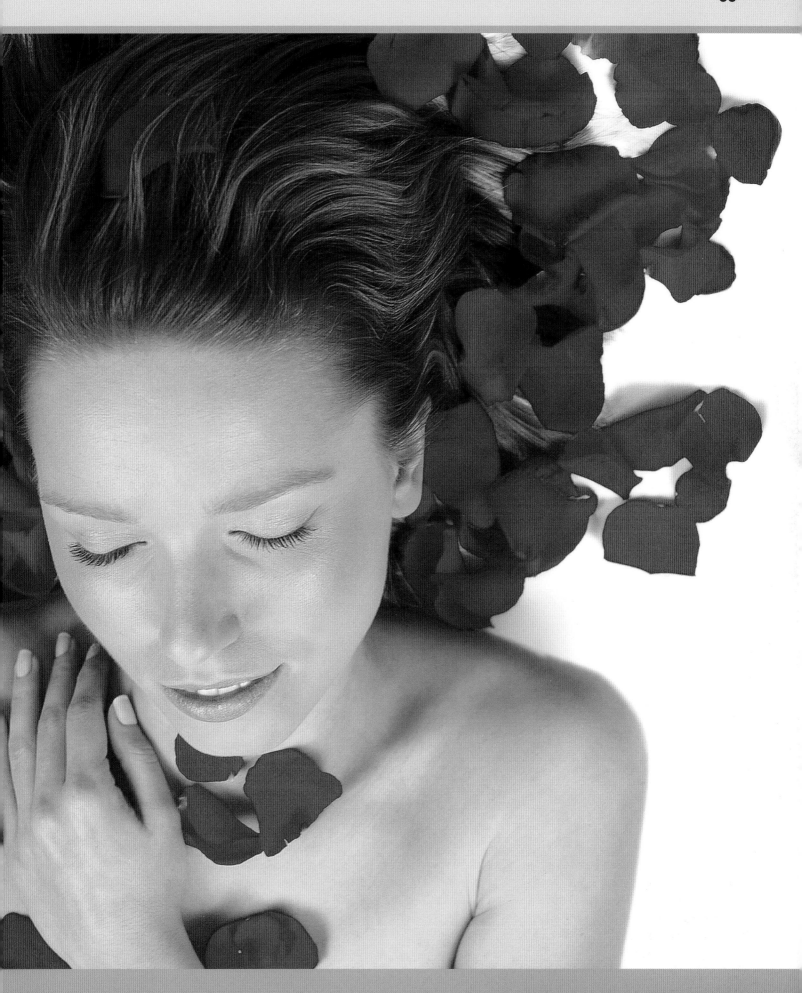

Finally, if the receiver experiences excessive perspiration and a feeling of being cold all over, this is a very unusual and overly strong reaction to the treatment. It is a sign of over-stimulation, which is probably not your fault as the receiver may be extremely sensitive or going through a very difficult time, or both. However, if it does occur, do not panic or abruptly break off the treatment. Speak to the receiver very calmly, giving him or her lots of reassurance, and gently hold the hands or feet. You may use light, stroking movements as you ask the receiver to take a few deep breaths. Offer the receiver a glass of water and tissues if necessary. Be a good listener if the receiver wants to talk, but do not force him or her to do so if the receiver does not want to discuss his or her problems. I must emphasise that this sort of reaction is extremely rare.

Possible reactions between treatments

The receiver may experience certain physical and emotional reactions between reflexology treatments.

Physical reactions

The following possible physical reactions are primarily due to the stimulation of the systems of elimination.

- An increase in the frequency of bowel movements; stools may also be more bulky and of a different colour.
- An increase in urination; urine may be cloudy or have an unpleasant smell.
- Vaginal discharge.
- Nasal secretions, sneezing or coughing.
- A sore throat.
- Watery eyes.
- Toothache.
- An increase in skin activity: spots, rashes and similar blemishes may appear, but will clear up quickly, and the skin will then look clearer and more glowing.
- An increase in perspiration as toxins are eliminated
- Short bouts of fever.
- Initial tiredness followed by increased vitality and renewed energy.
- Frequent dreaming.
- Deeper and more restful sleep.
- A need to drink more water to flush away toxins.
- A temporary flaring-up of previous illnesses that have been suppressed before they finally disappear.

▼ **Energy and vitality will increase following a series of treatments.**

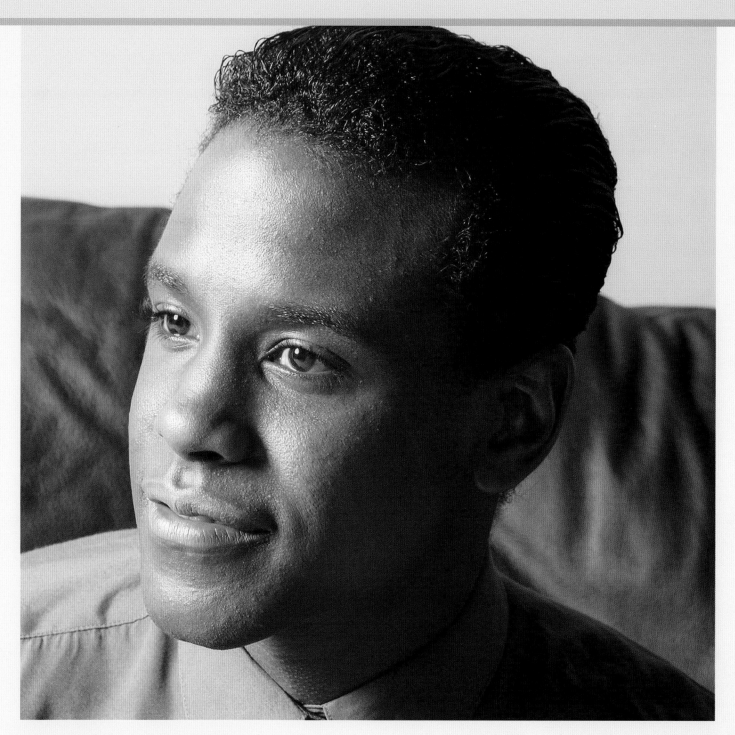

▲ Feel confident and more focused after reflexology.

Emotional reactions

After a reflexology treatment, the receiver may experience the following emotional reactions.

- A state of deep relaxation.
- The ability to think more clearly.
- Increased positivity and confidence.
- A more loving, compassionate and trusting state.

- Reduced fear and anxiety and an increased ability to cope with stress.
- Improved concentration.
- Increased patience and calmness.

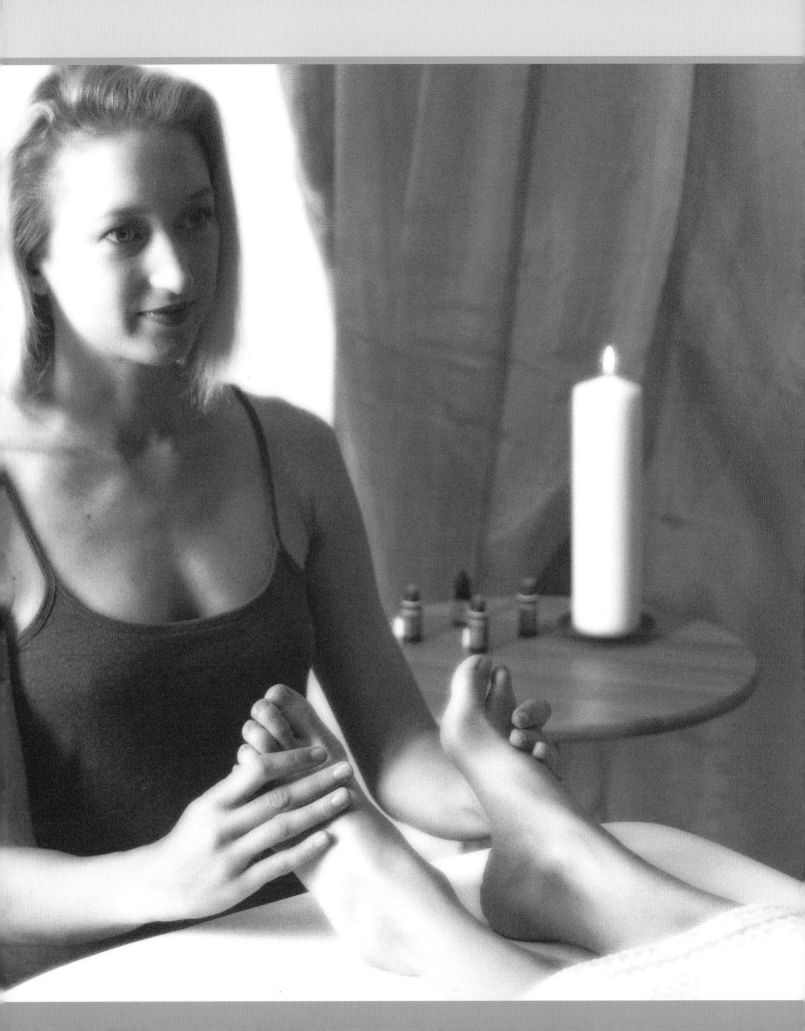

CHAPTER ONE

Foot reflexology

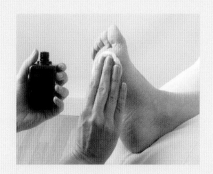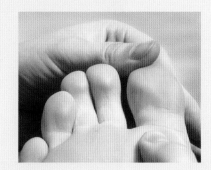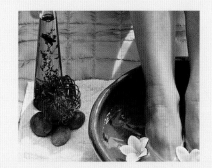

Foot reflexology is a simple, natural and non-invasive therapy which will enable you to achieve the most amazing results.

The bony structure of the feet

There are 26 bones in each foot:

- 14 phalanges, phalanges being the bones of the toes. There are three phalanges in each toe, apart from the big toe, which has only two.
- 5 metatarsals. The metatarsals meet with the phalanges, and there is one metatarsal for each toe.
- 7 tarsal bones: three cuneiforms (called the medial, intermediate and lateral cuneiforms), the cuboid, the navicular, the talus and the calcaneus (the heel bone), which is the largest bone in the foot.

The bones in the feet make up a quarter of the bones in the body.

There are three arches in the feet: a medial longitudinal arch, a lateral longitudinal arch and a transverse arch.

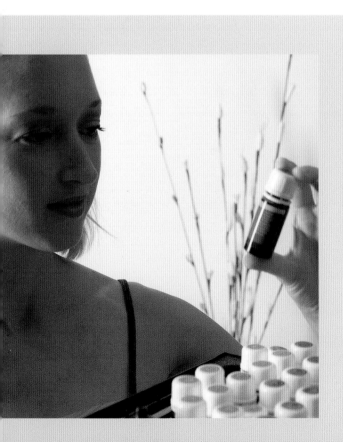

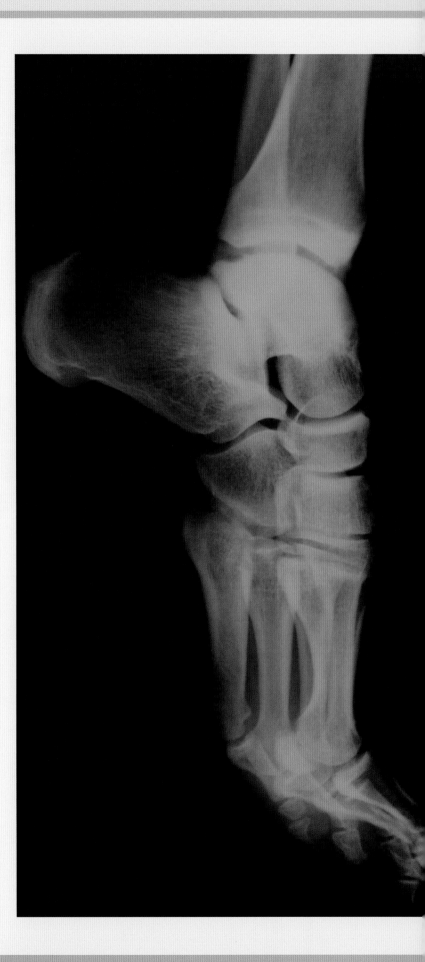

Preparing for a foot reflexology treatment

Although a reflexology treatment can be carried out anywhere, and at any time, you should ideally try to create a pleasing and relaxing environment in which both giver and receiver can enjoy some peace and tranquillity.

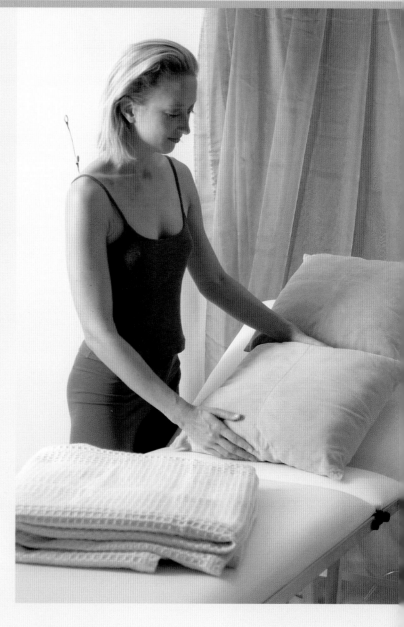

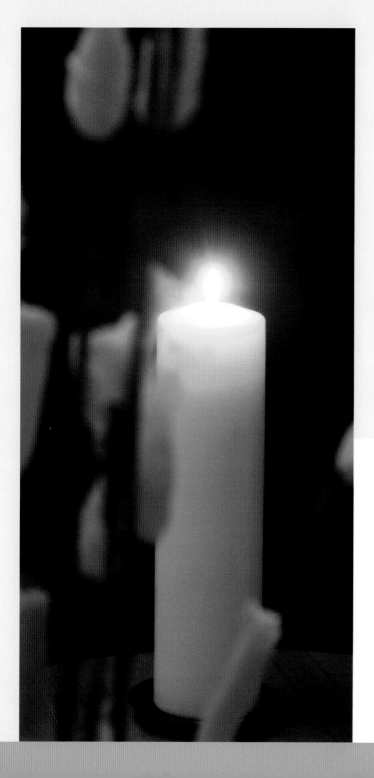

Choose a quiet room in which you will not be disturbed. Take the telephone off the hook or put on the answering machine and tell your family (especially any children) that you do not wish to be disturbed. Choose a room in which you can dim the lighting – a dimmer switch is excellent for this – or perhaps light a few candles. Depending on what time of the year it is, you may need to warm the room prior to the reflexology session. Have a blanket on hand with which to cover your partner, as well as several pillows. Note that some people like to listen to music during treatments, whereas others prefer silence. It is a good idea to keep conversation to a minimum during the session, both to allow the receiver to relax deeply so that healing can take place and to enable you to focus fully on giving the treatment and to enhance your intuition.

A few crystals placed around the room add a thoughtful touch to the surroundings. A piece of purple amethyst will transmute negativity, while rose quartz encourages love and contentment. The receiver may like to hold a crystal in each hand, in which case polished or shaped stones, such as heart-shaped crystals, are particularly suitable.

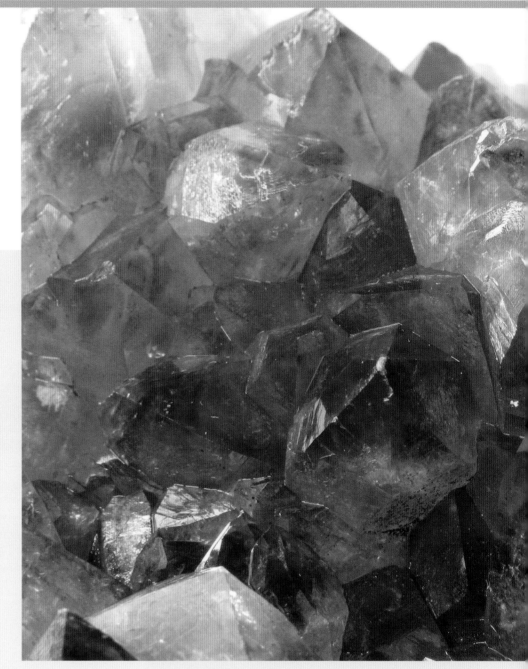

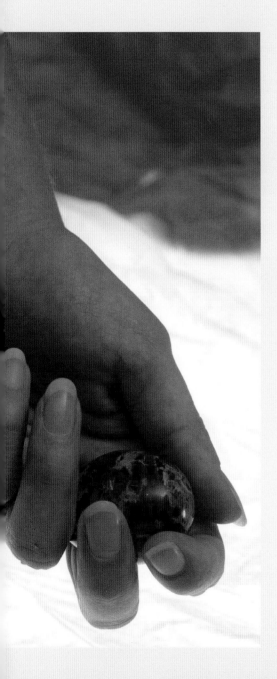

Essential oils may be diffused into the room to create a healing atmosphere. Clay burners are inexpensive and easy to use: just fill the bowl on top with water and add a few drops of your favourite essential oil or oils before heating the bowl to create the desired atmosphere. When selecting an essential oil, bear the following oils and their properties in mind:

- lavender, geranium or clary sage calm the mind
- bergamot or grapefruit help to lift depression
- juniper or cypress assist in the detoxification of the body, mind and spirit
- frankincense helps to soothe deep wounds and encourages the receiver to let go of the past
- rosemary or black pepper stimulate the mind and restore confidence
- jasmine or ylang-ylang are powerful aphrodisiacs that help to heal relationships

Positions for treatment

A foot reflexology session will work best if both the receiver and giver are relaxed and comfortable.

Regarding where the receiver should be positioned, the following options are all acceptable:

- a massage couch (a professional reflexologist will use a treatment table, but it is not necessary to invest in one; if you find yourself giving lots of treatments, you may then decide to purchase one, however)
- a reclining chair or sun-lounger
- a bed

Regardless of which of the above options you choose, you will also need several pillows or cushions to provide maximum comfort. Place one or two pillows or cushions under the receiver's head to support the neck and to allow you to observe his or her facial expressions. You should also place a pillow or cushion under the receiver's knees in order to make his or her back comfortable and relaxed.

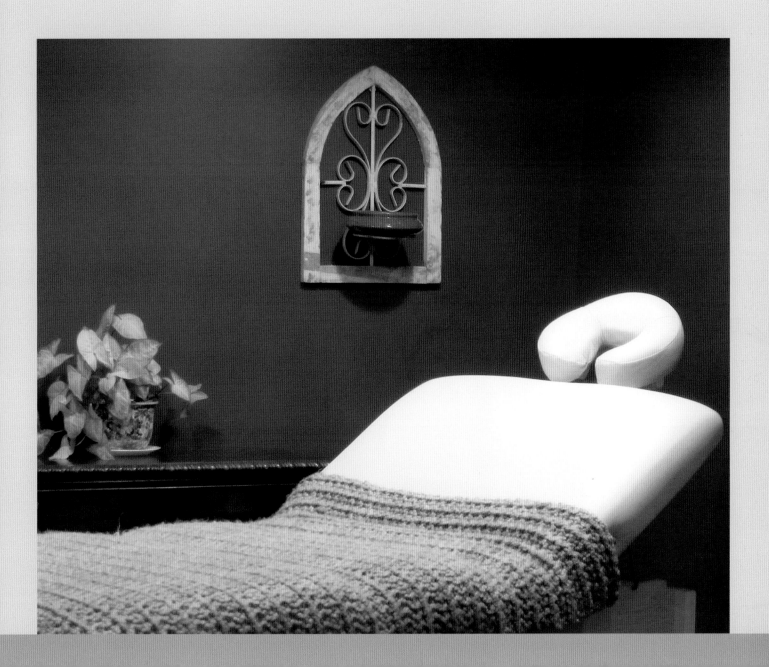

Remember to cover the receiver with a towel, sheet or blanket as his or her body temperature decreases as the treatment progresses. This also preserves the receiver's modesty, encouraging him or her to relax completely. As the giver, you will need a chair (swivel chairs are ideal) or stool to sit on. You need to be able to reach the receiver's feet easily without straining or creating any tension in your back, neck or shoulders.

Other points

There are a few other points to remember before starting a reflexology session:

- always wash your hands before and after giving a reflexology treatment
- make sure that your nails are short and clean
- take off your jewellery as rings, bracelets and watches can all scratch the receiver

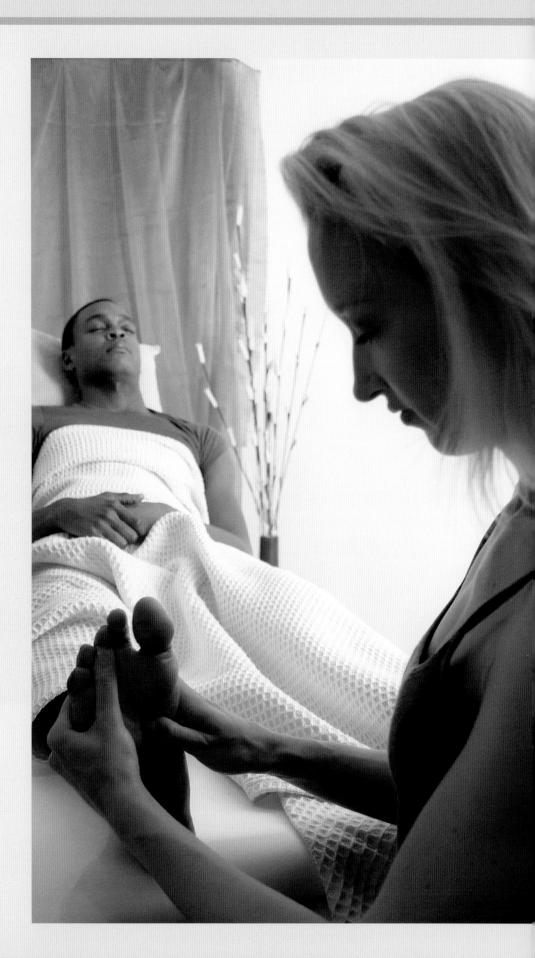

A physical examination of the feet: what the feet can tell you

A healthy pair of feet will look evenly pink in colour, will appear relaxed and free of hard skin, corns and calluses, and will feel pleasantly warm, but not clammy. The muscle tone will be good, the nails strong, and the feet will be supple and flexible. Feet like this are seldom seen, however!

The feet not only reveal physical problems, but are an indication of our emotional state, which is why it is helpful to consider the following aspects when examining the feet.

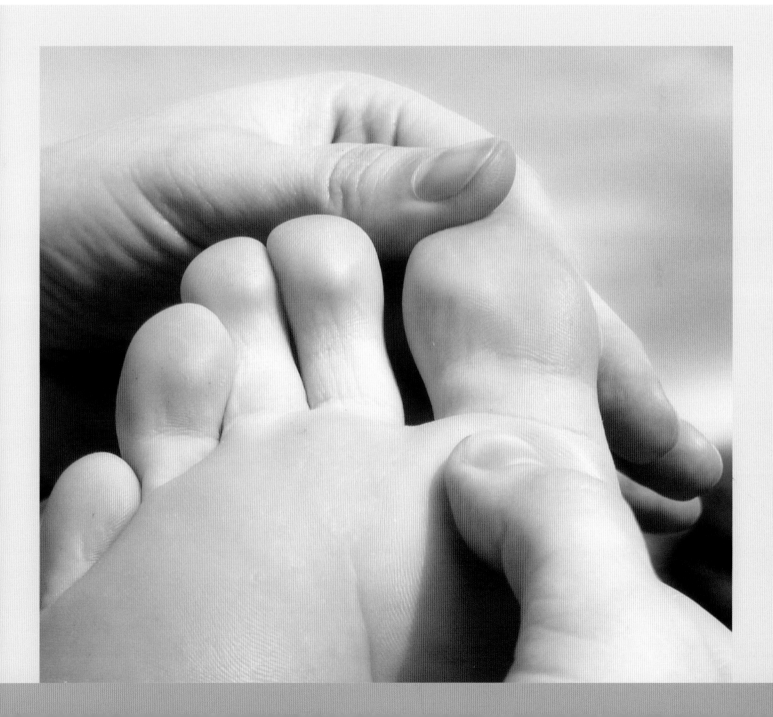

Skin colour

The skin colour of the feet can send certain messages.

- White feet indicate that circulation is poor. Feet that are drained of colour usually suggest exhaustion and tiredness.
- Red feet indicate blockages of energy to the reflexes. Anger and frustration can also cause the feet to turn red.
- Yellow feet indicate toxins in the body. Smoking can cause an intense yellowing over the lung area. Chemicals, medication and poor diet can all turn the feet yellow.
- Brown feet indicate a greater level of toxicity than yellow feet. Is the receiver fed up, or 'browned off', with life?
- Blue feet indicate poor circulation, and the feet may even turn purple with congestion. Emotional trauma can also make the feet appear 'black and blue'.
- Green tinges on the feet not only indicate areas of toxicity, but can also reveal envy and dissatisfaction with life.

Skin condition

The condition of the skin of the feet can tell you more about the receiver's wellbeing.

- Dry or peeling skin indicates dehydration and the need to drink more water. During a period of change, areas of skin can peel off the feet as the body lets go of the past to make way for the future.
- Hard skin impairs the flow of energy to the reflex areas. Areas of hard skin can also protect us from being hurt or suggest that we are hiding our true feelings.
- Corns and calluses also impair the energy flow to reflex areas. Continual pressure or friction can make areas of the feet callused (corns are smaller and develop on the toes, whereas calluses are usually found on the soles of the feet).

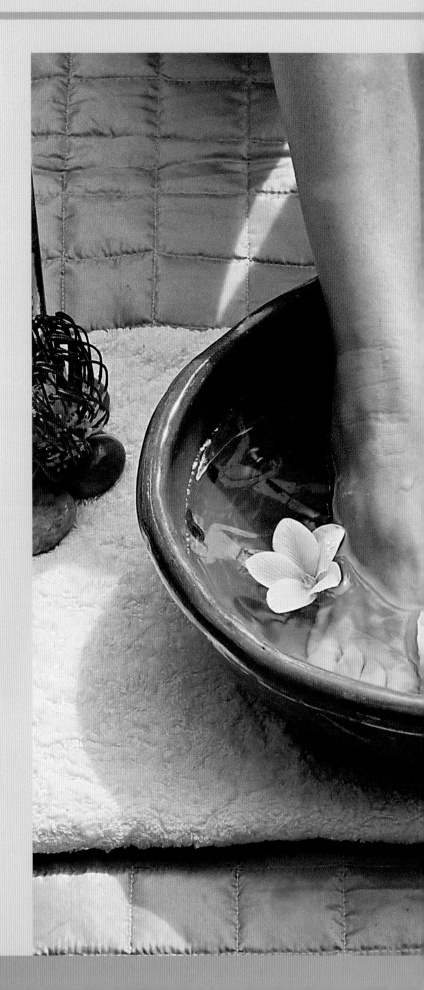

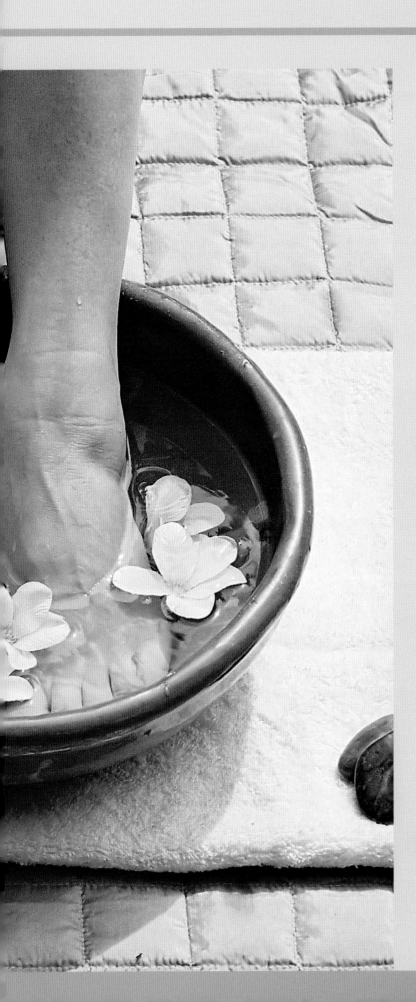

Foot odour

A 'cheesy' odour reveals the presence of toxins and a need for all of the systems of elimination to be stimulated.

An 'acetone' odour is also an indication that the systems of elimination, particularly the urinary system, are overburdened.

The nails

Don't forget to look at the nails for clues as to the receiver's wellbeing.

- Pinkish nails reveal a good state of health.
- White, blue or purple nails indicate poor circulation.
- Soft or thin nails may reveal a nutritional imbalance. They can also indicate a weak constitution and are often seen in sensitive individuals with a delicate nervous system.
- Thicker nails reveal vitality and physical strength. However, if they have become hard and discoloured, the reflex areas are blocked; such nails may also point to rigidity and stubbornness.
- Vertical ridges can indicate poor nutrition, tiredness and fatigue, as well as shock and trauma.
- Horizontal lines or indentations can also suggest trauma. They suggest changes in diet, too, and if there is more than one indentation, it is likely that more than one dietary change has taken place. (Note that it takes over six months for a nail to grow.)
- White spots on the nails may indicate a weak constitution, trauma or a lack of zinc.
- Spoon-shaped nails can reveal an iron deficiency.
- Pitted nails can indicate a skin disorder, such as psoriasis.

Other points to look out for

Look out for the following indications that all is not well, too:

- swelling or puffiness in the feet (indicating congestion)
- a low skin temperature or sweatiness (coldness indicates poor circulation, whereas clamminess and sweatiness reveal that the body's systems are overburdened with toxins)
- verrucae
- athlete's foot
- flaccid, floppy feet (these may reveal a lack of energy and inner strength and a tendency to let others take charge)
- spongy feet (these may indicate a tendency to give in too easily to others' demands)
- tense feet (these suggest a need for relaxation and a feeling of being ill at ease with oneself)
- stiff toes (these can reveal rigidity, inflexibility and stubbornness)
- wrinkled and lined feet (these may point to a troubled and concerned individual)
- bony abnormalities, such as bunions, hammer toes and flat feet or particularly high arches
- scars

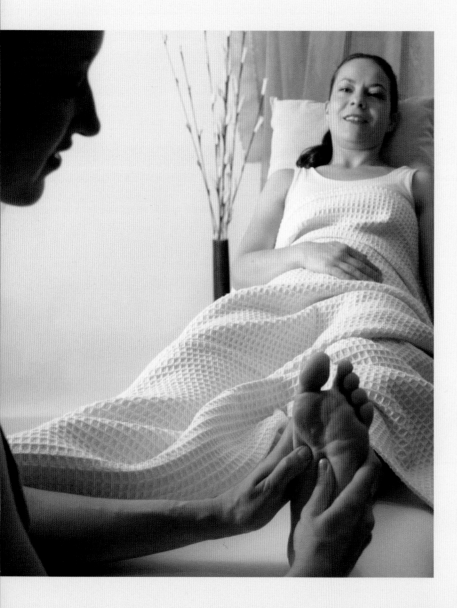

If you see anything unusual, remember that from the reflexologist's point of view the site of the abnormality is particularly important. For instance, any problem with the toes – whether it be corns, flaky skin, infections, bony deformities such as bent toes, or nail abnormalities – reveals that the reflex zones to the head are blocked. This could result in such disorders as sinusitis, headaches, problems with the teeth, hay fever, allergies, an inability to focus and concentrate, and so on. A small scar, puffiness or a bluish tinge over the area linked with the uterus or ovaries may indicate menstrual problems, such as irregular, scanty, heavy or painful menstruation, difficulties in conceiving or any other reproductive problem.

Remember! It does not matter what the abnormality is, but where it is!

Tense feet indicate a need for relaxation. ▶

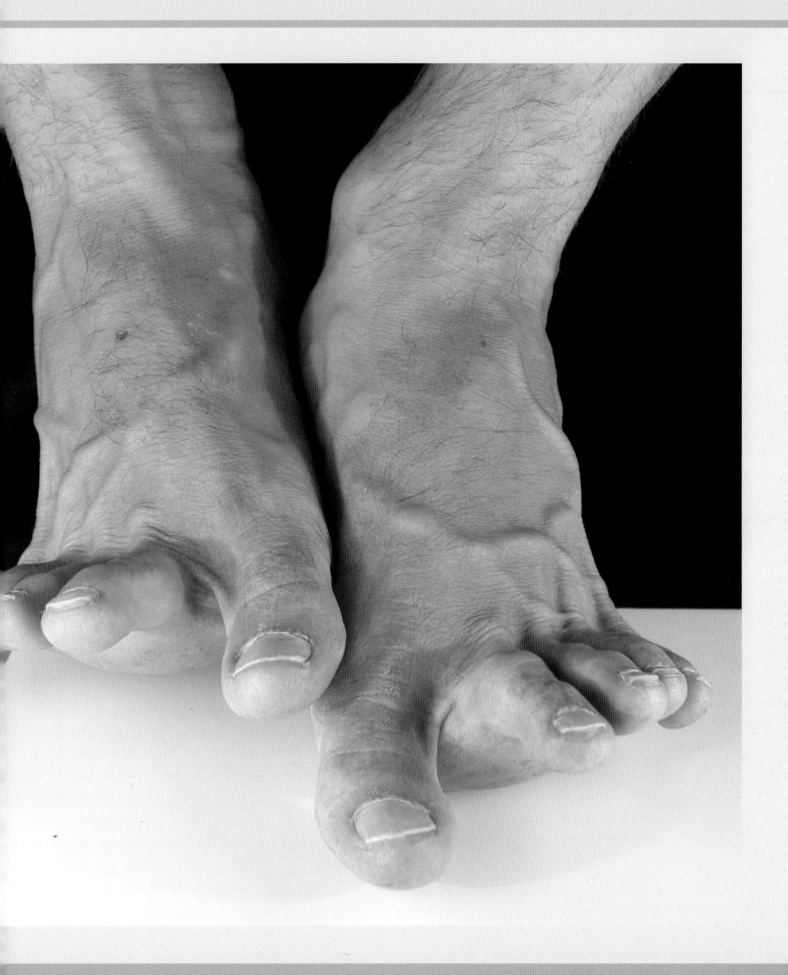

Cleansing the feet

After you have examined the receiver's feet, you may wish to cleanse them. Remember, however, to observe the feet first because after the feet have been cleansed, valuable information may be lost. So look first, then cleanse!

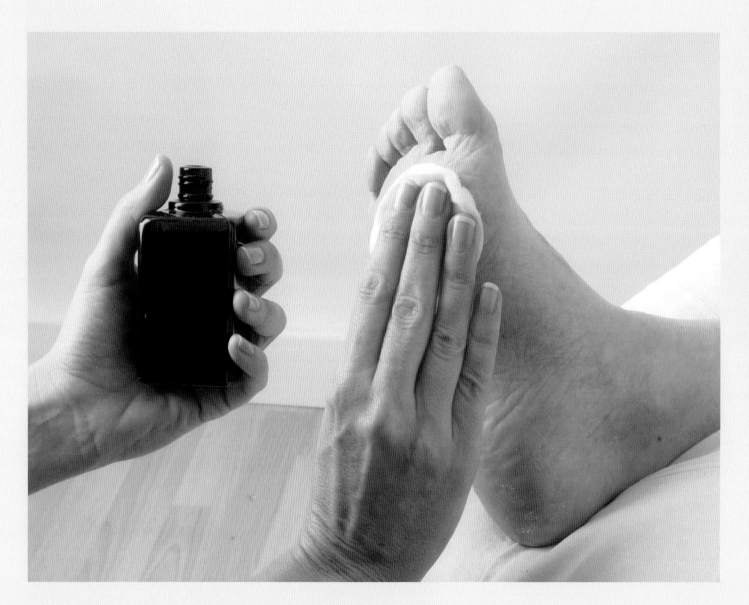

I like to cleanse and refresh the feet with rosewater, although any floral water, such as lavender or orange water, may be used. Use one cotton-wool pad or ball for each foot so that if there is an infection on one foot, you won't spread it to the other. You can also use surgical spirit to cleanse the feet, but be warned that the aroma is rather strong and not particularly appealing.

If you prefer, you can provide the receiver with a bowl of warm water in which to soak his or her feet. If you do this, why not add a few drops of essential oil to the bowl? Lavender is versatile and induces relaxation, while peppermint is perfect for cooling the feet during the summer months. If you have any fresh herbs growing in your garden, you could also add these to the water. There are many other fragrant possibilities, too!

Foot reflexology – basic techniques

There is a wide variety of treatment techniques used in reflexology. The ones most frequently used are described in this section.

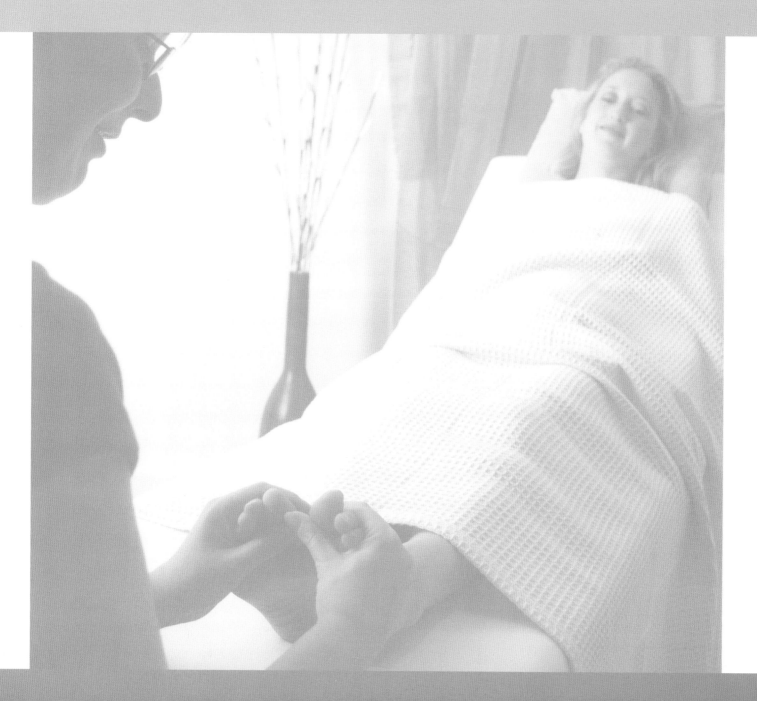

Supporting and holding techniques

There are many different ways in which to support and hold the feet during the treatment. By gently, yet firmly, supporting the receiver's feet properly, you are able to:

- instil trust and confidence
- make the treatment comfortable for both you and the receiver
- pinpoint and reach the reflex points and zones accurately and effectively.

Some of the most common holds are outlined below.

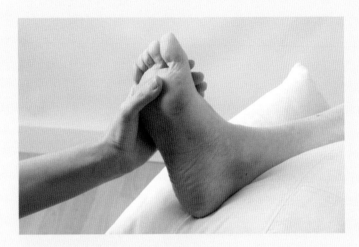

▲ Standard foot wrap

Lightly wrap the fingers of your hand over the upper third of the front of the foot, with your thumb resting gently on the ball of the foot. The outer aspect of the foot will rest gently in the palm of your hand.

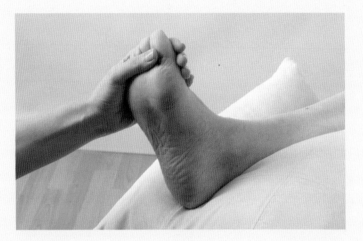

▲ High foot wrap

As a variation on the standard foot wrap technique, if you are working underneath the toes, or if you wish to bend the toes towards you, or away from you, then place your hand higher, so that your four fingers are positioned on the tops of the toes and your thumb rests on the underside of the toes.

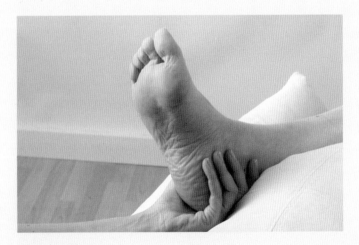

▲ Heel rest

The heel rest holding technique is particularly good when you are working on an area within the lower half of the foot, or when you are treating the inner or outer edge of the foot. Simply allow the receiver's heel to rest gently in the palm of your supporting hand.

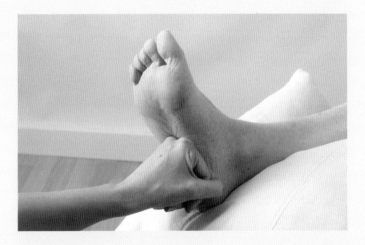

▲ Fist hold

For a fist hold, make a loose fist with your supporting hand and place it on the sole of the receiver's foot.

Flat of the hand hold ▶

You can also support the receiver's foot with the flat of your hand, either your palm or the back of your hand.

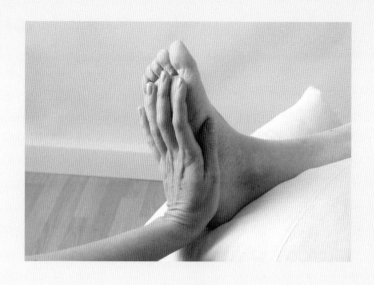

Basic foot reflexology treatment techniques

Many different treatment techniques are used in reflexology, and I will describe some of the ones that are used the most frequently. Note that the area that you are working on will largely determine the technique that you will use.

How much pressure?

The amount of pressure that you should use depends on the individual that you are working on, and should be adjusted accordingly. Generally, your touch should be firm, yet gentle – not too light or it will tickle, and not too firm or the receiver will try to pull his or her foot away from you. If you are working on a strong, fit adult, then a firmer pressure will be required than you would use if you were working on a frail, older person or a child.

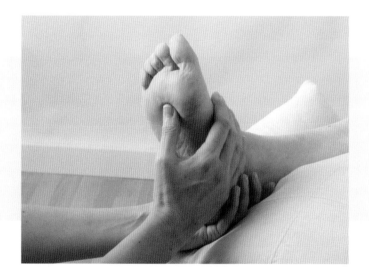

Although it is impossible to predict how much pressure it is best to use, I have noticed that stronger, earthier individuals like firmer pressure, whereas sensitive individuals prefer gentle pressure. (However, there will be times when they need a firmer touch.)
◀ Correct amount of pressure
▼ Too much pressure

It is important to remember that reflexology should never be painful for the receiver, but a wonderfully relaxing, delightful experience. On most occasions, the receiver will drift off to sleep.

Always observe the receiver's facial expressions or reactions during the treatment, and do not be afraid to ask for feedback about the amount of pressure that you are applying. Try to tune in to the pressure that the receiver requires – trust your intuition!

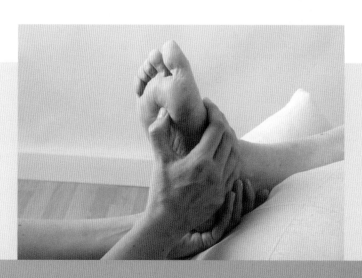

The thumb walking or caterpillar walking technique

The thumb walking or caterpillar walking technique is the most commonly used technique in reflexology, and is used on the majority of the reflexes. It is particularly useful for working on a large area of the foot. As the name of the technique suggests, the thumb 'walks' over the area of the foot being treated.

The basis of the thumb walking technique is the bending of the first joint of the thumb to an angle of about 45°. The following exercise is excellent for beginners.

Let's practice

Step 1 ▶

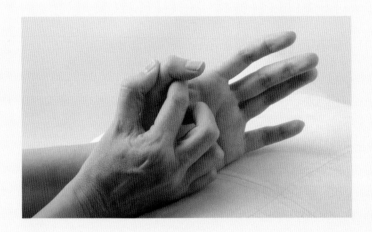

Using your index finger and thumb, hold your other thumb just underneath the first joint. This will stabilise it and prevent the other joint from bending. Now bend and straighten the joint several times. Then swap hands and bend your other thumb repeatedly. If you are right-handed, you may well find that your right thumb bends more easily than your left one, but don't worry about this as it won't be long before both thumbs are equally proficient at performing the movement. Now practise bending the first joint of each thumb without providing stabilisation.

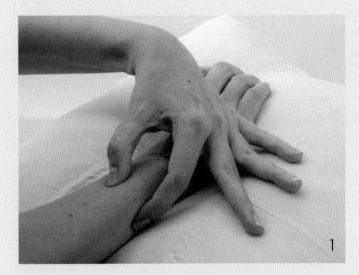

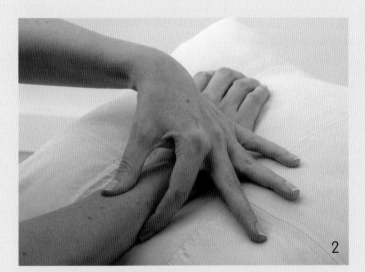

▲ **Step 2**
Once your thumbs are bending easily, place the outer edge of one of them either on your forearm or on your leg. (If you are unsure about which is the outer, and which is the inner, edge of your thumb, place your hand, palm facing downwards, on a flat surface, such as a table. The outer edge is the one that is touching the flat surface. By using the outer edge of your thumb, you will prevent your nail from pressing into the receiver's foot.)

▲ Now start to walk your thumb along your arm towards the elbow; then try this caterpillar walking technique on your other arm. You should take only tiny steps and should not bend and unbend your thumb fully, otherwise the receiver will feel it as being stiff and intrusive. Your thumb should bend at an angle of about 45°.

Step 3 The next step is to try caterpillar walking on your practice partner. Before you start, ensure that the receiver is positioned correctly (see pages 41-2). Although we are only practising, he or she will appreciate being relaxed and comfortable.
We will practise walking up each of the five zones on the sole of the foot. This zone walking is a treatment in itself, and can be used as a general boost for all of the systems of the body. The professional reflexologist will sometimes perform zone walking when a full treatment is not appropriate.

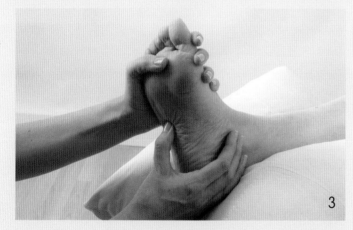

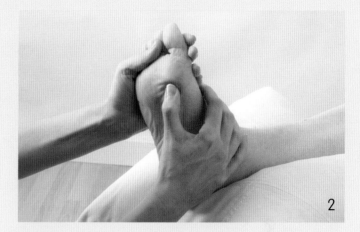

▲ Wrap your supporting hand around the receiver's foot, with your fingers on top and your thumb underneath. Position the thumb of your other hand at the bottom of zone 1 (i.e., in line with the big toe). Now caterpillar walk from the heel of the foot up, towards the big toe.

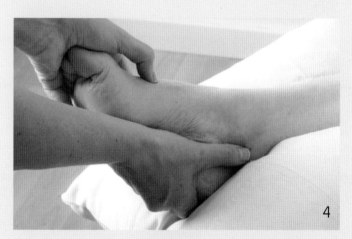

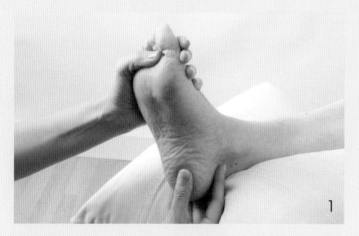

▲ Next, work upwards, from the base of the heel in zone 2 towards toe two, and then continue to caterpillar walk along zones 3, 4 and 5.

▲ Now try zone walking on the dorsum (top) of the foot. Rest the receiver's heel in your supporting hand and place the fingers of your supporting hand on the sole, with your thumb positioned on top, and pull the receiver's foot towards you slightly. Use your thumb to caterpillar walk down zone 1, from the big toe towards the ankle. Then caterpillar walk down zones 2, 3, 4 and 5.

Repeat this movement several times, both to give a general boost to all of the body's systems and to clear the zones. Now try caterpillar walking along the zones of the other foot. This technique is of prime importance in reflexology, and because it will take practice to perfect your techniques, it is vital to keep trying.

Tips
You may find the following tips helpful.

1 Ensure that you are using the outer edge of your thumb.
2 Bend only the first joint of your thumb, to an angle of approximately 45°, and do not flex it completely.
3 Keep the pressure that you are applying steady and constant.
4 Only ever caterpillar walk forwards, not backwards or sideways.
5 Do not grip the receiver's hand too firmly.

The finger walking technique

The finger walking technique is similar to the thumb walking technique, except that it involves the bending of the first joint of one or more fingers. It is a gentler technique, and is applied mainly to the dorsum (top) of the foot, which is more bony and sensitive than the sole of the foot.

Let's practice

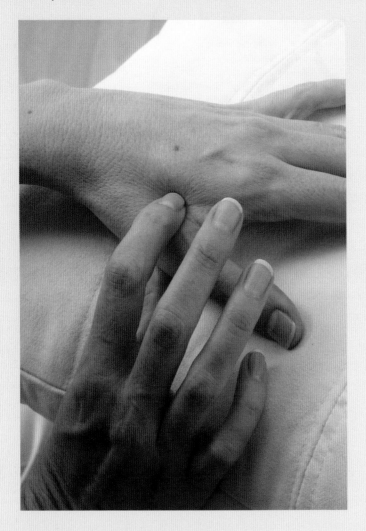

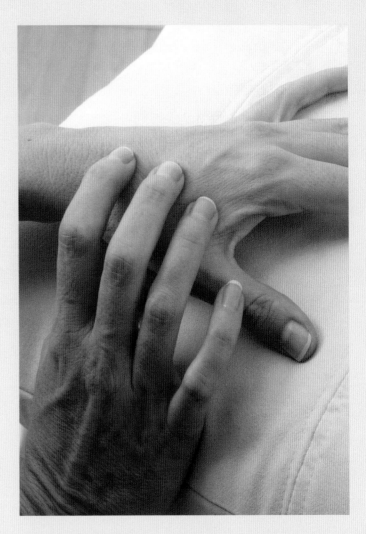

▲ **Step 1: single finger walking**
First of all, it is recommended that you practise finger walking on the top of your own hand. Try single finger walking across the top of your hand first. Gently walk your index finger across the top of your hand. Do several rows of finger walking until you reach the wrist.

▲ **Step 2: multiple finger walking**
Now try finger walking using more than one finger. Try walking two fingers across the top of your hand first, then use three fingers and, finally, use all four fingers. (You may find this technique easier when you are using more than one finger.)

Step 3: time to practise on your partner ▼ ▶

Support the receiver's foot by resting his or her heel in the palm of your hand. First of all, try to walk down the foot using just one finger of the other hand. Then place the tips of all four fingers on top of the foot, with your thumb on the sole, and walk all four fingers in unison across the top.

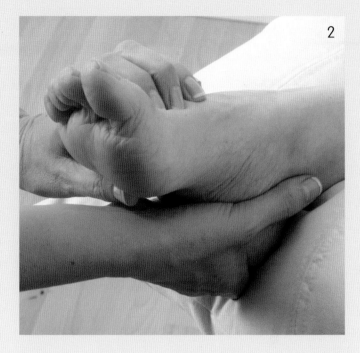

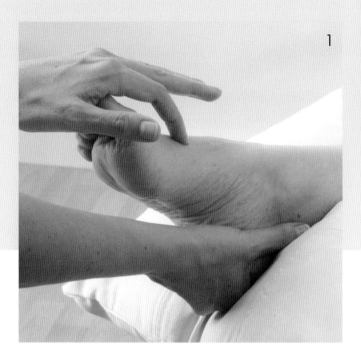

A variation ▶

A variation on this technique is two-handed finger walking. This movement is incredibly relaxing and gives a boost to all of the systems of the body. Place the fingertips of both hands on top of the foot, just above the toes, with your thumbs on the sole. Finger walk across the top of the foot until your fingertips meet up in the middle. Repeat this procedure several times, covering the entire dorsum (top) of the foot.

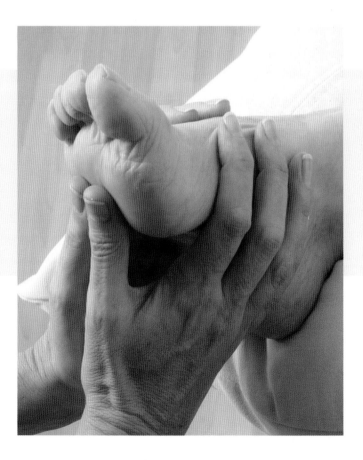

Tips

You may find the following tips helpful.

1 Apply gentle pressure.
2 Keep your movements constant and even.
3 Avoid digging your nails into the receiver's skin.
4 Keep your steps small.
5 Walk your fingers forwards.

The hook in and back up technique

The hook in and back up technique is often likened to a bee inserting its sting. It is particularly useful for accurately pinpointing reflex points that are small, specific and deep. The hook in and back up technique would never be used over a large area. To perform this technique, place the outer edge of your flexed thumb on the reflex, push it in and then pull your thumb back, across the point.

Let's practice

Step 1 ▼

First of all, practise this technique on your hand. Place your thumb on the palm of your other hand, with your fingers resting gently on the back of your hand (not gripping it). Bend the first joint of your thumb, press it into your hand firmly (hook in)

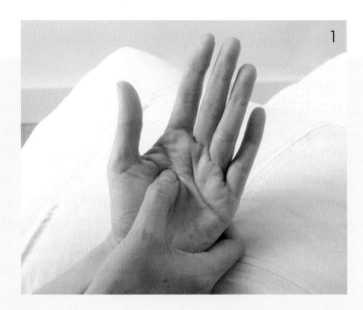

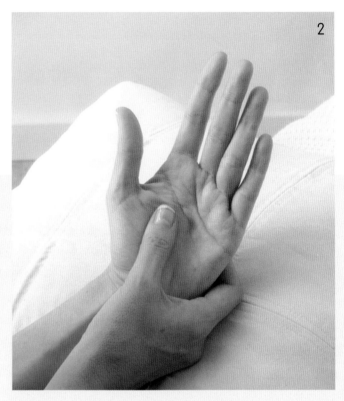

▲ and then pull it back, across the point (back up).

Step 2 ▶

Now practise the technique on the receiver's foot. Bend the first joint of your working thumb and then place the tip of your thumb on your chosen reflex point (for example, on the centre of the big toe, which reflects the pituitary gland, which it is vital to treat in cases of hormonal problems). Press firmly into the reflex point (hook in) and then pull your thumb back, across the point (back up).

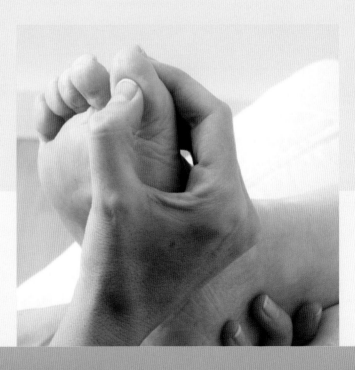

Tips

You may find the following tips helpful.

1 Avoid pressing in with your nail.
2 Do not grip the foot too tightly.

The pressure circle technique

Pressure circles are usually performed using the pad of the thumb, although the pad of a finger may be used if necessary. This technique is particularly useful for treating sensitive reflexes on the foot, enabling them to become unblocked and balanced.

Tips

You may find the following tips helpful.

1 Keep your circling movement slow and even.
2 Do not dig into the receiver's foot with your thumb.

Let's practice ▼

Support the receiver's foot by gently resting their heel in the palm of your hand. Place the flexed pad of your working thumb on your chosen reflex point (for instance, that of the thyroid gland), press it into the area and circle over it several times, keeping your thumb in contact with the point. After just a few pressure circles, any tenderness at that point should have subsided.

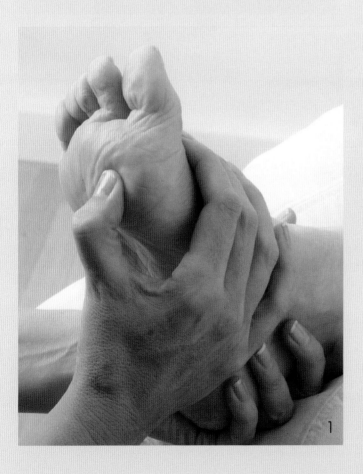
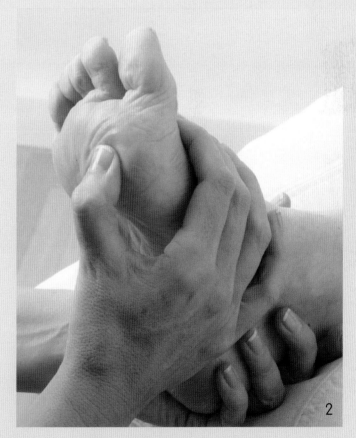

The press and release technique

The press and release technique is particularly suitable for treating small reflex points. The palmar surface of the thumb pad is used.

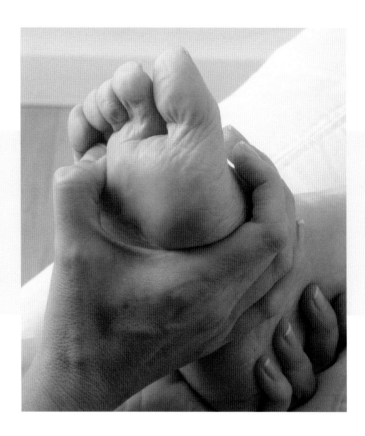

Let's practice ▶

Support the receiver's foot in the heel of your hand. Place the pad of your thumb on the chosen reflex point (such as the ear reflex, which is located between toes four and five), press it into the point for a few seconds and then release the pressure. Repeat several times.

Tips

You may find the following tips helpful.

1 Do not press in with your nail.
2 Maintain a steady pressure.

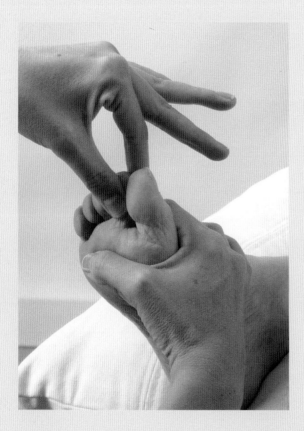

The press and hold technique

My press and hold technique is highly effective when pain relief is required, for instance, if the receiver is suffering from toothache or earache, or when a joint, such as a shoulder or knee, is painful and troublesome. This technique will enable you to decrease the pain and sensitivity in a specific area. It normally involves the combined use of your thumb and index finger.

Let's practice

Support the receiver's foot by wrapping your fingers around the dorsum (top) of the foot and positioning your thumb just under the base of the toes. Place the pad of the thumb of your working hand on the bottom of the toe and the tip of your index finger on the top of the toe. Gently squeeze your finger and thumb towards each other (but do not pinch) and maintain this pressure for up to 20 seconds, until any tenderness subsides. In this illustration, we are working on one of the reflexes for the teeth.

Tips

You may find the following tips helpful.

1 Do not pinch the area being worked on.
2 Try to apply equal pressure with both your thumb and index finger as you press and hold the reflex.

The rotation on a point technique

The rotation on a point technique is useful for treating a small reflex, and involves pinpointing an area and then rotating the receiver's foot around it. The pad of the thumb is usually employed in this technique, but you may use a finger if you prefer.

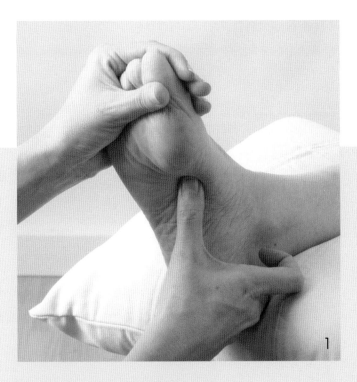

Let's practice ▶ ▼

Place the fingers of your supporting hand across the dorsum (top) of the foot, close to the base of the toes, and position your thumb so that it is resting across the ball of the foot. Use the pad of your working thumb to locate the relevant point (such as the adrenal reflex). Use your supporting hand to flex the foot gently and slowly down, onto your thumb, keeping your thumb stationary as you circle the foot around the point several times.

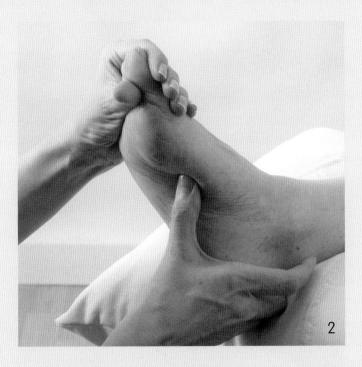

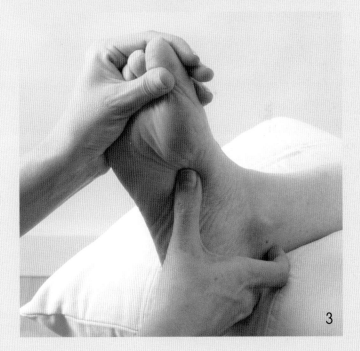

Tips

You may find the following tips helpful.

1 Do not grip the receiver's foot tightly with your holding hand.   2 Do not press your thumb or finger too firmly into the area.

3 For maximum comfort and effectiveness, always circle the foot slowly around the point.

The sliding technique

The sliding technique is particularly useful when treating the reflex for the spine (on the inner aspect of the foot), where it is often used in combination with caterpillar walking. The thumb is most commonly used for 'sliding', but the index finger is also suitable.

Let's practice ▼

We will be treating the inner aspect (medial border) of the foot, which relates to the spine. Support the receiver's foot under the heel with your holding hand.

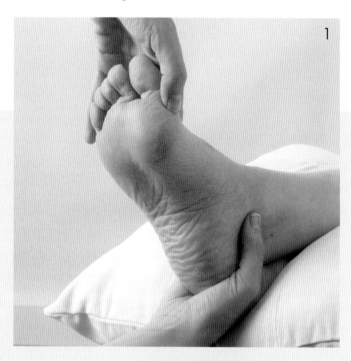

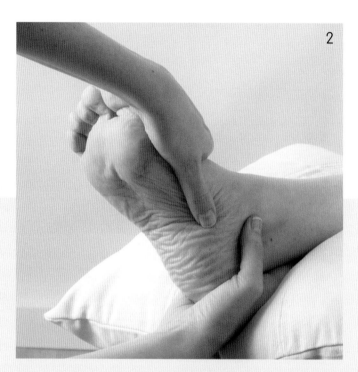

Gently press your working thumb on the inner edge of the foot at the base of the toenail (which represents the upper part of the spine) and slowly slide it all of the way down the inside of the foot, maintaining the pressure.

Then change hands and hold the top of the foot with your fingers, with your thumb positioned on the sole, under the base of the toes. Press your working thumb on the bottom of the inner edge of the foot and slide it upwards from the bottom of the heel.

Tips

You may find the following tips helpful.

1 Ensure that you slide your thumb forwards.
2 Try to slide slowly and smoothly and avoid making any jerky actions.
3 Keep the pressure constant.

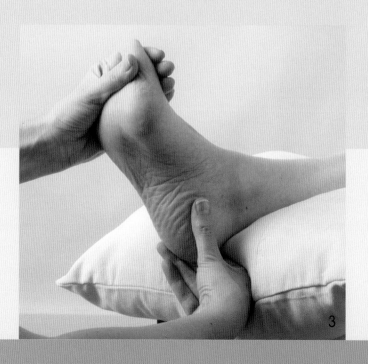

The kneading technique

The kneading technique is suitable for thicker, less sensitive areas of the sole of the foot, where you wish to apply deep pressure over a large area.

Let's practice ▶

This technique is often performed on the sole over the heel area, as well as just below the base of the toes. To work on the area under the base of the toes, wrap your holding hand around the upper part of the receiver's foot, with your thumb positioned underneath and your fingers on top. Make a loose fist with your working hand, place it on the receiver's foot, and use a gentle, circular action over the thicker, upper part of the sole and then knead the heel area.

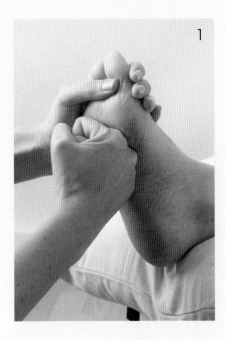
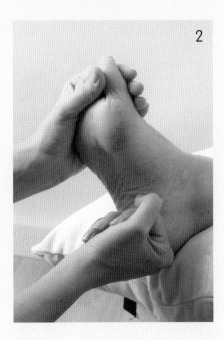

Tips

You may find the following tips helpful.
1   Do not apply too much pressure.
2   Make sure that you have removed any rings.

The rubbing technique

The rubbing technique is useful when you wish to bring warmth to an area, to decongest a reflex or to de-stress and energise. Various parts of your hands may be employed for rubbing. For instance, the palms of both hands would be used when working on the inner and outer edges of the foot, whereas the index fingers would be used to rub the toes. Rubbing creates friction, and therefore generates warmth.

Let's practice ▶

Step 1: rubbing the sides of the foot
Place one palm on the inside edge of the foot and the other on the outside edge and rub your hands alternately up and down the sides of the foot. Feel the warmth!

Step 2: rubbing a toe
Place your index fingers on either side of your chosen toe and then rub it gently, moving your index fingers in opposite directions.

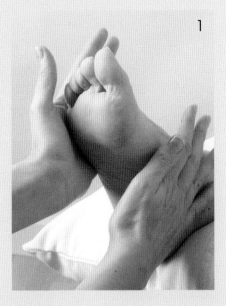
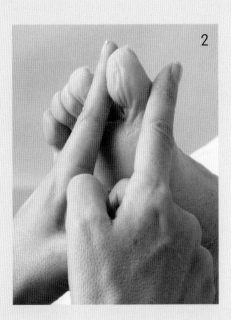

Tips

You may find the following tips helpful.
1   Do not rub too vigorously.
2   Keep your hands or fingers relaxed.

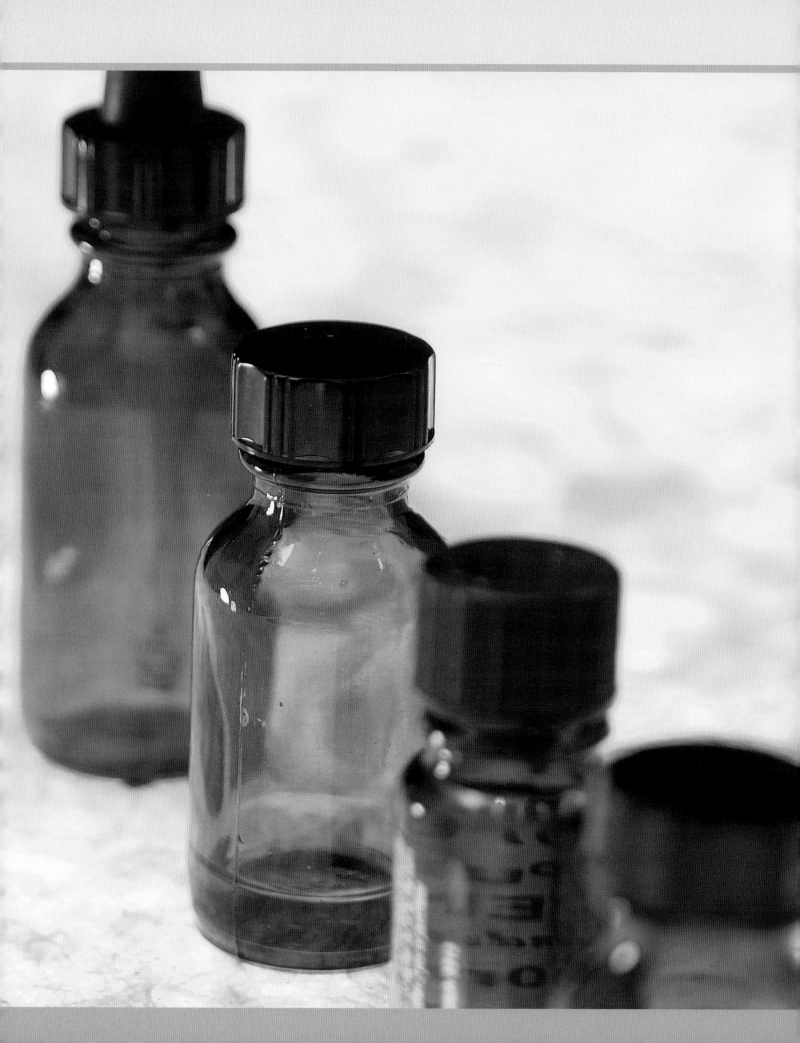

Foot reflexology – the sequence

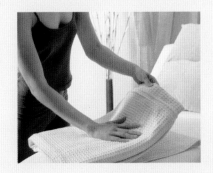 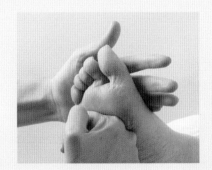 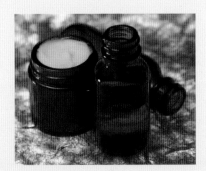

This section will enable you to carry out a complete reflexology routine. Detailed instructions and colour photographs will guide you gently first of all through a relaxation sequence, and then through the reflexes of the feet step-by-step. Your confidence and expertise will soon grow! Detailed colour foot charts can be found at the back of this book and you may wish to familiarise yourself with them before giving a treatment.

How long should the treatment take?

The length of a reflexology session can vary, depending on the receiver's age, fitness and sensitivity. (Please refer to pages 29-31 for advice on contraindications and cautions.) But in the case of a healthy individual, a treatment will normally take about 45 minutes. (The routine will obviously take you longer to work through at first because you are learning a new skill, but you will be surprised how quickly you speed up.) Do not think that a longer treatment is more effective, however, because if you provide treatment for too long, the reflexes can be overstimulated.

How often should I provide treatment?

Providing treatment once a week to begin with would achieve excellent results. Note that it is necessary to leave time between treatments in order to allow healing to take place.

How many sessions will be needed?

Just one session of reflexology is a wonderful experience for the receiver. You will be amazed by its effects, and the receiver will definitely want more! Providing approximately six sessions initially, and then one session per month in order to maintain health and prevent any problems from occurring, is ideal. This is not always possible, of course, in which case give or receive a treatment whenever you can.

How quickly will I see results?

Remarkably, results are sometimes seen after just one session of reflexology, although it may take a few sessions before the full benefits become evident. Do not be discouraged if results are not immediately obvious, however, for this does not mean that the treatment is not working. Keep persevering, for you will eventually succeed!

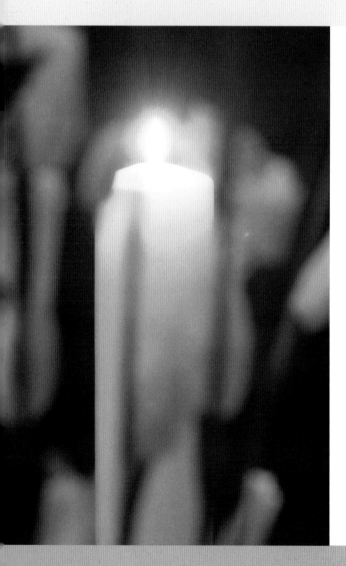

A reflexology checklist

Prior to the reflexology session, ensure the following.

1   Ensure that you have created the right ambience (see pages 39-40).

2   Ensure that the receiver is comfortable, with pillows under his or her head and one under the knees. If you wish, keep a small, rolled-up towel to hand to place under the foot that you are working on.

3   Ensure that you are positioned comfortably.

4   Ensure that you have removed any jewellery.

5   Ensure that your nails are short and your hands are clean.

6   Ensure that you have checked for any contraindications.

7   Ensure that you have carried out a physical examination of the receiver's feet.

8   Ensure that you have refreshed the receiver's feet.

9   Ensure that you have washed your hands.

10 Ensure that you feel relaxed and full of positivity. Consciously try to clear your mind and take a few deep breaths to release any tension. Try to be serene, peaceful and loving.

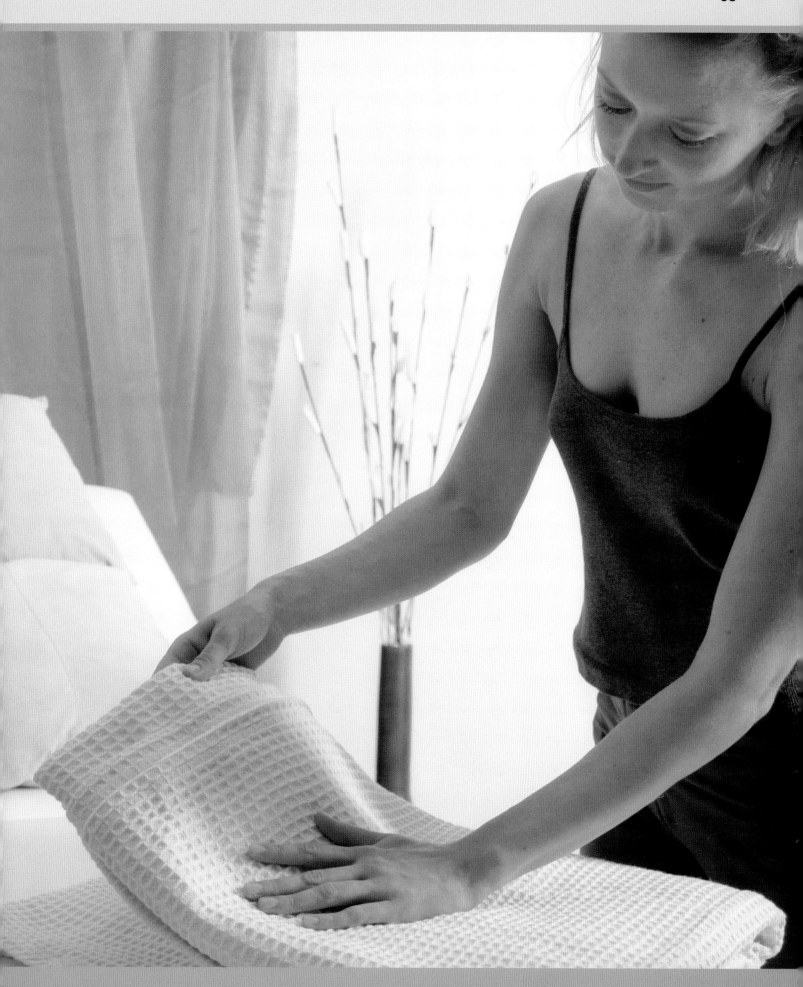

The relaxation sequence

Relaxation techniques are recommended for use prior to a specific reflexology treatment as they:

- encourage initial relaxation;
- build up a relationship of trust between giver and receiver;
- put both of you at ease;
- loosen muscular tension in the feet so that they are easier to work on;
- provide the perfect opportunity for you to judge how much pressure is needed.

Relaxation techniques may also be used during the reflexology routine gently to disperse any toxins released during treatment. And when used at the end of a session, they provide a wonderful 'dessert'.

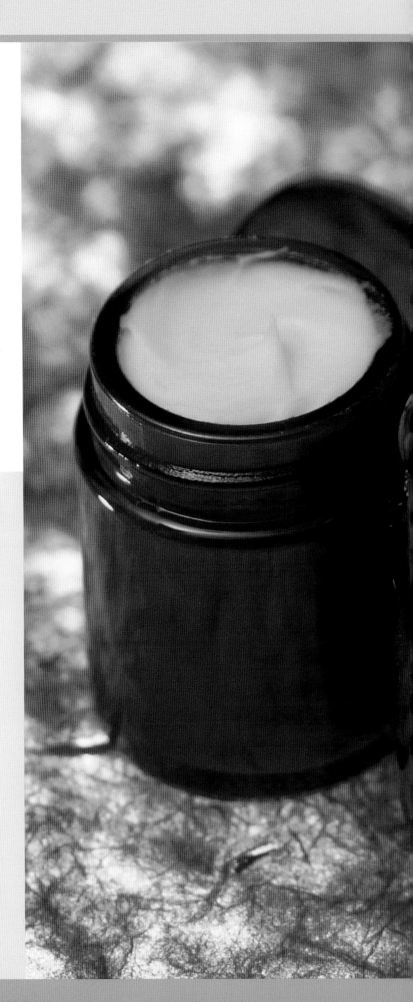

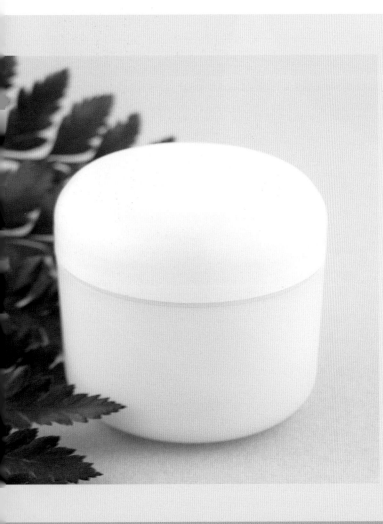

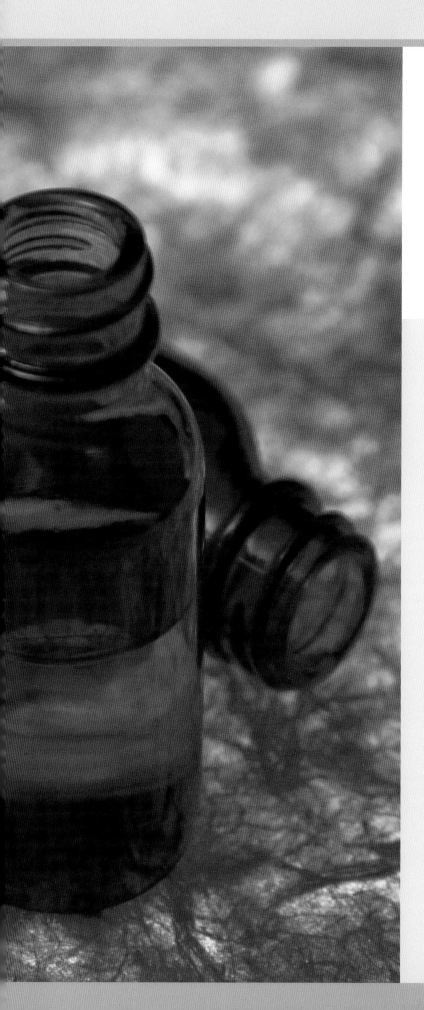

Should I use oils or creams?

Do not use oils or creams either prior to or during the reflexology treatment, otherwise the receiver's feet and your hands will become oily, causing them to slip and slide and making it difficult for you to feel the reflex points.

You can use oils or creams for your final relaxation movements at the end of a treatment, however. You can make the most wonderful blended oils or creams tailored specially to the individual, and if this interests you, please refer to pages 235-41.

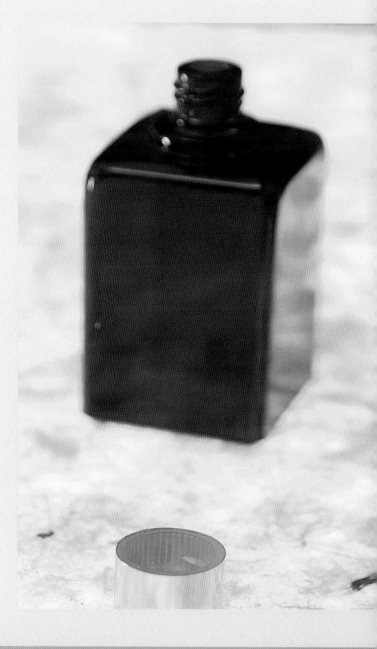

Relaxation sequence – right foot

It is not necessary to use all of the relaxation techniques described here, just as many as you wish.

These techniques are very flexible, and it is not essential to use them in a set order. But whichever ones you eventually choose, try to ensure that you always work on all areas of the foot, i.e., the sole, the dorsum (top) and the sides of the foot. It is also advisable to use the joint-loosening techniques.

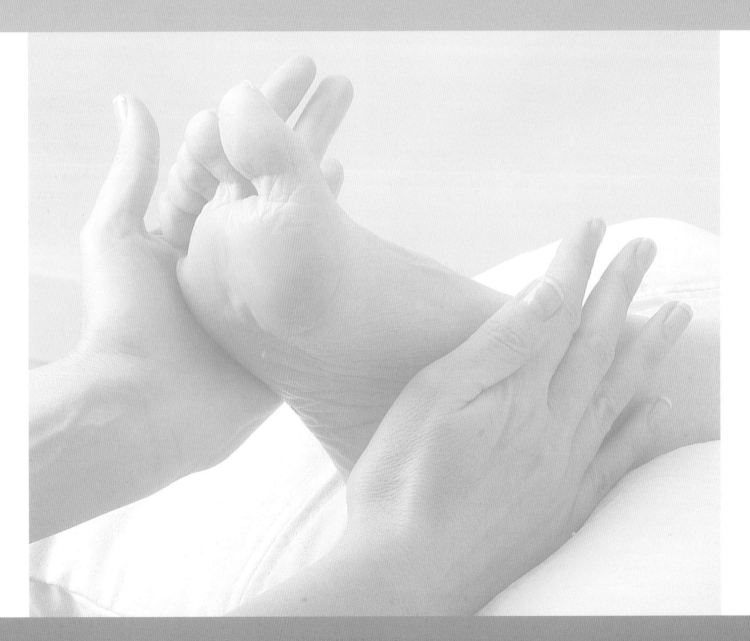

Opening moves

Relaxation movement 1: greeting the foot ▶

Place one palm on top of the receiver's foot and the other palm on the sole and gently hold the foot between your hands for about 30 seconds, or until you both become relaxed. This initial contact not only relieves tension, but also enables you to tune in to the receiver.

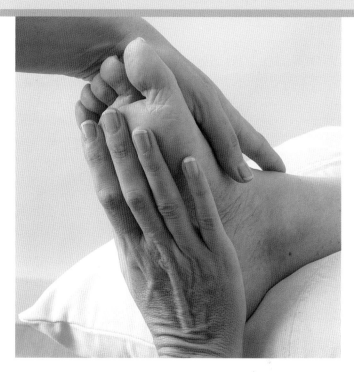

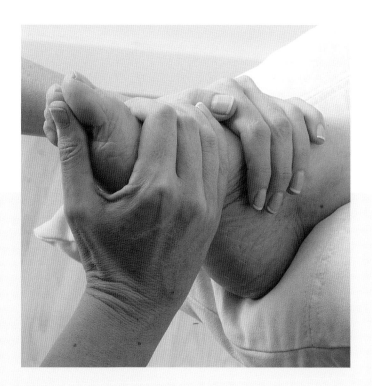

◀ Relaxation movement 2: stroking the foot

Place both hands on top of the receiver's foot and then gently stroke it, moving upwards, from the toes towards the ankle. When you reach the ankle, move smoothly around the anklebones and then glide your hands back to their starting point, without applying any pressure. Your movements should be gentle at first in order to release tension, but you should then start to increase the pressure to stimulate the circulation and to help to disperse any retained fluid, especially around the ankles.

There are many variations on this stroking movement, and all are valid. Try to develop your own stroking movements, ones that you feel happy with. For instance, try stroking the receiver's foot with one hand on top of the foot and one underneath it.

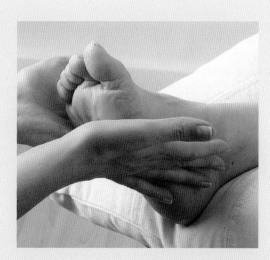

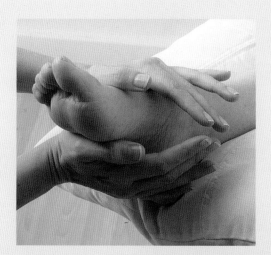

Working the sole

Relaxation movement 3: opening the sole of the foot ▶ ▼

The opening the sole of the foot technique involves using your thumbs to slide across the sole of the receiver's foot. Place both thumbs at the bottom of the sole of the foot, with one positioned slightly higher than the other and your fingers resting on the dorsum (top) of the foot. Slide your thumbs out, towards the sides of the foot, and then glide them back towards one another, allowing them to reverse their position (i.e., if your left thumb was higher when you started, the right thumb should now be higher). Repeat this movement until you reach the base of the toes, and then work all of the way back down again. Repeat until the sole feels soft and supple.

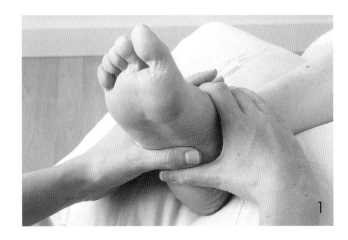

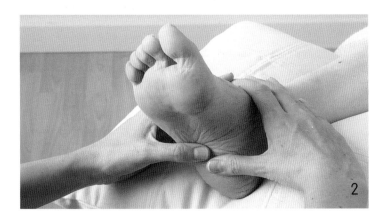

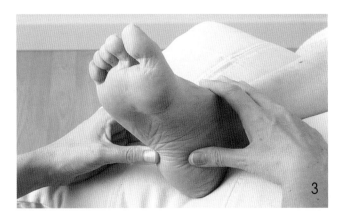

▼ **Relaxation movement 4: stretching the sole of the foot**

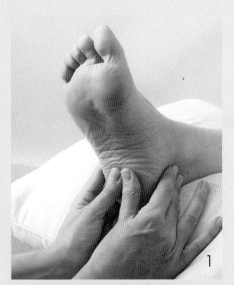

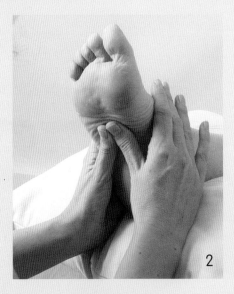

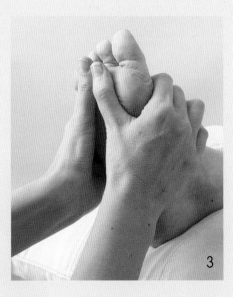

Now place both hands roughly in the middle of the bottom of the receiver's foot. Pull your thumbs up the foot, working towards the toes. Repeat this movement several times to stretch the sole of the foot gently.

Relaxation movement 5: kneading the foot ▶
This kneading the foot movement is often called 'metatarsal kneading' as it involves using the fist to work into the metatarsals of the feet. Wrap your holding hand across the top of the receiver's foot, with your fingers on top and your thumb underneath. Make a loose fist with your other hand and place it on the heel area. Now knead your fist into the area using a gentle, circular motion.

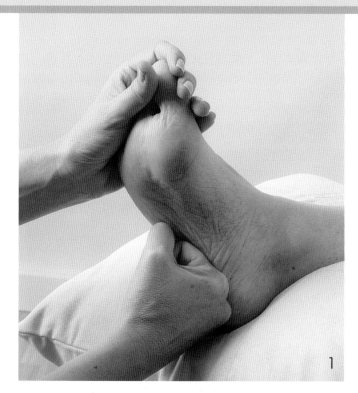

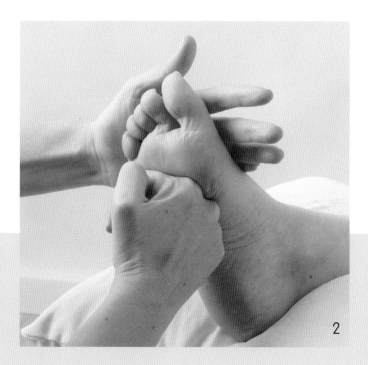

◀ Work upwards, towards the ball of the foot, and as you knead the upper part of the sole, move your supporting hand slightly so that the whole of your palm is on top of the foot. Metatarsal kneading is excellent for releasing muscular tension, loosening joints and decongesting the sole of the foot.

Relaxation movement 6: fist sliding ▶
Gently support the receiver's foot either by resting the heel in the palm of your hand, or by wrapping your supporting hand around the top of the foot. Make a loose fist with your other hand and place it on the heel area. Slide your fist slowly up the foot, towards the toes, and then gently stroke the foot with the back of your hand as you return to your starting position. Repeat several times.

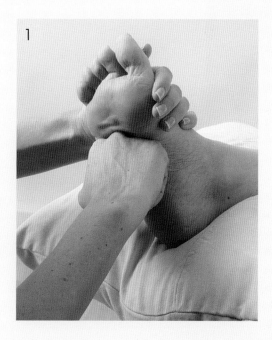

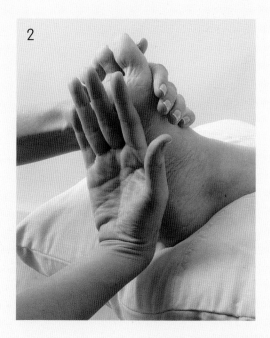

Working the dorsum (top) of the foot

Relaxation movement 7: ▶
finger circling on the dorsum
Place the pads of all of your
fingers on the top of the
receiver's foot, just below the
toes, with your thumbs on the
sole. Now make tiny, circular
movements with your fingers,
moving from the toes upwards,
towards the ankle. Continue to
circle all around the anklebones
and then gently glide your
hands back to your starting
position. Repeat several times.

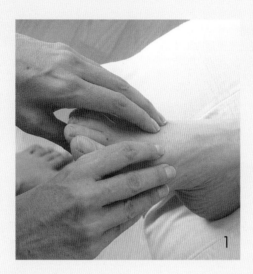

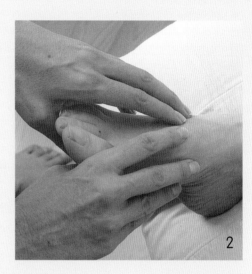

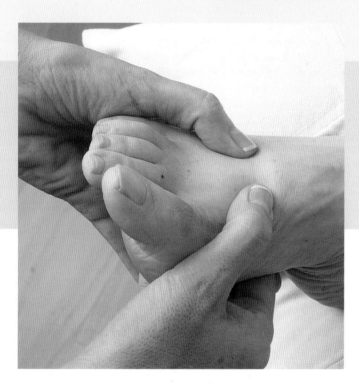

◀ **Relaxation movement 8: thumb circling on the dorsum**
This relaxation movement is very similar to the last movement.
Place your thumbs on the top of the receiver's foot, just below the
bases of the toes, and perform circular movements with them as
you move them down, towards the ankle, before gently gliding
your hands back up the foot.

Relaxation movement 9: finger sliding on the dorsum ▶
Support the receiver's foot with your holding hand and place
the fingertips of your other hand on the top of the foot.
Gently slide your fingers down the foot, moving towards the
ankle, and then glide them back again. Repeat several times to
loosen up the top of the foot.

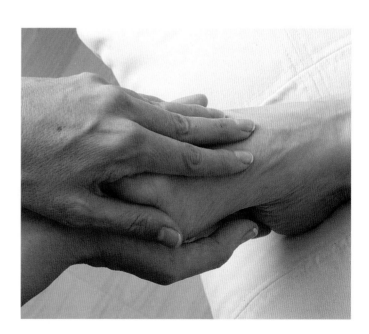

Working the sides of the feet

▼ Relaxation movement 10: stroking the spine

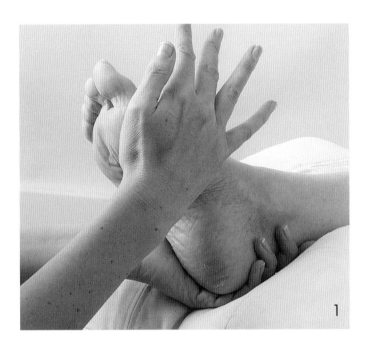

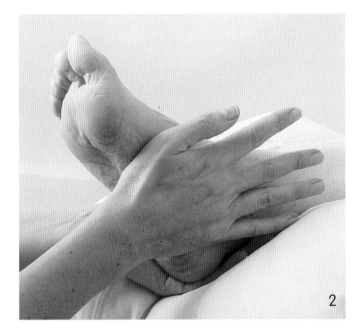

Gently cup the heel of the receiver's foot with your supporting hand. Now use the heel of your working hand to stroke down, along the inside of the foot, before gently gliding back again. Repeat several times to loosen up the inside of the foot (which corresponds to the spine).

Relaxation movement 11: sliding the ▶ spine

Once again, support the receiver's foot under the heel. Place your working thumb at the base of the toenail on the inner edge of the foot and then slide it slowly down the inside of the foot. Now hold the top of the foot, place your working thumb on the bottom of the inner edge of the foot and slide it up, towards the big toe. Repeat several times.

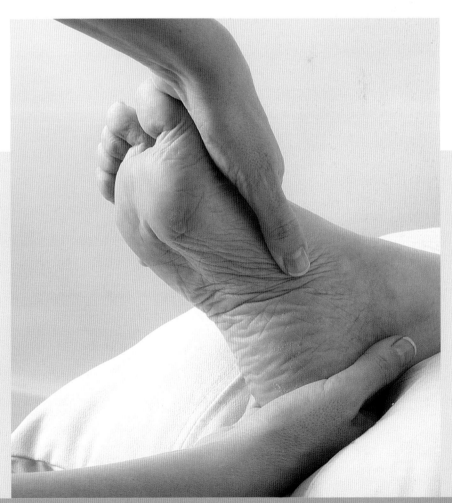

Relaxation movement 12: twisting the spine   ▼ ▶
Place the palm of one hand on the inside of the receiver's foot
and the other on the outside. Now use the heels of your hands
to pull the outside of the foot towards you as you push the
inside of the foot away from you and then vice versa. You will
really feel the sides of the feet loosening. This technique is a
must for people who suffer from back problems as it helps to
mobilise the spine.

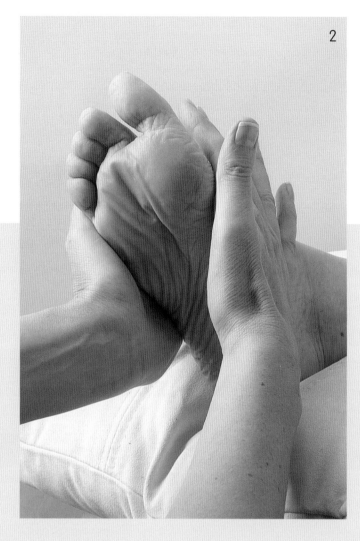

2

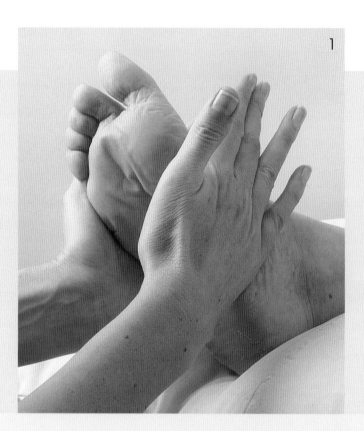

1

Relaxation movement 13: ▶
rubbing the sides of the foot
Place one palm on the inside of the receiver's
foot and one on the outer edge of the foot.
Now rub your hands alternately up and down
the sides of the foot.

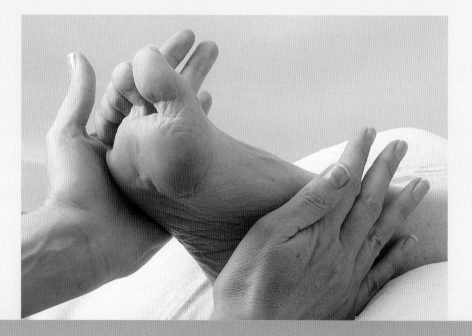

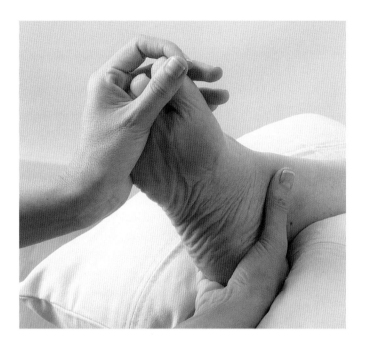

Loosening the joints

◀ **Relaxation movement 14: loosening the ankle**
Support the receiver's foot under the heel, with your thumb resting on one side of the ankle and your fingers on the other. Gently hold the top of the foot with your working hand and then slowly circle the ankle clockwise and then anti-clockwise. The amount of movement will vary, depending on the individual: expect a wider range of movement from a healthy, young adult than from an arthritic, elderly person. This movement is great for increasing mobility in the hips and pelvis.

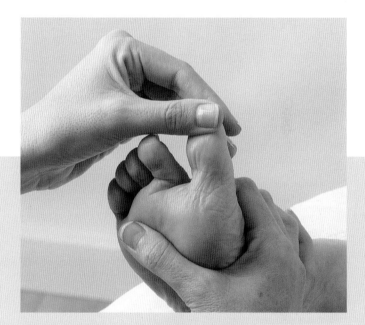

Relaxation movement 15: loosening the toes ▶
Support the receiver's foot, with your thumb placed on the sole and your fingers on the dorsum (top). Using your other thumb and index finger, gently and slowly rotate each toe in a clockwise direction, and then in an anticlockwise one. This technique will not only help to keep the toes flexible, but can also loosen the neck (whose reflex is in the big toe) and unblock the sinuses (whose reflexes are in the other toes).

As a variation on this technique, place your thumb on the sole of the foot and your fingers on the top and then use your working hand to rotate all of the toes at once.

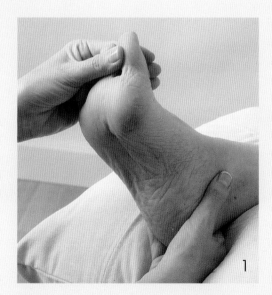

1

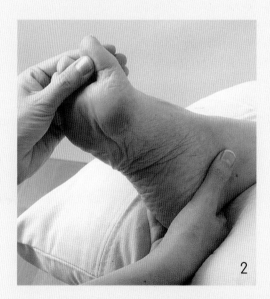

2

Final moves

▼ **Relaxation movement 16: the Achilles' stretch**

Gently clasp the receiver's heel in the palm of one hand and place the other hand on the top of the foot. Moving slowly and gently, pull the receiver's heel towards you and hold this position for a few seconds before gradually releasing the stretch (1).

Now gently, but firmly, push the receiver's foot away from you and then pull it down, towards you (2).

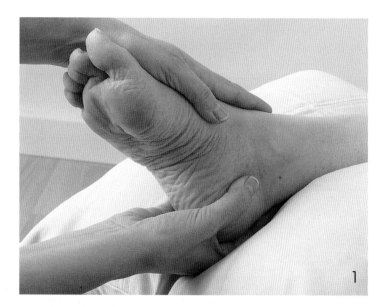

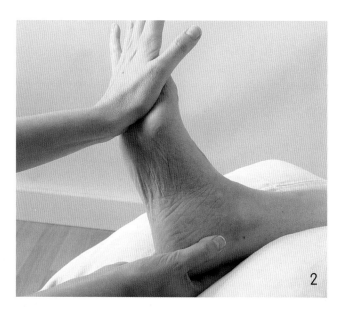

▼ **Relaxation movement 17: the solar plexus release**

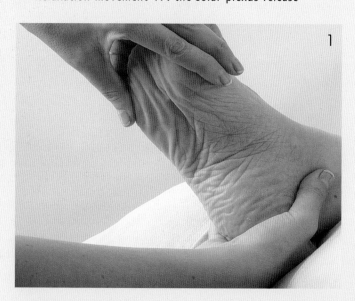

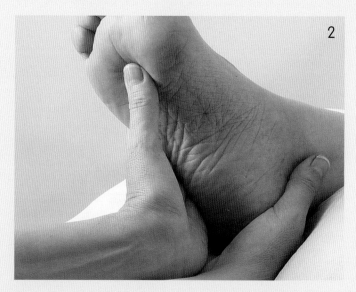

Support the receiver's foot under the heel and place the pad of the thumb of your working hand on the solar plexus reflex area, which is located roughly in the middle of the diaphragm line, just below the ball of the foot. (A good way of finding the solar plexus reflex area is to place one hand over the top of the upper part of the foot and to squeeze it gently – a hollow will then appear, which is the solar plexus reflex (1).)

Now move your thumb very gently in a circular direction three times. This technique is marvellous for relieving stress and tension (2).

The reflexes of the right foot

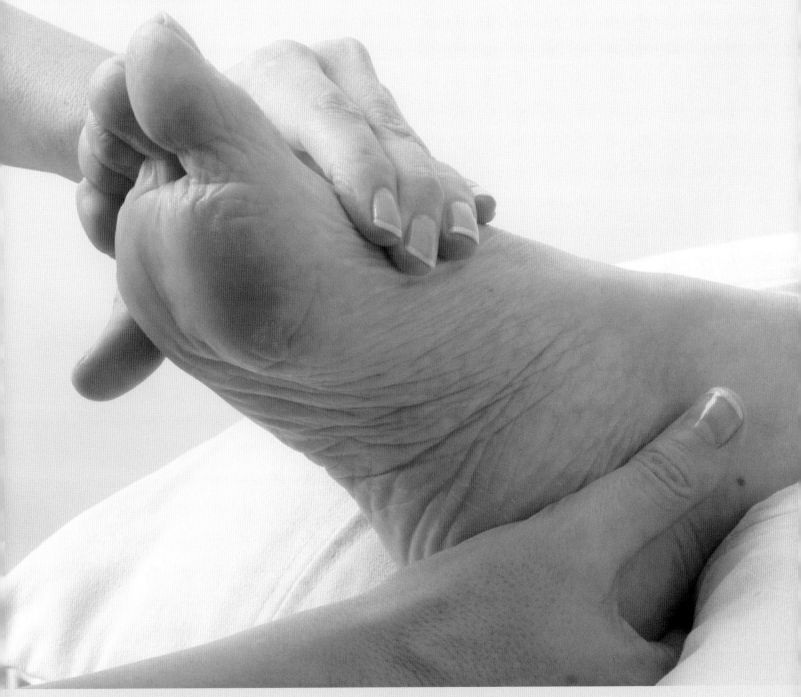

Areas treated when working on the head and neck reflexes include:

- the head and brain
- the pituitary gland, pineal gland and hypothalamus
- the occiput, mastoid and temple
- the right ear and right Eustachian tube
- the face

- the neck
- the vocal chords
- the tonsils
- the throat

- the sinuses
- the teeth and gums
- the upper lymphatics
- the right eye

The big toe

The head and brain reflex

Disorders eased by treating the head and brain reflex include:

- headaches and migraines
- mental congestion
- amnesia
- fainting
- multiple sclerosis
- poor co-ordination
- scalp problems
- lack of confidence and self-esteem

- lack of concentration
- memory defects
- neuralgia
- Bell's palsy (facial paralysis)
- stroke and paralysis
- the after-effects of anaesthetics
- learning difficulties, e.g., dyslexia
- depression

- the inability to think clearly
- Alzheimer's disease
- loss of balance
- Parkinson's disease
- epilepsy
- baldness
- Attention Deficit Disorder (ADD)
- a lack of intuition and a closed mind

Step 1 ▶

Wrap the fingers of your left hand over the front of the receiver's toes, with your thumb under the toes. Place your right thumb on the outer edge of the base of the big toe and caterpillar walk up the outside, over the top and down the inside of the big toe. Repeat several times.

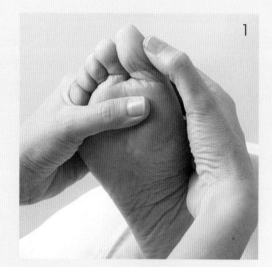

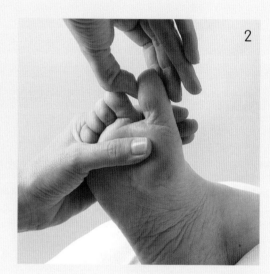

Step 2 ▶

Now use your right thumb to caterpillar walk up the back of the big toe, from the base to the tip. Caterpillar walk up the big toe for as many rows as you need to cover the entire area.

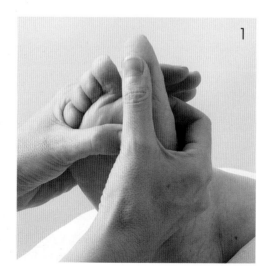

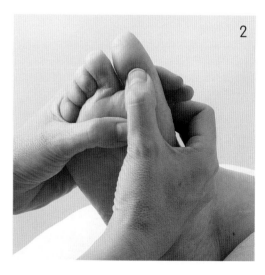

The pituitary gland reflex

Disorders eased by treating the pituitary gland reflex include:

- hormonal imbalances
- premenstrual syndrome (PMS)
- scanty, heavy or painful menstruation
- difficulties conceiving
- the menopause

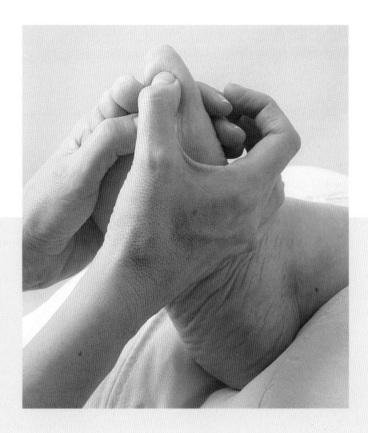

Step 3 ▶

The pituitary gland reflex is located approximately in the centre of the widest part of the pad of the big toe. Note that it is often a little off-centre, but that a slight lump is sometimes visible, indicating the location of this reflex. Wrap the fingers of your left hand over the front of the receiver's toes, with your thumb positioned underneath them. Use your right thumb to perform the hook in and back up technique on the pituitary gland reflex: press in firmly with your thumb (hook in) and then pull it back, across the point (back up).

The pineal gland and hypothalamus reflexes

Disorders eased by treating the pineal gland and hypothalamus reflexes include:

- Seasonal Affective Disorder (SAD)
- sleep problems
- mood swings; hormonal imbalances
- a lack of insight, intuition or vision

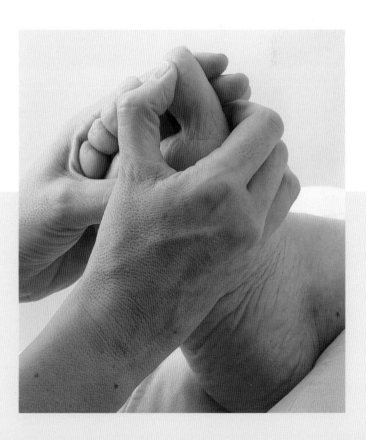

Step 4

The pineal gland and hypothalamus reflexes are situated very close to the pituitary gland reflex. First support the receiver's foot, as described in the previous step. Now move your working thumb very slightly upwards, rock it over to the left and perform several pressure circles over the pineal area. Then rock your thumb over to the right and make several pressure circles over the hypothalamus reflex.

The occiput, mastoid and temple reflexes

Disorders eased by treating the occiput, mastoid, and temple reflexes include:

- headaches
- ear problems

Step 5 ▶ ▼

Position your right thumb at the base of the receiver's big toe and perform three tiny caterpillar-walks upwards, towards the top of the toe, pressing into the occiput reflex (this point is usually located just below the slight protrusion) and releasing three times. Take one more step and press into the mastoid reflex (just above the protrusion) and release three times, then take two steps and press and release to treat the temple reflex.

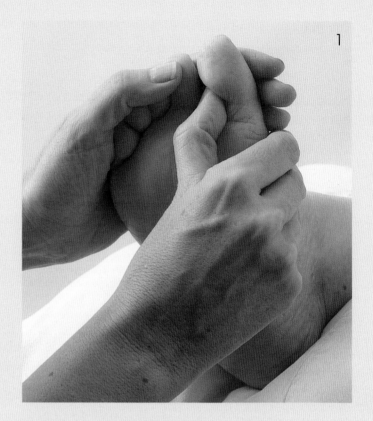

Occiput

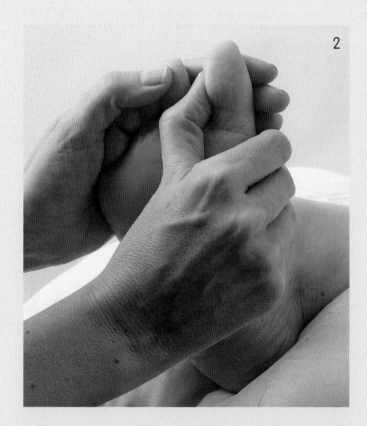

Mastoid

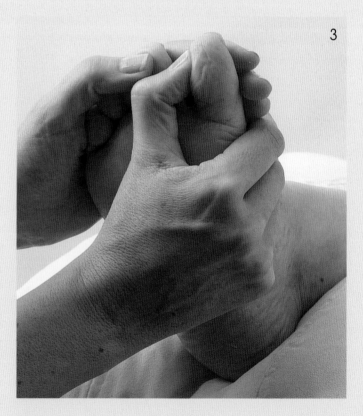

Temple

The face reflex

Disorders eased by treating the face reflex include:

- eye problems, e.g., conjunctivitis
- Bell's palsy (facial paralysis)
- sinusitis

- nasal problems
- facial neuralgia
- facial acne

- jaw problems
- teeth and gum problems

▼ Step 6

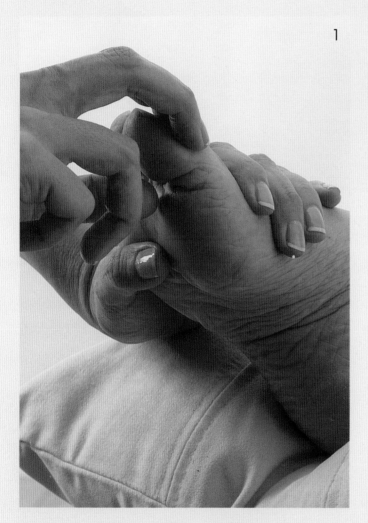

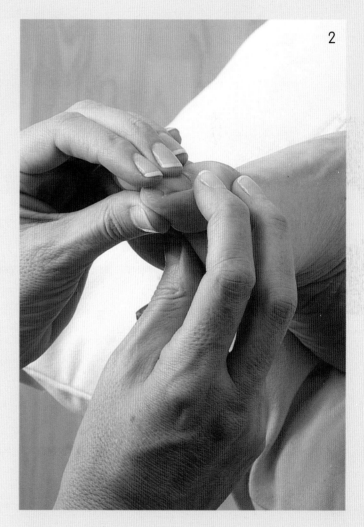

Wrap your left hand around the upper part of the receiver's foot, with your thumb positioned underneath and your fingers on the dorsum (top). Place your working index and middle fingers on the front of the big toe, just below the nail, and then walk down the big toe. Repeat several times. You may also use your index finger only, or even three fingers, to perform this movement, depending on the size of the toe and your fingers.

If you prefer, you may caterpillar walk across the face reflex. With your thumb positioned on the back of the big toe for support, use two or three fingers to caterpillar walk across the front of the toe.

The neck reflex

Disorders eased by treating the neck reflex include:

- aches and pains in the neck
- a lack of mobility in the neck
- whiplash injuries
- arthritis in the neck
- throat problems, such as tonsillitis and problems with the adenoids, pharynx and larynx, when working across the front of the neck reflex

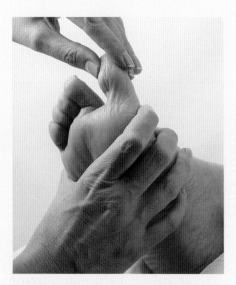

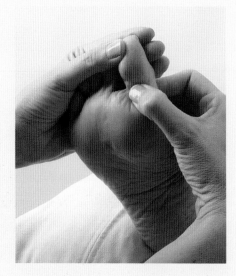

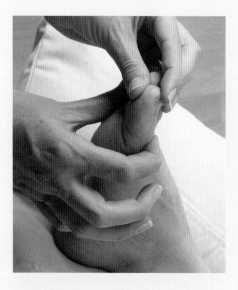

▲ Step 7

To find out how mobile the receiver's neck is, gently grasp his or her big toe between the thumb and forefinger of your working hand and slowly move the toe clockwise and then anti-clockwise. You may hear grinding noises as you do this, or else the big toe may not move very far (do not force it!), indicating problems with the neck.

▲ Step 8

To treat the back of the neck, place your fingers on the front of the receiver's toes, with your thumb positioned underneath, and gently push back the toes. Use your right thumb to caterpillar walk across the back of the big toe, moving from the outside to the inside.

▲ Step 9

To treat the front of the neck, use your index finger to caterpillar walk across the front of the big toe. This is a good area to work on if the receiver has throat problems.

The vocal cords reflex

Disorders eased by treating the vocal cords reflex include:

- vocal cord problems
- laryngitis
- pharyngitis
- tonsillitis
- tracheitis
- difficulty expressing oneself
- a 'lump' in the throat
- an inability to say what one thinks
- speech problems
- an over-use of the voice

Step 10 ▶

Support the receiver's foot with your right hand and place the index finger of your left, working hand on the front of the foot, between the big toe and the second toe, positioning your thumb on the sole behind your index finger. Use your index finger to circle gently over the vocal cords reflex.

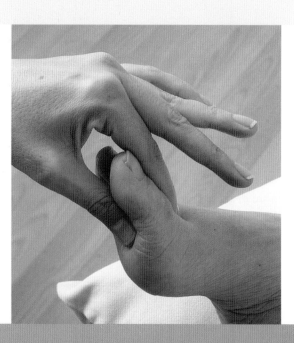

The small toes

The sinus reflexes

Disorders eased by treating the sinus reflexes include:

• sinus problems   • allergies   • catarrh   • hay fever   • rhinitis   • colds   • a loss of the sense of smell   • nasal polyps

Step 11 ►

The sinus reflexes are located on the back and sides of the small toes. To work on the backs of the toes, support the receiver's right foot between the thumb and fingers of your left hand, gently pulling back the toes. Use your right thumb to caterpillar walk up the back of each toe. Note that you may need to caterpillar walk for two or three rows on each toe to completely cover the area (1). Alternatively, you may use your thumb to caterpillar walk down the back of each toe (2).

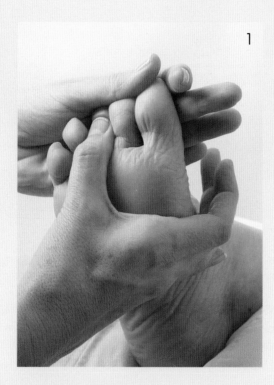
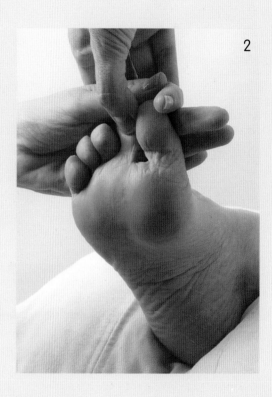

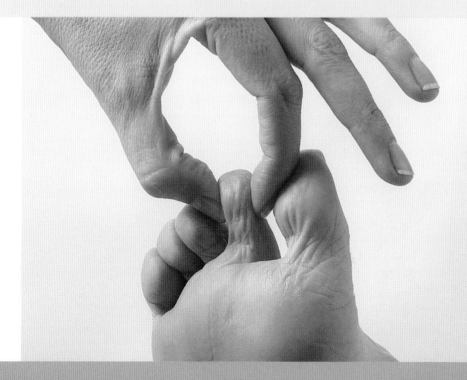

◄ Step 12

To treat the sides of a toe, you will need to work from the top of the receiver's foot. Position your thumb on one side of the toe and your index finger on the other and then caterpillar walk from the top to the base of the toe, repeating this procedure for each small toe in turn. Alternatively, assume the same position, but simply slide your thumb and index finger down each toe instead.

The teeth and gum reflexes

Disorders eased by treating the teeth and gum reflexes include:

- toothache
- abscesses
- painful or sensitive teeth
- pain after dental procedures
- gum problems
- teething

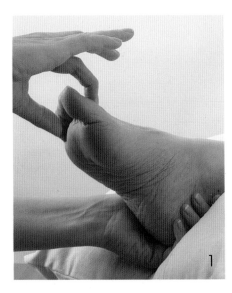 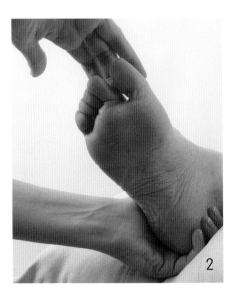 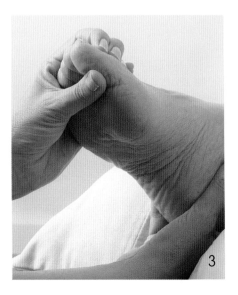

▲ Step 13

The reflexes for the teeth are located on the front of all of the toes. Support the receiver's foot using your left hand, either with your fingers on top and your thumb on the bottom or by resting the heel in the palm of your hand, and place your right index finger on the top of the big toe, just below the nail. Finger walk down the big toe, performing as many rows as you need in order to cover the area completely. Note that you are giving a general treatment to all of the teeth and gums when finger walking down the big toe. Now finger walk down toe two to treat the incisors and canine teeth; down toe three to treat the premolars; down toe four to treat the molars; and down toe five to treat the wisdom teeth (1 and 2).

An alternative way of treating the teeth is to finger walk across the fronts of the toes in both directions (3).

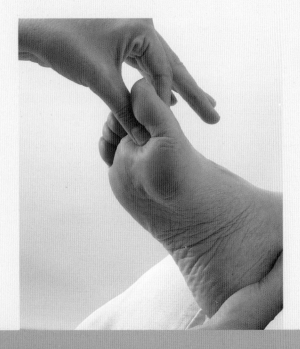

The upper lymphatic reflexes

Disorders eased by treating the upper lymphatic reflexes include:

- a poor immune function, e.g., if a person suffers from recurrent infections
- myalgic encephalomyelitis (ME)
- a toxic lymphatic system (which is often due to poor diet and a lack of exercise)
- ear, nose and throat problems
- acne (this technique will help to drain the head and neck area)

◀ Step 14

The reflex areas for the upper lymphatics are located in the webbing between the toes. Support the receiver's foot by either cupping the heel or by wrapping the fingers of your left hand over the front of the foot, with your thumb positioned underneath. Use your left thumb and index finger to squeeze the webbing between each of the toes gently. Repeat several times.

Reflexes for the right ear and Eustachian tube, and the right eye

Disorders eased by treating the reflexes for the right ear and Eustachian tube, and the right eye include:

- earache
- glue ear
- balance problems
- tinnitus
- sore eyes
- hay fever
- conjunctivitis

- ear infections
- hearing problems
- vertigo or dizziness
- watery eyes
- itchy eyes
- blocked tear ducts
- glaucoma

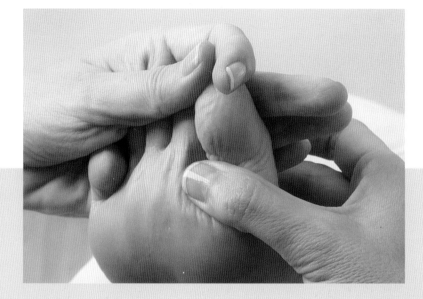

Step 15 ▶
Support the receiver's right foot between the thumb and fingers of your left hand and gently pull back the toes. Place your right thumb at the base of toe two and caterpillar walk across the ridge leading from toe two to toe five.

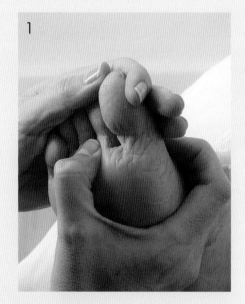

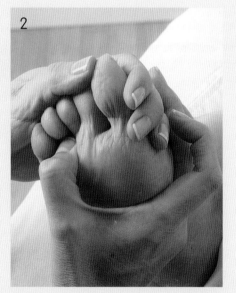

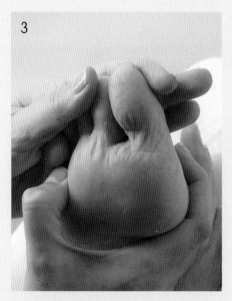

▲ Step 16
To work more specifically on the right eye, caterpillar walk across the ridge again, but this time, stop between the second and third toes and press and release the eye reflex point. Perform pressure circles over the area if it is particularly sensitive.

Continue caterpillar walking and then stop between toes three and four and press and release the Eustachian tube reflex. Perform pressure circles over the area if it is particularly sensitive.

Now continue to caterpillar walk along the ridge and press into the ear reflex located between toes four and five.

The spine

The spinal reflexes

Disorders eased by treating the spinal reflexes include:

- backache
- muscle spasm
- arthritis of the spine
- stiffness and lack of mobility
- disc problems

Step 17 ▶

The spinal reflexes are located along the inner aspect of each foot. First of all, we will stroke the spine. Gently cup the heel of the receiver's foot with your left, supporting hand. Use the heel of your right hand to stroke down the inside of the foot before gliding gently back again. Repeat several times.

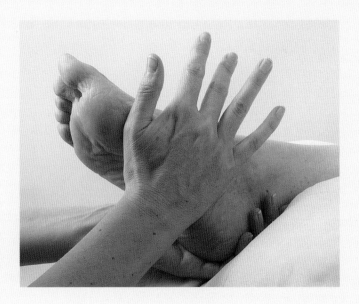

Step 18 ▶

Still supporting the receiver's foot under the heel, place your working thumb at the base of the toenail on the inner edge of the foot and then slide it slowly down the inside of the foot (1). Now wrap your holding hand around the top of the foot, place your working thumb on the bottom of the inner edge of the foot and then slide it up the inner aspect of the foot towards the big toe (2).

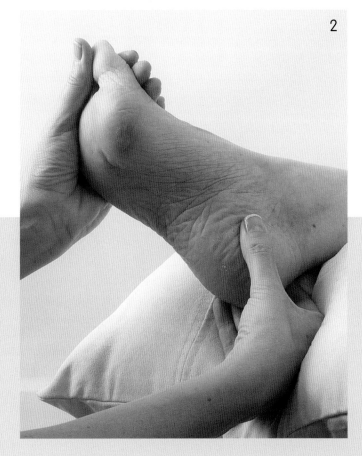

2

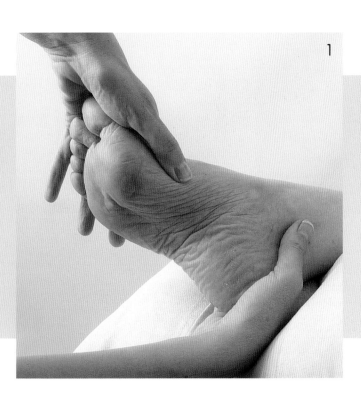

1

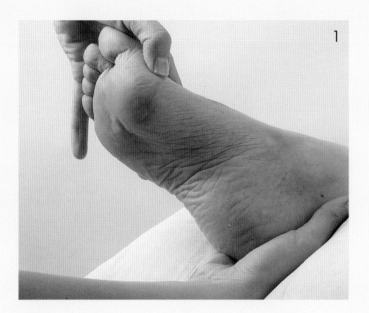

1

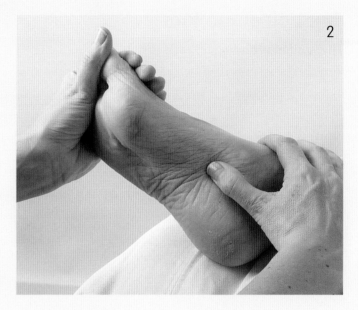

2

▲ **Step 19**
Continuing to support the receiver's foot under the heel with
your right hand, place your left thumb on the inner aspect of the
foot at the base of the nail bed. Caterpillar walk down the inner
edge of the foot, following the curve of the bone. As you
caterpillar walk down the foot, you are treating the cervical area
(the neck), the thoracic area (the middle of the back) and the
lumbar area (the lower back).

To change hands, wrap your left, holding hand around the top of
the foot, place your right thumb at the base of the heel and
caterpillar walk back up, towards the big toe.

If you discover any areas that feel hard, gritty, spongy or just
different, perform gentle pressure circles over them.

Step 20 ▶
The following technique helps to release fear and anxiety, especially
that which has been experienced while in the womb. (The tips of the
big toes are thought to represent the moment of conception, the
spinal reflex, the time spent in the womb and the ankle, birth.)
Supporting the receiver's right foot under the heel, lightly place the
tip of the third finger of your working hand on the top of the big
toe and rest it there for a few moments. Using an exceptionally
feather-light touch, slowly stroke your finger down the spinal reflex
and under the anklebone. Rest it here for a few moments before
repeating the movement three or more times.

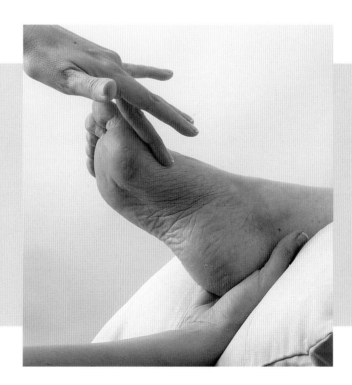

The ball of the foot

The shoulder and chest reflexes

Areas treated when working on the shoulder and chest reflexes include:

- the thyroid gland
- the right shoulder
- the parathyroid glands
- the diaphragm
- the thymus gland
- the solar plexus
- the right lung
- the ribs, sternum and right breast

The thyroid gland, parathyroid glands and thymus gland reflexes

Disorders eased by treating the thyroid gland, parathyroid glands and thymus gland reflexes include:

- thyroid problems, nervousness and weight problems (the thyroid gland reflex)
- osteoporosis, muscle-twitching and arthritis (the parathyroid glands reflex)
- a poor immune function (the thymus gland reflex)

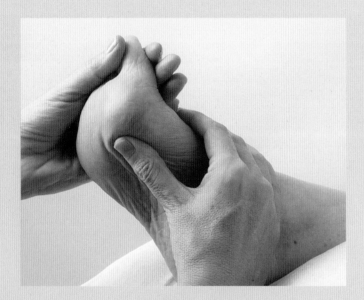

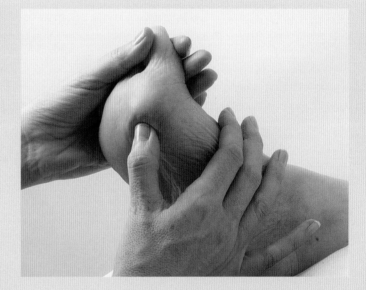

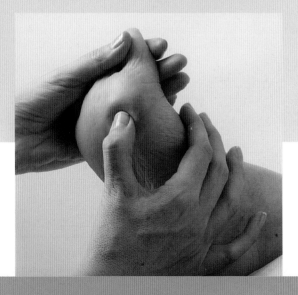

Step 21 ▲

Wrap your left hand around the receiver's foot to provide support. Place your right thumb on the diaphragm line, just below the pad of the big toe, and caterpillar walk along the diaphragm line. Then turn your thumb and caterpillar walk on the area of the ball of the foot between the big toe and the second toe. Repeat several times.

◀ **Step 22**

Return to the diaphragm line and caterpillar walk up the ball of the foot several times, until you have completely covered the ball of the foot beneath the big toe.

Step 23 ▶

Place the flat pad of your working thumb in the centre of the pad of the area on which you have worked in order to locate the thyroid gland reflex. Perform three pressure circles.

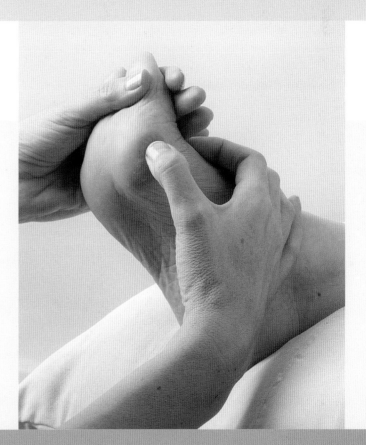

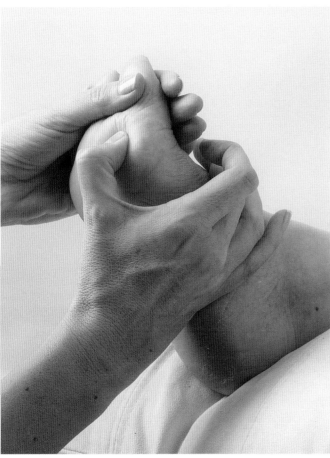

◀ **Step 24**

Move your thumb slightly to the left and upwards to locate the parathyroid glands reflex. Then perform three pressure circles.

Step 25 ▶

Return your thumb to the thyroid gland reflex area and move it slightly to the right and down to find the thymus gland reflex. Now perform three pressure circles over the area.

The right lung reflex

Disorders eased by treating the right lung reflex include:

- lung problems
- bronchitis
- fear and anxiety
- difficulty in expressing emotions
- coughs and colds
- hyperventilation
- panic attacks
- chest infections
- a lack of self-esteem
- shallow breathing
- exhaustion from nurturing others
- asthma
- hysteria
- the effects of smoking
- emphysema
- emotional dependence

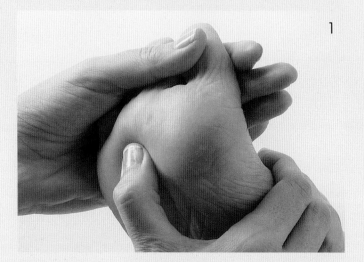 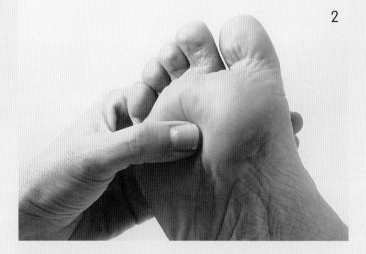

▲ **Step 26**

Wrap your left, holding hand around the top of the receiver's foot and gently push back the toes, away from you. Place your right, working thumb on the diaphragm line and caterpillar walk upwards, in vertical strips, towards the base of toes two, three and four to treat the lung area (1). Alternatively, you may support the heel of the foot in the palm of your hand and use your working thumb to caterpillar walk in horizontal rows across the foot (2).

The right shoulder reflex

Disorders eased by treating the right shoulder reflex include:

- tension and pain in the shoulder
- a frozen shoulder
- arthritis
- a lack of mobility
- shouldering too much responsibility

Step 27 ▶

The shoulder reflex is found in zone 5, under the little toe, as well as on the lateral edge of the foot, at the base of the little toe. Support the receiver's foot with your right hand. Place your left thumb on the sole and your index finger on the top of the foot, just under the little toe, and gently squeeze your thumb and finger together three times. While maintaining the pressure, rotate your thumb and index finger using a circular motion (this is equivalent to rotating the shoulder!). Now move your working thumb to the lateral edge of the foot, to the base of the little toe, and perform pressure circles over the area. Because the shoulders are usually tense, grittiness and congestion can often be felt here.

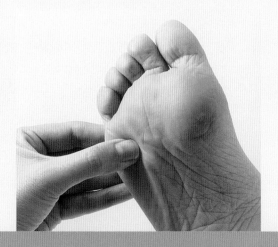

Reflexes for the right lung, ribs, sternum and right breast

Disorders eased by treating the reflexes for the left lung, ribs, sternum and right breast include:

- all respiratory problems
- harmless breast lumps
- mastitis
- tension and anxiety
- palpitations and hyperventilation
- breast problems; e.g., tenderness prior to menstruation
- overwhelming emotions (it helps to get them off the receiver's chest)

Step 28 ▶
Support the receiver's foot forward with your left hand, gently pulling the toes towards you, and place the pads of your working fingers on the dorsum (top) of the foot, just below the base of the toes. Finger walk down the front of the foot, moving from the base of the toes to the diaphragm line, covering the area in vertical strips. You are treating the right lung and ribs. Alternatively, you may finger walk across the top of the foot to treat this area. Make a loose fist with your left hand, position it under the receiver's toes for support and then use two or three fingers to finger walk across the top of the foot.

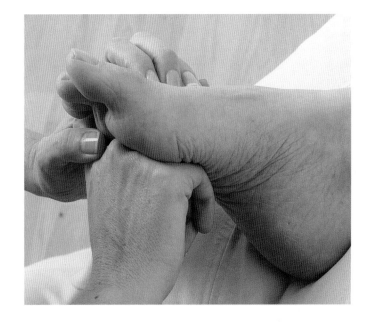

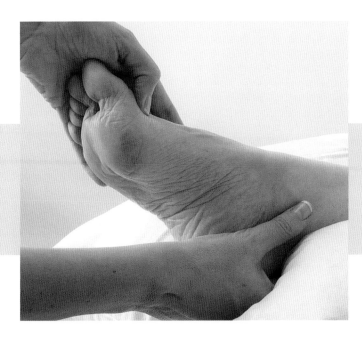

◀ Step 29
To treat the sternum reflex, support the receiver's foot with your right hand and place your working thumb just below the base of the big toe. Now perform gentle pressure circles over this area.

Step 30 ▶
To give the right breast reflex area extra attention, support the receiver's foot under the heel, place the thumb of your working hand on the ball of the foot and your fingers on the top and then perform large, circular movements over the top of the foot.

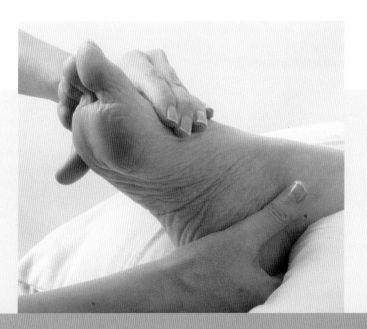

The diaphragm and solar plexus reflex

Disorders eased by treating the diaphragm and solar plexus reflex include:

- respiratory problems
- fear
- panic attacks
- hyperventilation

- stress and tension
- shallow breathing
- hysteria

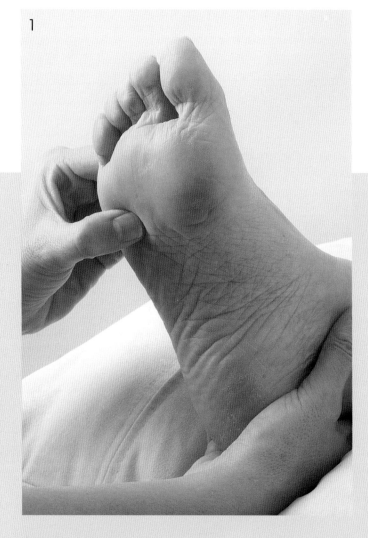

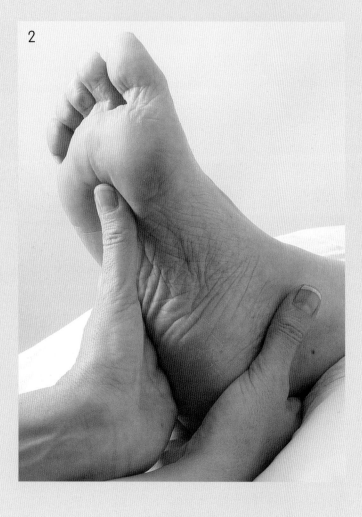

▲◄ Step 31

Support the receiver's foot with your right hand and place your left thumb under the ball of the foot. Caterpillar walk across the diaphragm line and, as you reach the centre, turn your thumb to face upwards before performing gentle pressure circles over the solar plexus reflex. (If you are working on a highly stressed person, this area may be sensitive, so do take care.) Then continue to walk across the diaphragm line to zone 1.

The reflexes of the abdomen

Areas treated when working on the reflexes of the abdomen include:

- the liver
- the pancreas
- the appendix
- the right adrenal gland

- the gallbladder
- the duodenum
- the ileocaecal valve
- the right kidney, ureter and bladder

- the stomach
- the small intestine
- the large intestine (ascending and transverse colon)

The liver and gallbladder reflexes (the right foot only)

Disorders eased by treating the liver and gallbladder reflexes include:

- liver problems
- gallbladder problems
- digestive disturbances
- overindulgence in drink or food
- toxicity
- difficulties in breaking down fats

▶ **Step 32**

The reflexes for the liver and gallbladder are found on the right foot only, between the diaphragm line and waist line, and the area that the liver reflex occupies looks rather like a triangle. Hold the top of the receiver's foot with your right hand and bend the toes away from you to open up the reflex areas. Place the thumb of your left hand on zone 5, just below the diaphragm line, and caterpillar walk across the foot to zone 1.

For your next row, begin slightly lower down and caterpillar walk from zone 5 to zone 2. Then walk from zone 5 to zone 3, and, finally, from zone 5 to zone 4. You will then have described the shape of a triangle.

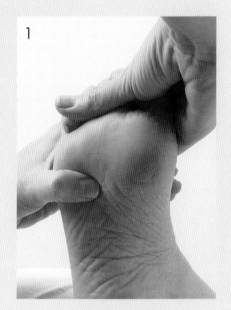

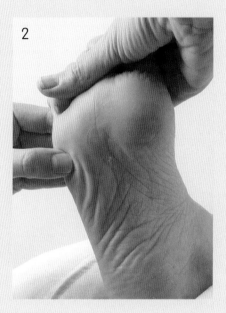

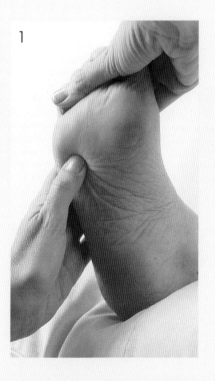

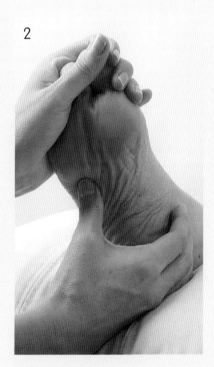

▶ **Step 33**

The gallbladder reflex is found approximately in line with the third and fourth toes. This reflex is small, not always easy to find and its position seems to vary slightly. It can feel like an indentation, a slight swelling or even a small lump. Once again, support the receiver's foot with your right hand, as described in the previous step, and use the pad of your left thumb either to press and release the gallbladder reflex or to perform several pressure circles over the area.

Alternatively, use the rotation on a point technique, which is very useful when treating small reflex areas, such as the gallbladder reflex. Hold the receiver's foot with your left hand and place your right thumb on the gallbladder reflex. Slowly flex the foot downwards, onto your right thumb, and then circle the foot around the point several times.

The stomach, pancreas and duodenum reflexes

Disorders eased by treating the stomach, pancreas and duodenum reflexes include:

- ulcers
- diabetes
- low blood sugar
- general digestive problems
- indigestion and heartburn
- stomach cramps

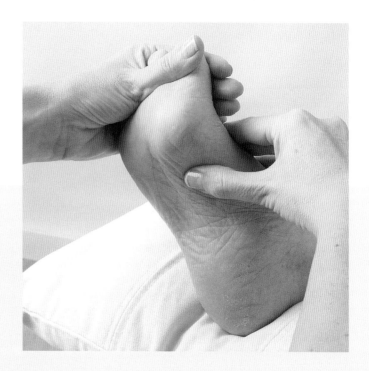

Step 34 ▶

The reflexes for the stomach, pancreas and duodenum are located between the diaphragm line and waist line, and occupy zones 1 and 2. Using your left hand to support the receiver's foot, place your right thumb just below the diaphragm line on the medial (inner) side of the foot. Caterpillar walk from zone 1 to 2 several times in horizontal rows until you reach the waist line. (If you wish, you may work the area in the opposite direction.)

The small intestine reflex

Disorders eased by treating the small intestine reflex include:

- all digestive disorders
- abdominal cramps
- bloating
- allergies

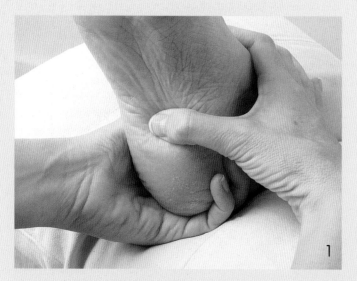

1

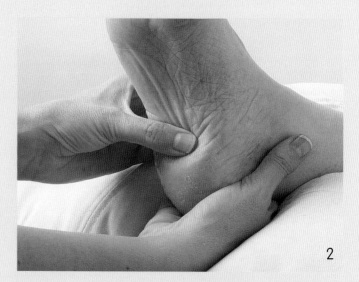

2

▲ Step 35

The reflex area for the small intestine lies between the waist line and the pelvic girdle line and covers zones 1 to 4. Supporting the receiver's foot with your left hand, place your right thumb in line with toe one, just below the waist line, and caterpillar walk across to zone 4. Continue to caterpillar walk in horizontal rows from zone 1 to zone 4 until you reach the pelvic girdle line (1).
Then change hands and caterpillar walk from zones 4 to 1 with your left thumb (2).

The appendix, ileocaecal valve and large intestine (ascending and transverse colon) reflexes

Disorders eased by treating the appendix, ileocaecal-valve and large-intestine (ascending and transverse colon) reflexes include:

- all digestive problems
- irritable bowel syndrome
- constipation
- diarrhoea

Step 36 ▶

Supporting the receiver's foot with your right hand, place your left thumb, tip pointing upwards, just above the pelvic girdle line between zones 4 and 5. You may feel a small, hollow spot, which is the reflex for the appendix. Perform several pressure circles over this area. Then move your thumb upwards very slightly to circle over the ileocaecal valve reflex.

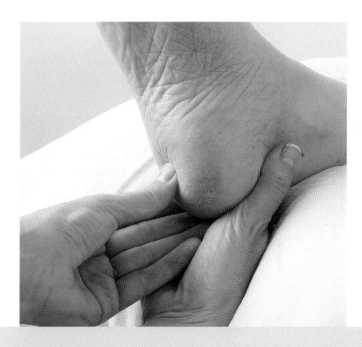

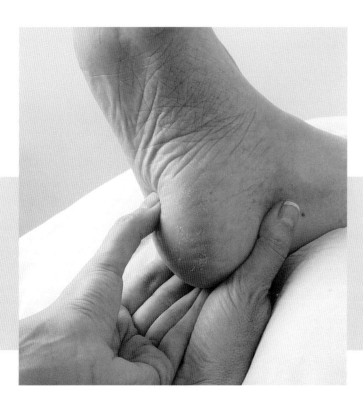

◀ Step 37

Now caterpillar walk up the foot (still between zones 4 and 5) towards the waist line to treat the ascending colon. Just below the waist line, perform three pressure circles to treat the hepatic flexure, which is where the colon turns before continuing as the transverse colon.

Step 38 ▶

Turn your thumb 90° to the right and caterpillar walk across the foot towards zone 1. You are now treating the transverse colon reflex.

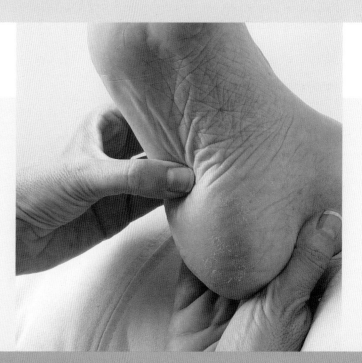

The right kidney, ureter and bladder reflexes

Disorders eased by treating the right kidney, ureter and bladder reflexes include:

- kidney problems
- bladder infections
- cystitis
- fluid retention
- incontinence

▼ Step 39

The right kidney reflex is located between zones 2 and 3 straddling the waist line. Supporting the receiver's foot with your right hand, place your left thumb, tip pointing towards the toes, on the right kidney reflex. Perform several pressure circles over the area.

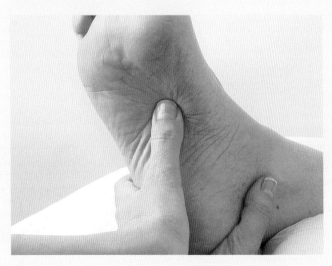

▼ Step 40

Now swivel your thumb around so that it is facing downwards and caterpillar walk down the foot on the ureter reflex towards the slightly puffy area of the medial (inner) edge of the foot, which is the bladder reflex.

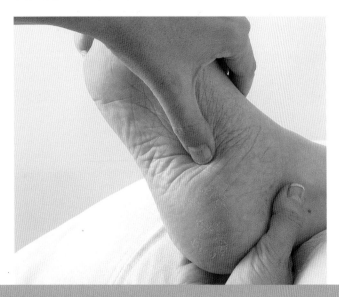

▼ Step 41

Perform pressure circles on the bladder reflex with your left thumb

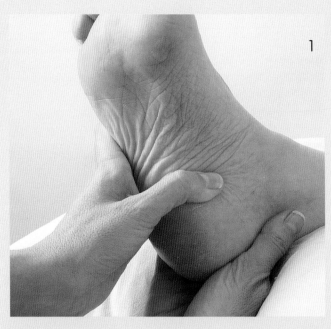

and then caterpillar walk over the area towards the toe.

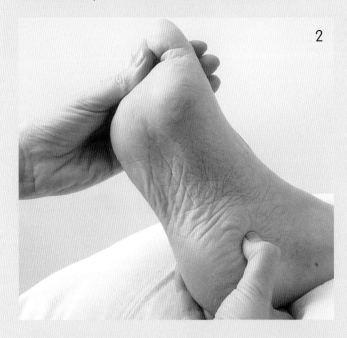

Caution

Always work from the right kidney reflex towards the bladder reflex (and never from the bladder reflex towards the right kidney reflex) to avoid the danger of transforming a bladder infection into a kidney infection.

The right adrenal gland reflex

Disorders eased by treating the right adrenal gland reflex include:

- nervous conditions
- allergies
- a lack of energy
- inflammatory disorders, such as irritable bowel syndrome and rheumatoid arthritis
- pain

▼ **Step 42**

The right adrenal gland reflex is found just above the right kidney reflex in zone 2. It is usually easily located as it is a tender point (because we all have stress in our lives!). Wrap your left hand around the top of the receiver's foot and use your right thumb either to press and release the right adrenal gland reflex or to hook in and back up. If the area is very tender, then perform several pressure circles over it.

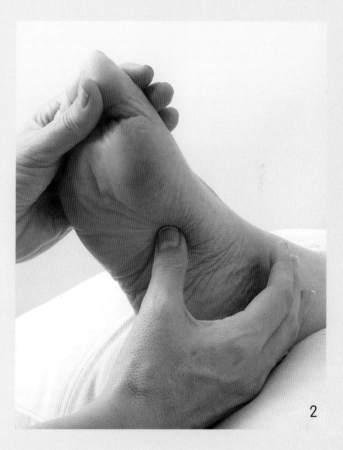

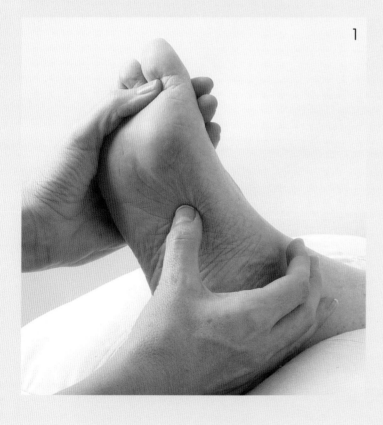

▲ Alternatively, use the rotation on a point technique. Supporting the receiver's foot with your left hand, place your right thumb on the right adrenal gland reflex. Use your supporting hand to flex the foot downwards, onto your thumb, and then circle the foot around the point several times.

The reflexes of the joints, sciatic nerve and pelvic muscles

Areas treated by working on the reflexes of the joints, sciatic nerve and pelvic muscles include:

- the right shoulder;
- the right hip
- the right arm;
- the sciatic nerve
- the right elbow
- the pelvic muscles
- the right knee

The reflexes of the joints

Disorders eased by treating the reflexes of the joints include:

- all joint problems
- arthritis
- sports injuries
- hip disorders
- a frozen shoulder
- tennis elbow
- housemaid's knee
- sprains and strains
- cartilage and ligament problems

Step 43 ▼ ▶

The reflexes for the joints are found along the lateral side (outer edge) of the foot. To give a general treatment to the joints, cup the receiver's heel in your left hand and use your right thumb to caterpillar walk down the outside of the foot, working from the base of the little toe to the heel.

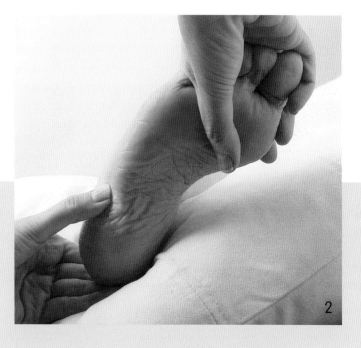

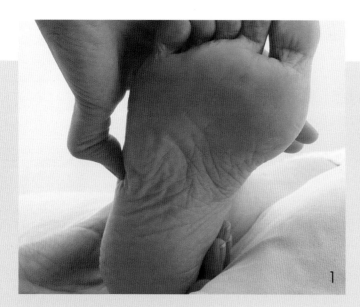

Then hold the top of the foot with your right hand and use your left thumb to caterpillar walk up the outer edge of the foot, moving from the heel area to the little toe

Step 44 ▶

To give a more specific treatment to the individual joints, first support the receiver's heel in your right hand. Now place your left, working thumb on the outer edge of the foot, at the base of the little toe, and either perform pressure circles to treat the shoulder or, alternatively, thumb walk over this reflex several times.

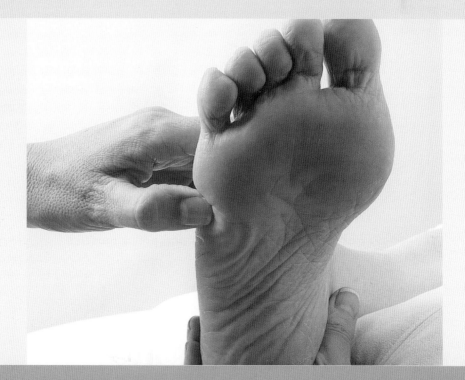

Step 45 ▶

Continue by performing three small caterpillar walks; in doing this, you are treating the arm. Now perform three pressure circles to treat the elbow. Alternatively, caterpillar walk upwards, onto the foot slightly, to treat the elbow reflex.

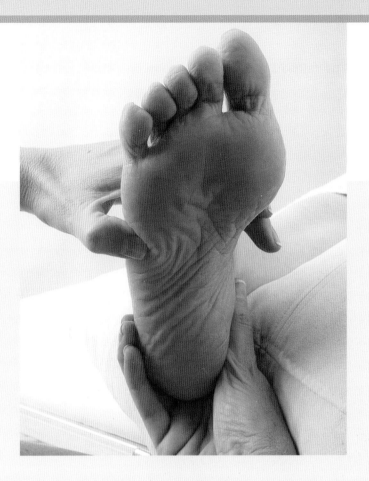

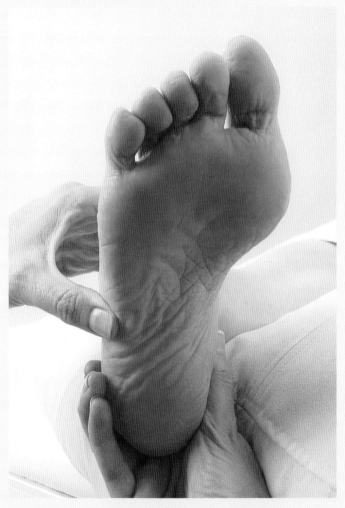

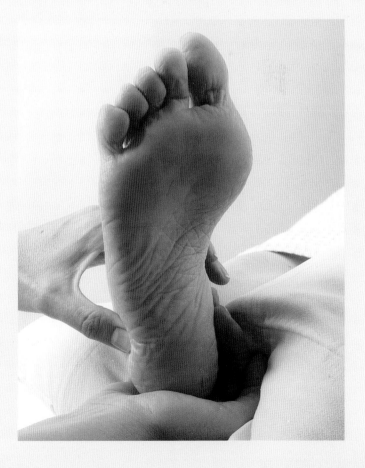

▲ Step 46

Continue to caterpillar walk along the outer edge of the foot until you reach the protrusion that is the knee reflex. Either perform several pressure circles, depending upon how much 'grittiness' you find, or caterpillar walk over the area, which is shaped like a half moon.

Step 47 ▶

Next to the knee reflex, you will find the hip reflex. Perform pressure circles on this, then use your thumb or fingers to caterpillar walk over this half moon-shaped reflex.

The reflexes of the sciatic nerve and pelvic muscles

Disorders eased by treating the reflexes of the sciatic nerve and pelvic muscles include:

- sciatica
- lower back problems
- disc problems
- hip problems
- tightness in the muscles of the buttocks and pelvis

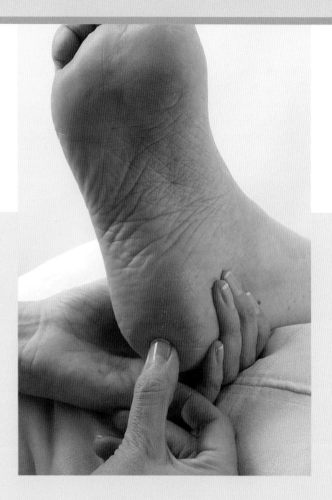

▶ **Step 48**

To treat the muscles of the pelvis, cup the receiver's foot with your left hand. Make a loose fist with your right hand and then, moving in a circular direction, gently work your knuckles into the heel area below the pelvic girdle line. Alternatively, either caterpillar walk from the base of the heel up to the pelvic girdle line to cover the area completely or else caterpillar walk across the heel in horizontal rows.

▼ **Step 49**

When treating the sciatic nerve reflex, first wrap your supporting hand around the receiver's foot and then use the palm of your working hand to stroke and squeeze the calf muscles at the back of the leg.

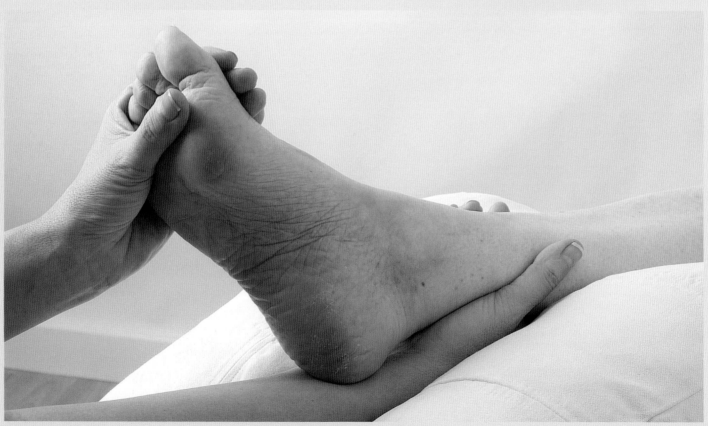

▶ **Step 50**

 Now support the receiver's right foot with your left hand and position your right thumb, tip pointing downwards, above the inner anklebone. Caterpillar walk down the side of the Achilles tendon, moving towards the heel.

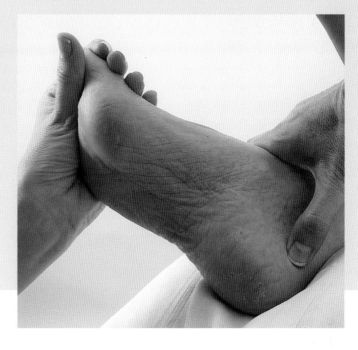

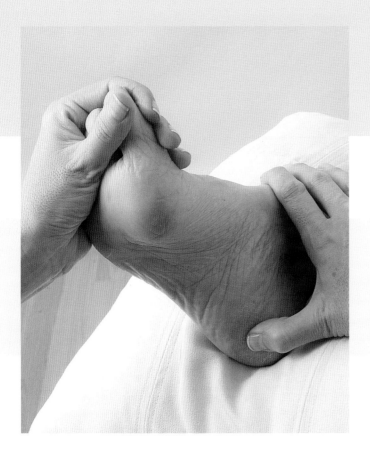

◀ **Step 51**

Continue to caterpillar walk across the sciatic nerve reflex on the heel pad.

▶ **Step 52**

Finally, caterpillar walk up the other side of the Achilles tendon. You should be able to treat the complete sciatic nerve reflex with your right thumb only, but change hands if you find this uncomfortable.

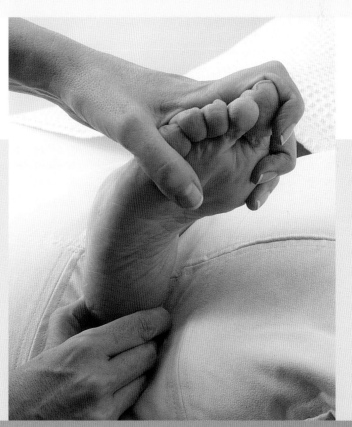

The reflexes of the reproductive organs and lymph nodes of the groin

Areas treated by working on the reflexes of the reproductive organs and lymph nodes of the groin include:

- the right ovary or right testicle;
- the lymph nodes of the groin
- the right fallopian tube or the vas deferens;
- the uterus or prostate gland.

Disorders eased by working on the reflexes of the reproductive organs and lymph nodes of the groin include:

- all menstrual problems
- premenstrual tension (PMT)
- the menopause;
- an accumulation of toxins;
- infertility problems
- prostate problems

Step 53 ▶

To locate the right ovary reflex (in the case of a female receiver) or the right testicle reflex (if the receiver is male), first draw an imaginary, diagonal line running from the receiver's outer anklebone to the heel and then locate the midpoint. Hold the top of the receiver's foot with your right hand, place your left thumb or index finger on the reflex and then perform gentle pressure circles over the area.

Caution

If the receiver is pregnant, then leave out these areas if there is a history of miscarriage. (A fully qualified reflexologist may treat these reflexes, however.) If a female receiver has an intrauterine device (IUD) fitted, then gently stroke the uterus reflex area rather than pressing on it.

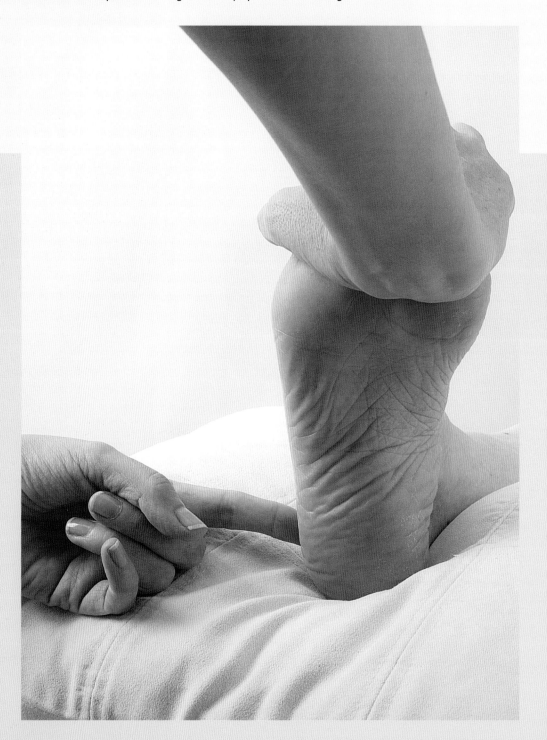

▶ **Step 54**

Thumb or finger walk across the top of the receiver's foot to a point midway between the inner anklebone and the heel. This is the reflex for the right fallopian tube (if the receiver is female) or the vas deferens (if the receiver is male). However, this is also the reflex for the lymphatic nodes of the groin, and since the lymphatic nodes are often clogged up due to poor diet, lack of exercise and stress, a tender area will usually reveal a toxic lymphatic system. Caterpillar walk over this area several times if the reflex for the lymphatic nodes seems congested, which will be indicated by puffiness or 'grittiness'.

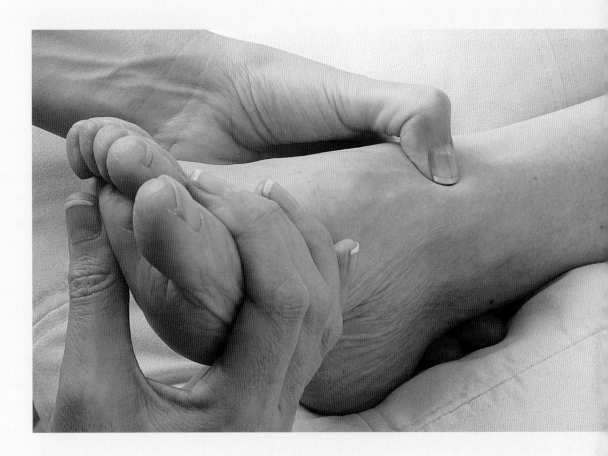

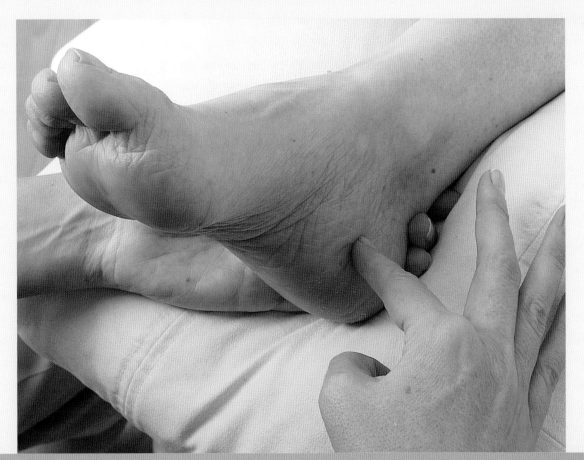

◀ **Step 55**

Place your right thumb or index finger on the uterus reflex (if the receiver is female) or the prostate reflex (if the receiver is male), which is located midway between the inner anklebone and the heel, and then perform gentle pressure circles over the area.

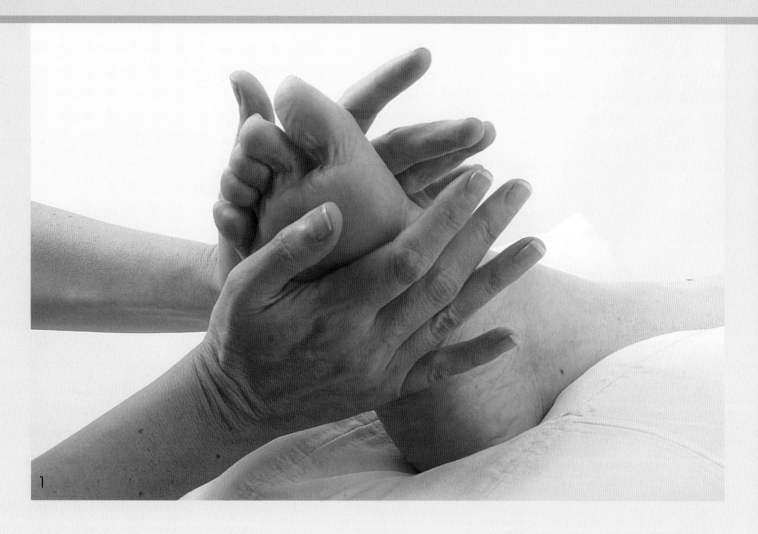

To finish

To finish, stroke the receiver's right foot with both hands several times, both to ensure that all of the toxins have been dispersed and to relax the foot fully. Then gently clasp the receiver's foot between both hands and cover it up.

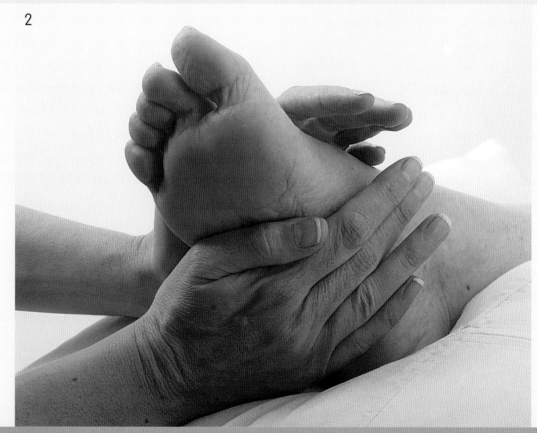

Relaxation sequence – left foot

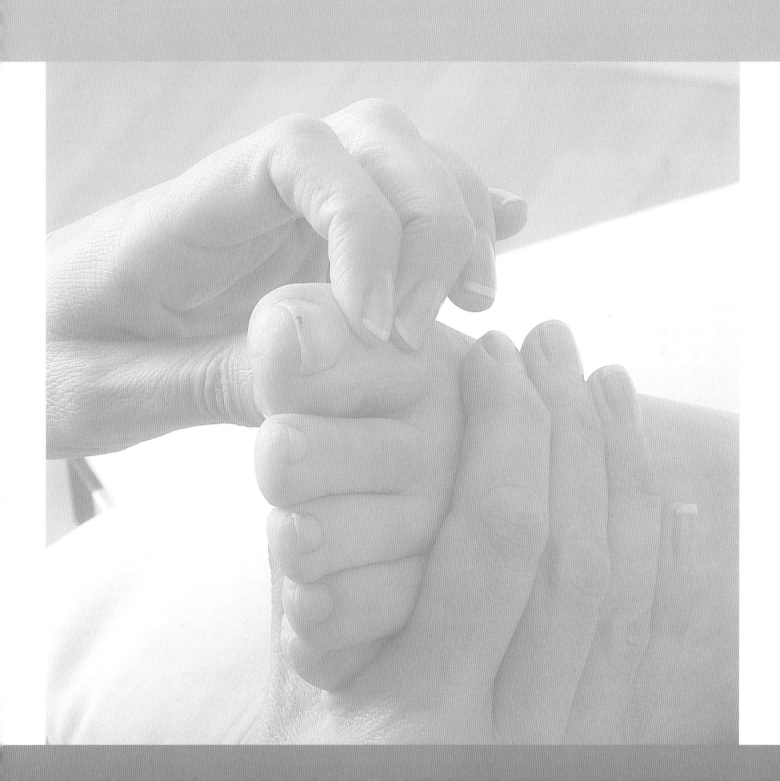

Uncover the receiver's left foot and then perform your favourite relaxation techniques on it, ensuring that you cover the sole, top and sides of the foot.

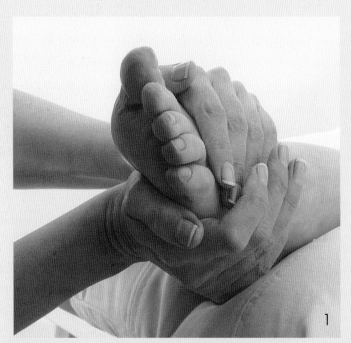

▲ Stroking the foot

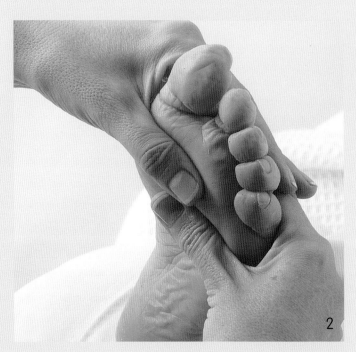

▲ Opening the foot

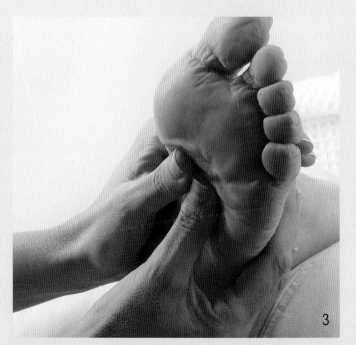

▲ Stretching up the sole

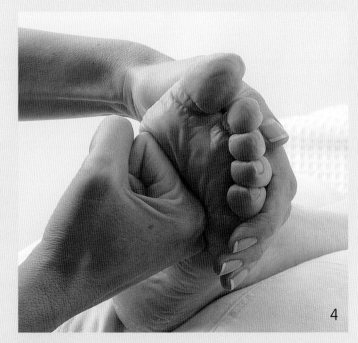

▲ Kneading

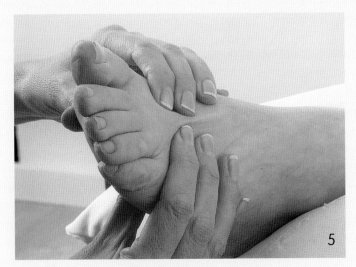

▲ Finger circling on the top of the foot

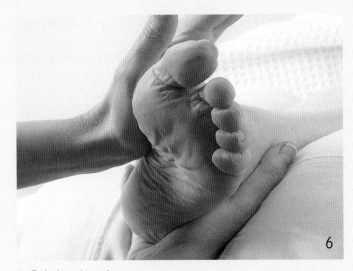

▲ Twisting the spine

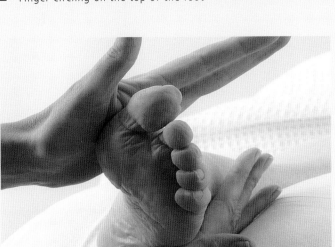

▲ Rubbing the sides of the foot

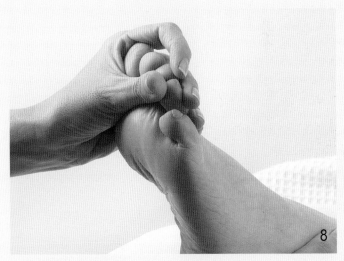

▲ Loosening the ankle

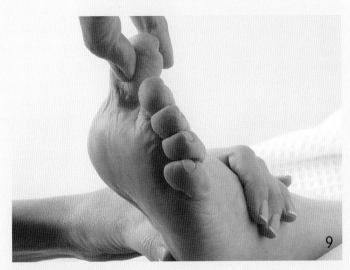

▲ Loosening the toes

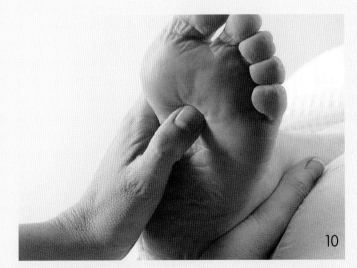

▲ The solar plexus release

The reflexes of the left foot

The head and neck reflexes

Areas treated when working on the head and neck reflexes include:

- the head and brain
- the face
- the tonsils
- the upper lymphatics

- the pituitary gland, pineal gland and hypothalamus
- the neck
- the sinuses
- the left ear and Eustachian tube

- the occiput, mastoid and temple
- the vocal cords
- the teeth and gums
- the left eye

The big toe

The head and brain reflex

Disorders eased by treating the head and brain reflex include:

- headaches and migraines
- mental congestion
- amnesia
- fainting
- multiple sclerosis
- poor co-ordination
- scalp problems
- lack of confidence and low self-esteem

- a lack of concentration
- memory defects
- neuralgia
- Bell's palsy (facial paralysis)
- stroke and paralysis
- the aftereffects of anaesthetics
- learning difficulties, e.g., dyslexia
- depression

- the inability to think clearly
- Alzheimer's disease
- loss of balance
- Parkinson's disease
- epilepsy
- baldness
- Attention Deficit Disorder (ADD)
- a lack of intuition and a closed mind

Step 1 ▶

Wrap the fingers of your right hand over the front of the receiver's toes, with your thumb positioned under the toes. Place your left thumb on the outer edge of the base of the big toe and caterpillar walk up the outside, over the top and down the inside of the big toe. Repeat several times.

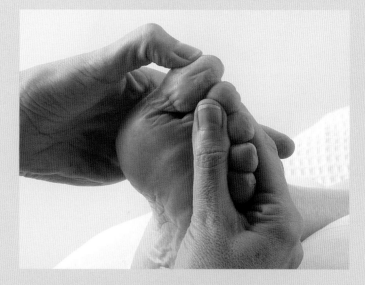

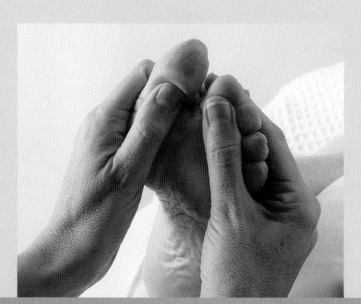

◄ Step 2

Now use your left thumb to caterpillar walk up the back of the big toe, moving from the base to the tip. Caterpillar walk for as many rows as you need to cover the entire area.

The pituitary gland reflex

Disorders eased by treating the pituitary gland reflex include:

- hormonal imbalances
- premenstrual syndrome (PMS)
- scanty, heavy or painful menstruation
- difficulties conceiving
- the menopause

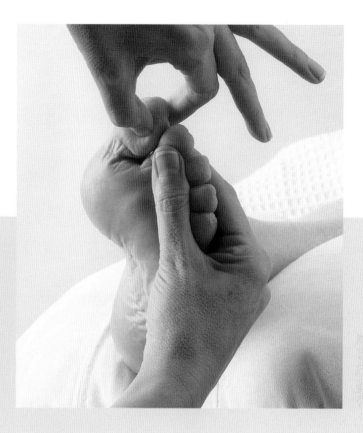

Step 3 ▶

The pituitary gland reflex is located approximately in the centre of the widest part of the pad of the big toe. Note that it is often a little off-centre, but that a slight lump is sometimes visible, indicating the location of this reflex. Wrap the fingers of your right hand over the front of the receiver's toes, with your thumb positioned underneath. Use your left thumb to perform the hook in and back up techniques on the pituitary gland reflex: press in firmly with your thumb (hook in) and then pull it back, across the point (back up).

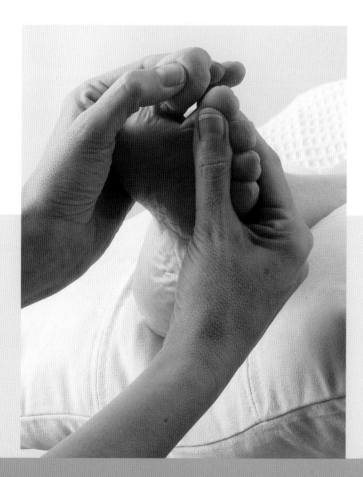

The pineal gland and hypothalamus reflexes

Disorders eased by treating the pineal gland and hypothalamus reflexes include:

- Seasonal Affective Disorder (SAD)
- sleep problems
- mood swings
- hormonal imbalances
- a lack of insight, intuition or vision

◀ Step 4

The pineal gland and hypothalamus reflexes are very close to the pituitary gland reflex. Support the receiver's foot, as outlined in the previous step. Then move your working thumb very slightly upwards, rock it over to the right and perform several pressure circles over the pineal area. Then rock your thumb over to the left and make several pressure circles over the hypothalamus reflex.

The occiput, mastoid and temple reflexes

Disorders eased by treating the occiput, mastoid, and temple reflexes include:

- headaches
- ear problems

Step 5 ▶ ▼

Position your working thumb at the base of the receiver's big toe and perform three tiny caterpillar walks upwards, towards the top of the toe, pressing into the occiput reflex (this point is usually located just below the slight protrusion) and releasing three times.

Take one more step and press into the mastoid reflex (just above the protrusion) and release three times, then take two steps and press and release to treat the temple reflex.

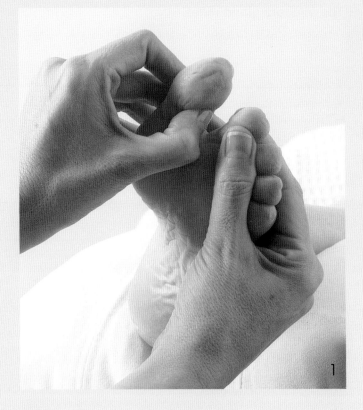

Occiput

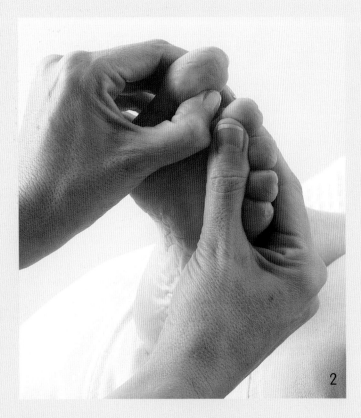

Mastoid

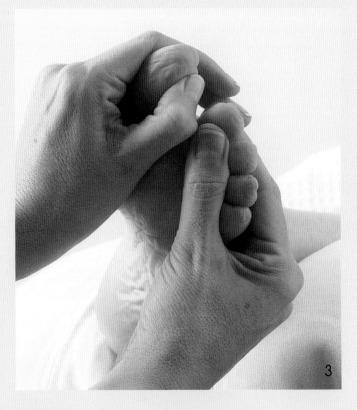

Temple

The face reflex

Disorders eased by treating the face reflex include:

- eye problems, e.g., conjunctivitis
- Bell's palsy (facial paralysis)
- sinusitis

- nasal problems
- facial neuralgia
- facial acne

- jaw problems
- teeth and gum problems

Step 6 ▼

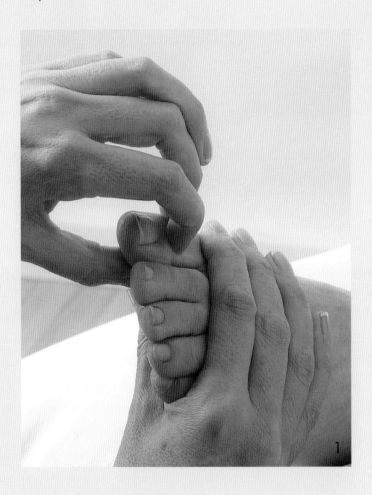

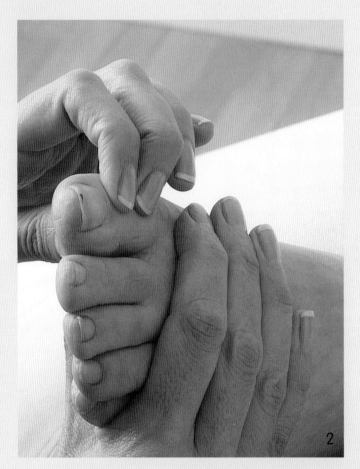

Wrap your right hand around the upper part of the receiver's foot, with your thumb positioned underneath and your fingers on the dorsum (top). Place your other index and middle fingers on the front of the big toe, just below the nail, with your thumb positioned underneath for support, and then caterpillar walk down the big toe. Repeat several times. You may also use your index finger only, or even three fingers, to perform this movement, depending on the size of the toe and your fingers.

If you prefer, you may caterpillar walk across the face reflex. With your thumb positioned on the back of the big toe for support, use two or three fingers to caterpillar walk across the front of the toe.

The neck reflex

Disorders eased by treating the neck reflex include:

- aches and pains in the neck
- whiplash injuries
- a lack of mobility in the neck
- arthritis in the neck
- throat problems, such as tonsillitis and problems with the adenoids, pharynx and larynx, when working across the front of the neck reflex

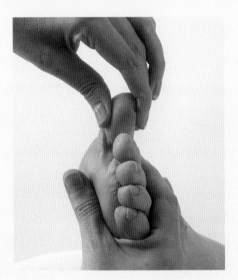

Step 7 ▲

To find out how mobile the receiver's neck is, gently grasp his or her big toe between the thumb and forefinger of your left hand and slowly move the toe clockwise and then anti-clockwise. You may hear grinding noises as you do this, or else the big toe may not move very far (do not force it!), indicating problems with the neck.

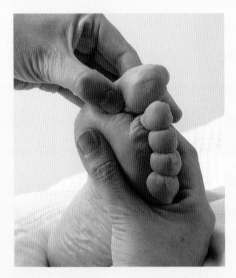

Step 8 ▲

To treat the back of the neck, place your fingers on the front of the receiver's toes, with your thumb positioned underneath, and gently pull back the toes. Use your left thumb to caterpillar walk across the back of the big toe, moving from the outside to the inside.

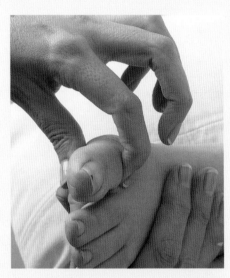

Step 9 ▲

To treat the front of the neck, use your index finger to caterpillar walk across the front of the big toe. This is a good area to work on if the receiver has throat problems.

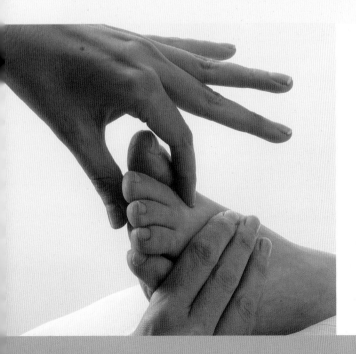

The vocal cords reflex

Disorders eased by treating the vocal cords reflex include:

- vocal cord problems
- pharyngitis
- difficulty expressing oneself
- speech problems
- an inability to say what one thinks
- laryngitis
- tracheitis
- a 'lump' in the throat
- an over-use of the voice

Step 10 ◄

Support the receiver's foot with your right hand and place the index finger of your left, working hand on the front of the foot, between the big toe and the second toe, positioning your thumb on the sole behind your index finger. Use your index finger to circle gently over the vocal cords reflex.

The small toes

The sinus reflexes

Disorders eased by treating the sinus reflexes include:

- sinus problems   • allergies   • catarrh   • hay fever   • rhinitis   • colds   • a loss of the sense of smell   • nasal polyps

Step 11 ▶

The sinus reflexes are located on the back and sides of the small toes. To work on the backs of the toes, support the receiver's left foot between the thumb and fingers of your right hand, gently back pulling the toes. Use your thumb to caterpillar walk up the back of each toe. Note that you may need to caterpillar walk along two or three rows on each toe to completely cover the area (1). Alternatively, you may use your thumb to caterpillar walk down the back of each toe (2).

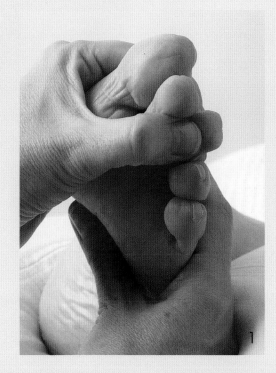
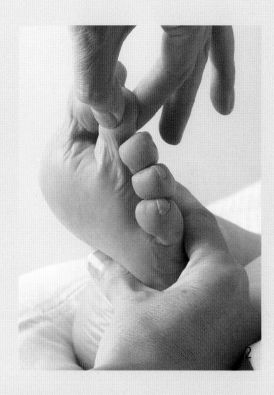

Step 12 ▶

To treat the sides of a toe, you will need to work from the top of the receiver's toe. Position your thumb on one side of the toe and your index finger on the other and then caterpillar walk from the top to the base of the toe, repeating this procedure for each small toe in turn. Alternatively, assume the same position, but simply slide your thumb and index finger down each toe instead.

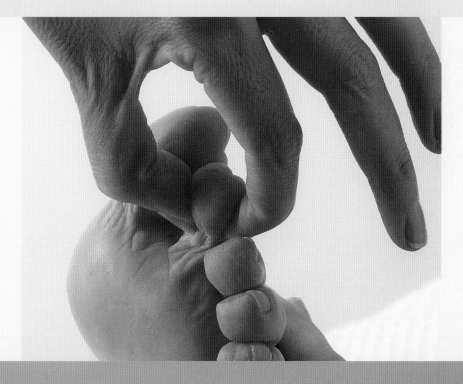

The teeth and gum reflexes

Disorders eased by treating the teeth and gum reflexes include:

- toothache
- abscesses
- painful or sensitive teeth
- pain after dental procedures
- gum problems
- teething

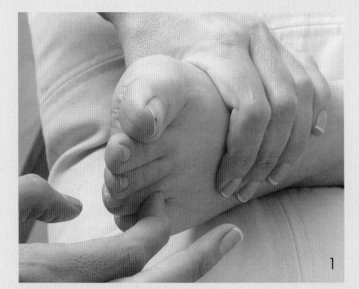 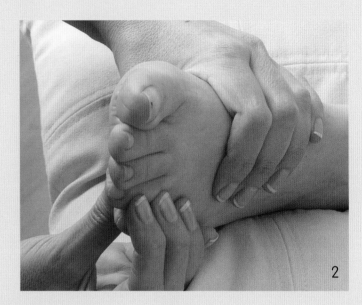

▲ **Step 13**

The reflexes for the teeth are located on the front of all of the toes. Support the receiver's foot using your left hand, with your fingers on top and your thumb on the bottom, and place your right index finger on the top of the big toe, just below the nail. Finger walk down the big toe, performing as many rows as you need in order to cover the area completely. Note that you are giving a general treatment to all of the teeth and gums when finger walking down the big toe. Now finger walk down toe two to treat the incisors and canine teeth; down toe three to treat the premolars; down toe four to treat the molars; and down toe five to treat the wisdom teeth (1).

An alternative way of treating the teeth is to finger walk across the fronts of the toes in both directions (2).

The upper lymphatic reflexes

Disorders eased by treating the upper lymphatic reflexes include:

- a poor immune function, e.g., if a person suffers from recurrent infections
- myalgic encephalomyelitis (ME)
- a toxic lymphatic system (which is often due to poor diet and a lack of exercise)
- ear, nose and throat problems
- acne (this technique will help to drain the head and neck area).

Step 14 ▶

The reflex areas for the upper lymphatics are located in the webbing between the toes. Support the receiver's foot by either cupping the heel or by wrapping the fingers of your right hand over the front of the foot, with your thumb positioned underneath. Use your left thumb and index finger to squeeze the webbing between each of the toes gently. Repeat several times.

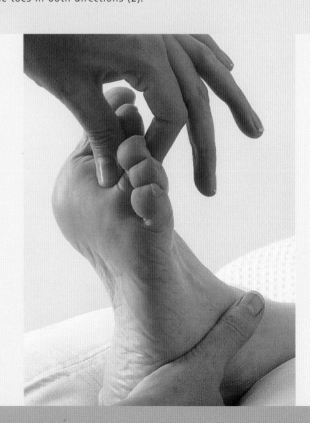

Reflexes for the left ear and Eustachian tube, and the left eye

Disorders eased by treating the reflexes for the left ear and Eustachian tube, and the left eye include:

- earache
- glue ear
- balance problems
- tinnitus
- sore eyes
- hay fever
- conjunctivitis
- ear infections
- hearing problems
- vertigo or dizziness
- watery eyes
- itchy eyes
- blocked tear ducts
- glaucoma

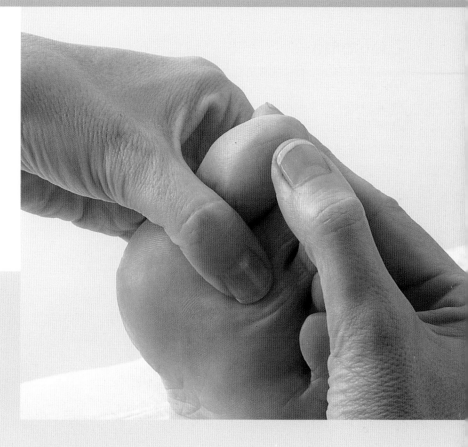

Step 15 ▶

Support the receiver's left foot between the thumb and fingers of your right hand and gently pull back the toes to make the area easier to reach. Place your left thumb at the base of toe two and caterpillar walk across the ridge leading from toe two to toe five.

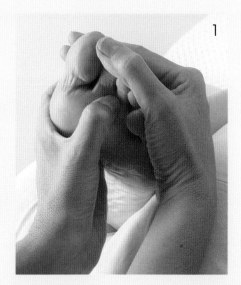

1

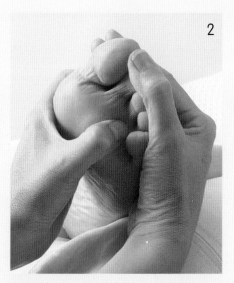

2

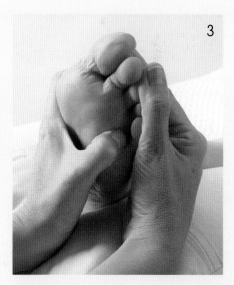

3

▲ Step 16

To work more specifically on the left eye, caterpillar walk across the ridge again, but this time, stop between the second and third toes and press and release the eye reflex point. Perform pressure circles over the area if it is particularly sensitive.

Continue caterpillar walking and then stop between toes three and four and press and release the Eustachian tube reflex. Perform pressure circles over the area if it is particularly sensitive.

Now continue to caterpillar walk along the ridge and press into the ear reflex located between toes four and five.

The spine

The spinal reflexes

Areas treated when working on the
spinal reflexes include:

- the cervical vertebrae
- the lumbar vertebrae
- the thoracic vertebrae
- the sacrum and coccyx

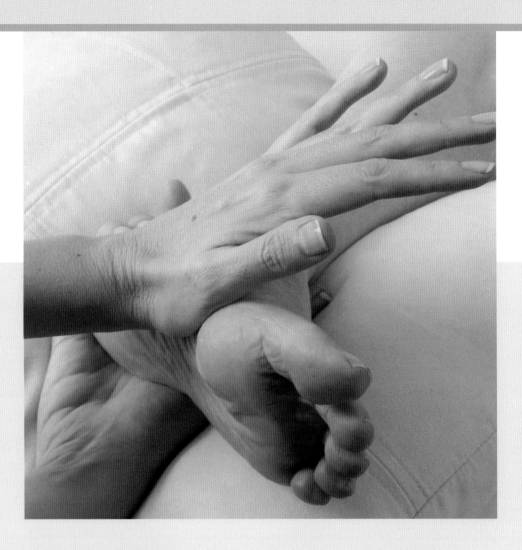

▶ **Step 17**
The spinal reflexes are located along
the inner aspect of each foot. First of
all, we will stroke the spine. Gently
cup the heel of the receiver's foot
with your right, supporting hand. Use
the heel of your left hand to stroke
down the inside of the foot before
gliding gently back again. Repeat
several times.

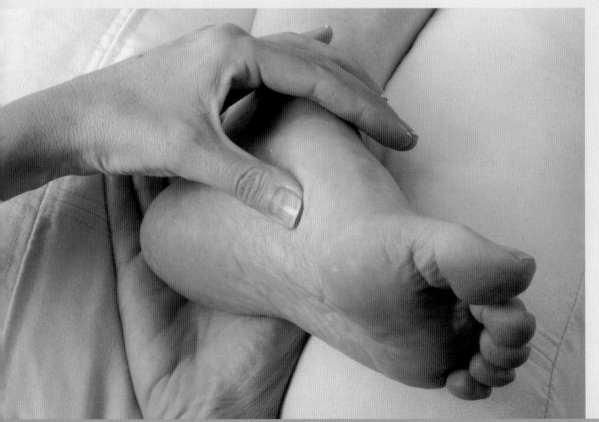

◀ **Step 18**
Still supporting the
receiver's foot under the
heel, place your working
thumb at the base of the
toenail on the inner edge of
the foot and then slide it
slowly down the inside of
the foot. Next slide your
working thumb up the inner
aspect of the foot towards
the big toe.

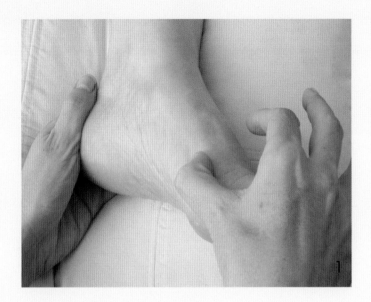

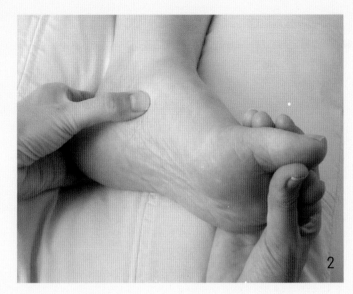

▲ **Step 19**

Continuing to support the receiver's foot under the heel with your left hand, place your right thumb on the inner aspect of the foot at the base of the nail bed. Caterpillar walk down the inner edge of the foot, following the curve of the bone. As you caterpillar walk down the foot, you are treating the cervical area (the neck), the thoracic area (the middle of the back) and the lumbar area (the lower back).

To change hands, wrap your right, holding hand around the top of the foot, place your left thumb at the base of the heel and caterpillar walk back up, towards the big toe.

If you discover any areas that feel hard, gritty, spongy or just different, perform gentle pressure circles over them.

Step 20 ▶

The following technique helps to release fear and anxiety, especially that which has been experienced while in the womb. (The tips of the big toes are thought to represent the moment of conception, the spinal reflex, the time spent in the womb and the ankle, birth.) Supporting the receiver's left foot, lightly place the tip of the third finger of your working hand on the top of the big toe and rest it there for a few moments. Using an exceptionally feather-light touch, slowly stroke your finger down the spinal reflex and under the anklebone. Rest it here for a few moments before repeating the movement three more times.

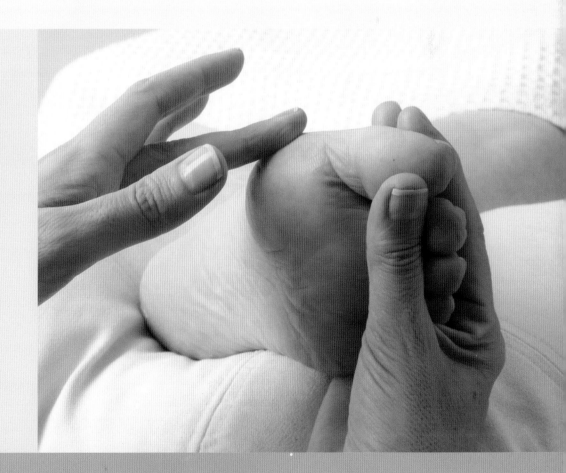

The ball of the foot

The shoulder and chest reflexes

Areas treated when working on the shoulder and chest reflexes include:

- the thyroid gland
- the parathyroid glands
- the thymus gland
- the left lung
- the heart
- the left shoulder
- the diaphragm
- the solar plexus
- the ribs, sternum and right breast

The thyroid gland, parathyroid glands and thymus gland reflexes

Disorders eased by treating the thyroid gland, parathyroid glands and thymus gland reflexes include:

- thyroid problems, nervousness and weight problems (the thyroid gland reflex)
- osteoporosis, muscle-twitching and arthritis (the parathyroid glands reflex)
- a poor immune function (the thymus gland reflex)

Step 21 ▶

Wrap your right hand around the receiver's foot to provide support. Place your left thumb on the diaphragm line, just below the pad of the big toe, and caterpillar walk along the diaphragm line. Then turn your thumb and caterpillar walk between the big toe and the second toe. Repeat several times.

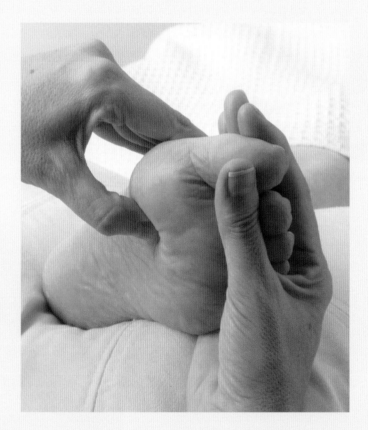

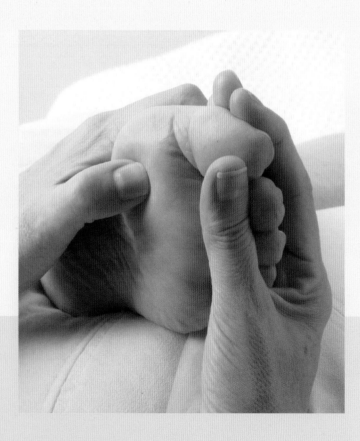

◀ **Step 22**

Return to the diaphragm line and caterpillar walk up the ball of the foot several times, until you have completely covered the ball of the foot beneath the big toe.

Step 23 ▶

Place the flat pad of your working thumb in the centre of the pad of the area on which you have worked in order to locate the thyroid gland reflex. Perform three pressure circles.

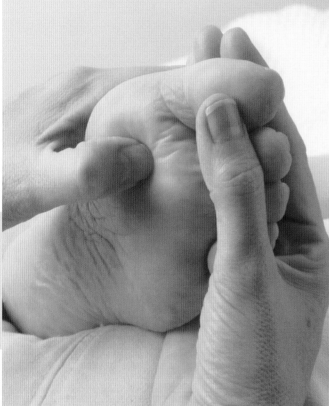

◀ **Step 24**

Move your thumb slightly to the right and upwards to locate the parathyroid glands reflex. Then perform three pressure circles.

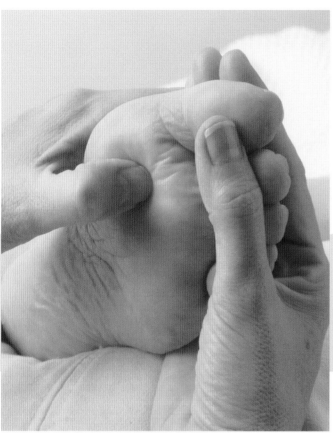

Step 25 ▶

Return your thumb to the thyroid gland reflex area and move it slightly to the left and down to find the thymus gland reflex. Now perform three pressure circles over the area.

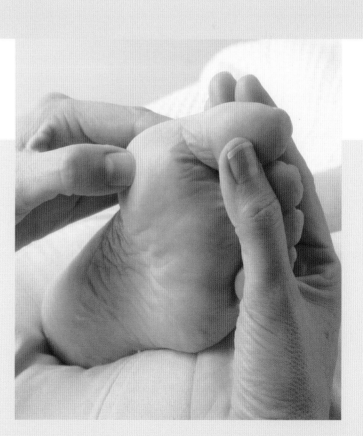

The left lung reflex

Disorders eased by treating the left lung reflex include:

- all lung problems
- bronchitis
- fear and anxiety
- difficulty in expressing emotions
- coughs and colds
- hyperventilation
- panic attacks
- chest infections
- a lack of self-esteem
- shallow breathing
- exhaustion from nurturing others
- asthma
- hysteria
- the effects of smoking
- emphysema
- emotional dependence

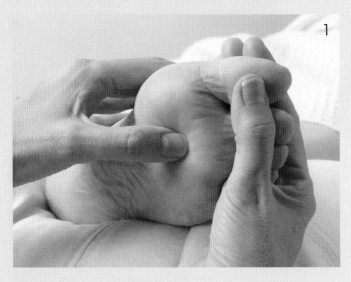
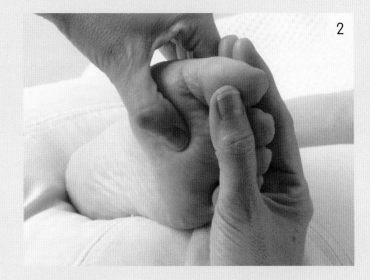

▲ **Step 26**

Wrap your right, holding hand around the top of the receiver's foot and gently push back the toes, away from you. Place your left, working thumb on the diaphragm line and caterpillar walk upwards, in vertical strips, towards the base of toes two, three and four to treat the lung area (1). Alternatively, you may caterpillar walk in horizontal rows across the foot (2).

The left shoulder reflex

Disorders eased by treating the left shoulder reflex include:

- tension and pain in the shoulder   • a frozen shoulder   • arthritis   • a lack of mobility   • shouldering too much responsibility

Step 27 ▶

The shoulder reflex is found in zone 5, under the little toe, as well as on the lateral edge of the foot, at the base of the little toe. Support the receiver's foot with your left hand. Place your right thumb on the sole and your index finger on the top of the foot, just under the little toe, and gently squeeze your thumb and finger together three times. While maintaining the pressure, now rotate your thumb and index finger using a circular motion (this is equivalent to rotating the shoulder!). Now move your working thumb to the lateral edge of the foot, to the base of the little toe, and perform pressure circles over the area. Because the shoulders are usually tense, 'grittiness' and congestion can often be felt here.

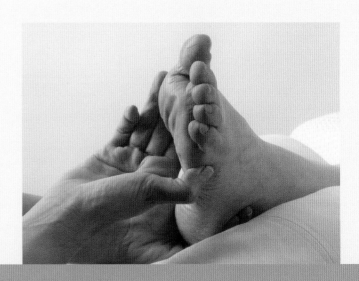

Reflexes for the left lung, ribs, sternum and left breast

Disorders eased by treating the reflexes for the left lung, ribs, sternum and left breast include:

- all respiratory problems
- harmless breast lumps
- mastitis
- tension and anxiety
- palpitations and hyperventilation
- breast problems; e.g., tenderness prior to menstruation
- overwhelming emotions (it helps to get them off the receiver's chest)

Step 28 ▶

Pull the receiver's foot forward with your left hand, gently pulling the toes towards you, and place the pads of your working fingers on the dorsum (top) of the foot, just below the base of the toes. Finger walk down the front of the foot, moving from the base of the toes to the diaphragm line, covering the area in vertical strips. You are treating the left lung, ribs. Alternatively, you may finger walk across the top of the foot to treat this area. Make a loose fist with your left hand, position it under the receiver's toes for support and then use two or three fingers to finger walk across the top of the foot.

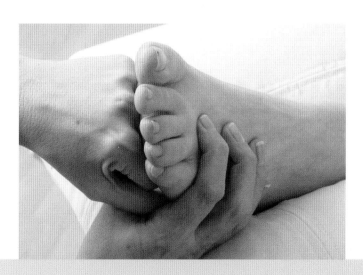

◀ Step 29

To treat the sternum reflex, support the receiver's foot with your right hand and place your left thumb or index finger just below the base of the front of the big toe. Now perform gentle pressure circles over this area.

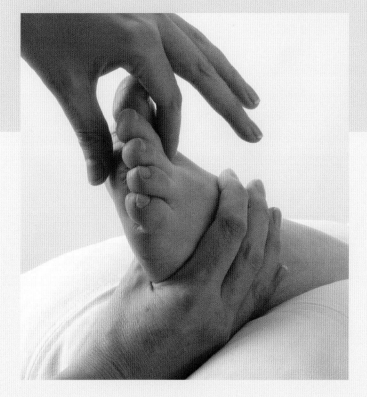

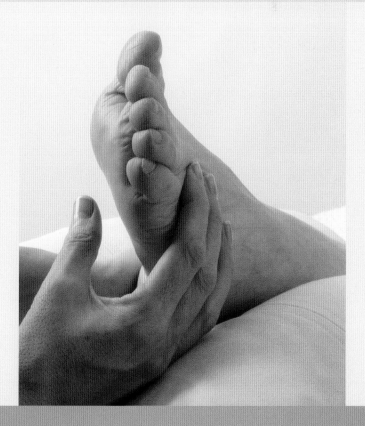

Step 30 ▶

To give the left breast reflex area extra attention, support the receiver's foot under the heel, place your fingers on the top and then perform large, circular movements over the top of the foot.

The heart reflex (the left foot only)

Disorders eased by treating the heart reflex include:

- palpitations
- heart problems
- blood pressure problems

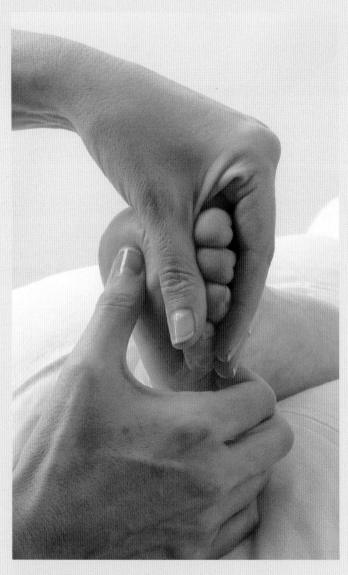

▲ **Step 31**
To treat the heart reflex, support the top of the receiver's foot with your left hand. Wrap your right hand around the upper third of the foot, with your thumb positioned on the sole and your fingers on the top. Use your thumb to massage the upper third of the sole of the foot, describing large circles.

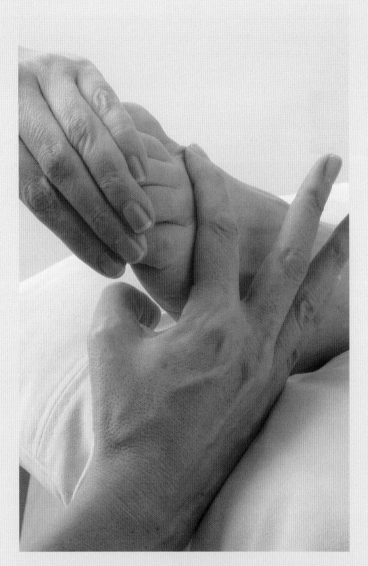

▲ Now pull the receiver's toes down, towards you, with your left hand and use your right index finger to massage the upper third of the top of the foot, again moving in a circular direction.

The diaphragm and solar plexus reflex

Disorders eased by treating the diaphragm and solar plexus reflex include:

- respiratory problems
- panic attacks
- stress and tension
- hysteria
- shallow breathing
- hyperventilation
- fear

Step 32 ▶
Support the receiver's foot under the heel and place your working thumb under the ball of the foot. Caterpillar walk across the diaphragm line and, as you reach the centre, turn your thumb to face upwards before performing gentle pressure circles over the solar plexus reflex. (If you are working on a highly stressed person, this area may be sensitive, so do take care.) Then continue to walk across the diaphragm line to zone 1. You may repeat this move in the other direction.

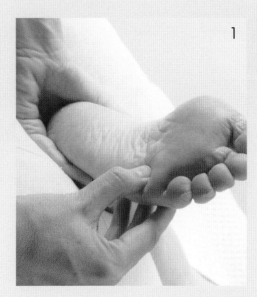
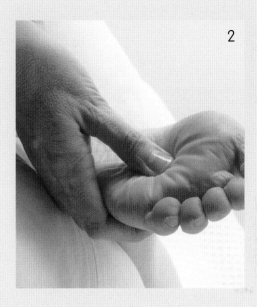

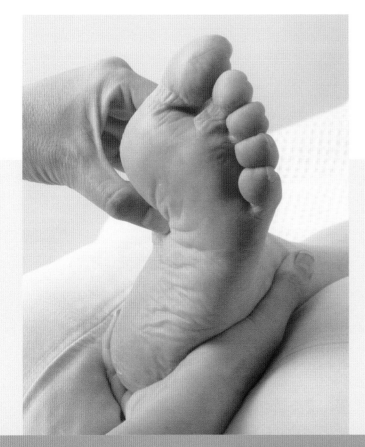

The stomach, pancreas and duodenum reflexes

Disorders eased by treating the stomach, pancreas and duodenum reflexes include:

- general digestive problems
- indigestion and heartburn
- stomach cramps
- ulcers
- diabetes
- low blood sugar

◀ **Step 33**
The reflexes for the stomach, pancreas and duodenum are located between the diaphragm line and waist line, and occupy zones 1 to 3. Using your right hand to support the receiver's foot under the heel, place your left thumb just below the diaphragm line on the medial (inner) side of the foot. Caterpillar walk from zones 1 to 3 several times in horizontal rows until you reach the waist line. (If you wish, you may work the area in the opposite direction using your right thumb.)

The reflexes of the abdomen

Areas treated when working on the reflexes of the abdomen include:

- the stomach
- the duodenum
- the rectum and anus
- the left kidney, ureter and bladder
- the large intestine (transverse and descending colon)

- the pancreas
- the spleen
- the small intestine
- the left adrenal gland

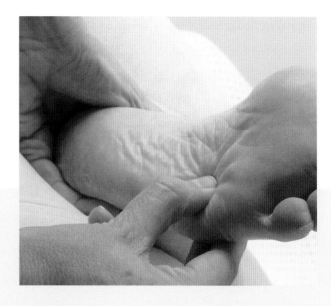

The spleen reflex (the left foot only)

Disorders eased by treating the spleen reflex include:

- a poor immune function

Step 34 ▶

Support the receiver's foot under the heel with your left hand. Place the pad of your right thumb just below the diaphragm line and caterpillar walk from zone 5 to zone 4, moving in horizontal rows until you reach the waist line.

The small intestine reflex

Disorders eased by treating the small intestine reflex include:

- all digestive disorders
- abdominal cramps
- bloating
- allergies

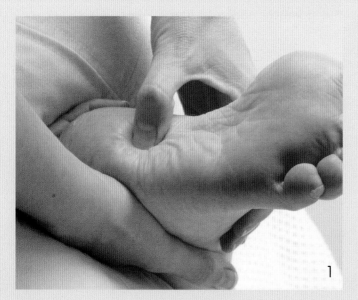

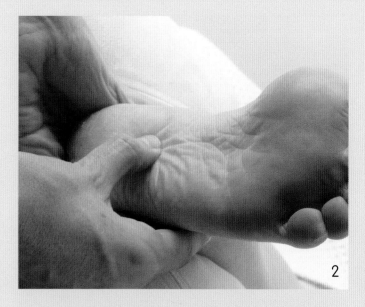

▲   Step 35

The reflex area for the small intestine lies between the waist line and the pelvic girdle line and covers zones 1 to 4. Supporting the receiver's foot with your right hand, place your left thumb in line with toe one, just below the waist line, and caterpillar walk across to zone 4. Continue to caterpillar walk in horizontal rows from zone 1 to zone 4 until you reach the pelvic girdle line (1).
You may change hands and caterpillar walk from zones 4 to 1 with your right thumb (2).

The large intestine (transverse and descending colon), rectum and anus reflexes

Disorders eased by treating the large intestine (transverse and descending colon), rectum and anus reflexes include:

- all digestive problems
- diverticulitis
- irritable bowel syndrome
- Crohn's disease
- constipation
- abdominal bloating
- diarrhoea
- allergies
- flatulence
- haemorrhoids

Step 36 ▶
Supporting the receiver's foot with your right hand, place your left thumb on the waist line and caterpillar walk across the transverse colon reflex to a location between zone 4 and zone 5. This is the splenic flexure reflex. Perform several pressure circles on this reflex.

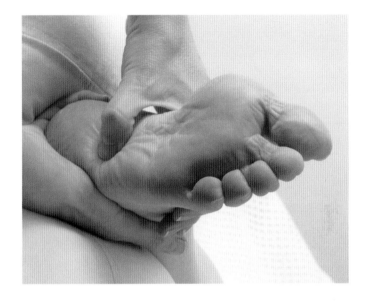

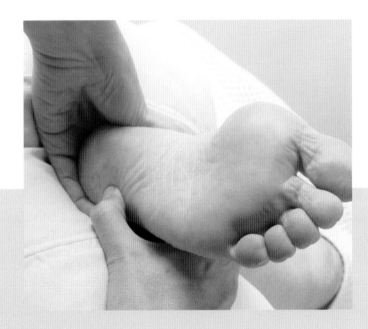

◀ Step 37
Now change hands and use your right thumb to caterpillar walk down the descending-colon reflex to the pelvic girdle line, where the sigmoid flexure reflex is located. Perform a few pressure circles on this reflex.

Step 38 ▶
Still using your right thumb, caterpillar walk across the foot towards zone 1, stopping between zones 3 and 4 to perform pressure circles on the sigmoid colon reflex (1).

Once your right thumb has reached the medial edge of the foot, just underneath the bladder reflex, perform several pressure circles on the reflex for the rectum and anus (2).

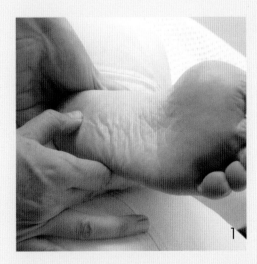

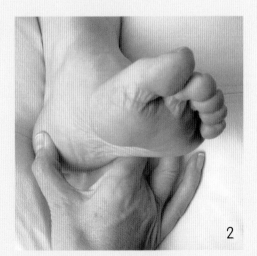

The left kidney, ureter and bladder reflexes

Disorders eased by treating the left kidney, ureter and bladder reflexes include:

- kidney problems
- fluid retention
- bladder infections
- incontinence
- cystitis

Caution

Always work from the left kidney reflex towards the bladder reflex (and never from the bladder reflex towards the left kidney reflex) to avoid the danger of transforming a bladder infection into a kidney infection.

Step 39 ▼

The left kidney reflex is located between zones 2 and 3 on the waist line. Supporting the receiver's foot with your left hand, place your right thumb, tip pointing towards the toes, on the left kidney reflex. Perform several pressure circles over the area.

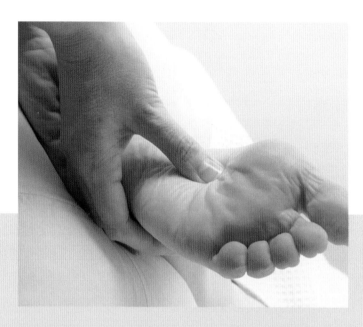

◄ Step 40

Now swivel your thumb around so that it is facing downwards and caterpillar walk down the foot on the ureter reflex towards the slightly puffy area of the medial (inner) edge of the foot, which is the bladder reflex.

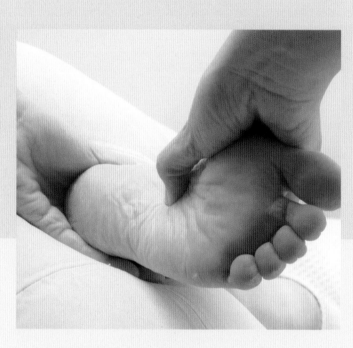

Step 41 ►

Perform pressure circles on the bladder reflex with your right thumb and then caterpillar walk over the area towards the toe.

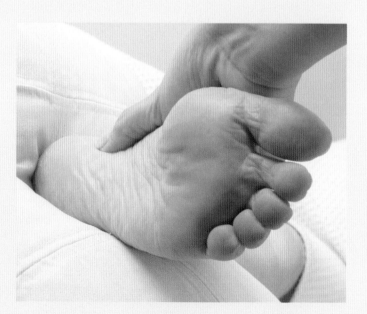

The left adrenal gland reflex

Disorders eased by treating the left adrenal gland reflex include:

- nervous conditions
- allergies
- a lack of energy

- inflammatory disorders, such as irritable bowel syndrome and rheumatoid arthritis
- pain

Step 42 ▶
The left adrenal gland reflex is found just above the left kidney reflex in zone 2. Cup your hand around the top of the receiver's foot or rest their heel in the palm of your hand and use your working thumb either to press and release the left adrenal gland reflex or to hook in and back up. If the area is very tender, then perform several pressure circles over it.

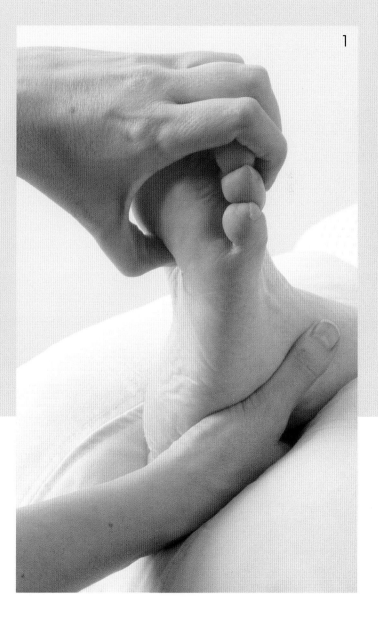

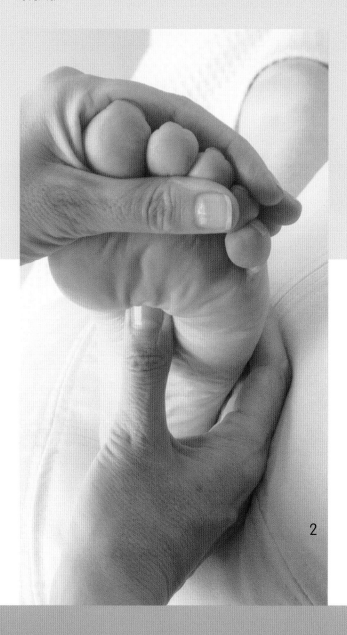

◀ Alternatively, use the rotation on a point technique. Supporting the receiver's foot with your left hand, place your right thumb on the left adrenal gland reflex. Use your supporting hand to flex the foot downwards, onto your thumb, and then circle the foot around the point several times.

The reflexes of the joints, sciatic nerve and pelvic muscles

Areas treated by working on the reflexes of the joints, sciatic nerve and pelvic muscles include:

- the left shoulder
- the left arm;
- the left elbow
- the left knee
- the left hip
- the sciatic nerve
- the pelvic muscles

The reflexes of the joints

Disorders eased by treating the reflexes of the joints include:

- all joint problems
- arthritis
- sports injuries
- hip disorders
- a frozen shoulder
- tennis elbow
- housemaid's knee
- sprains and strains
- cartilage and ligament problems

Step 43 ▶

The reflexes for the joints are found along the lateral side (outer edge) of the foot. To give a general treatment to the joints, cup the receiver's left heel in your supporting hand and use your working thumb to caterpillar walk down the outside of the foot, working from the base of the little toe to the heel.

Then hold the top of the foot with your left hand and use your right thumb to caterpillar walk up the outer edge of the foot, moving from the heel area to the little toe.

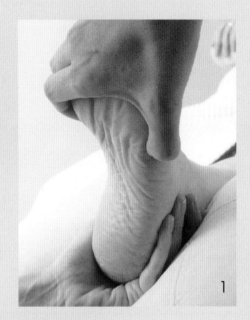

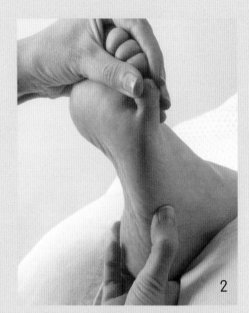

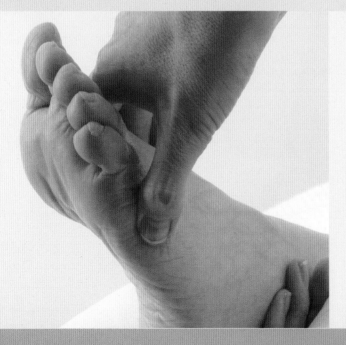

◀ Step 44

To give a more specific treatment to the individual joints, support the receiver's heel in your left hand and place your working thumb on the outer edge of the foot, at the base of the little toe, and either perform pressure circles to treat the shoulder or, alternatively, thumb walk over this reflex several times.

Step 45 ▶

Continue by performing three small caterpillar walks; in doing this, you are treating the arm. Now stop and perform three pressure circles to treat the elbow. Alternatively, caterpillar walk upwards, onto the foot slightly, to treat the elbow reflex.

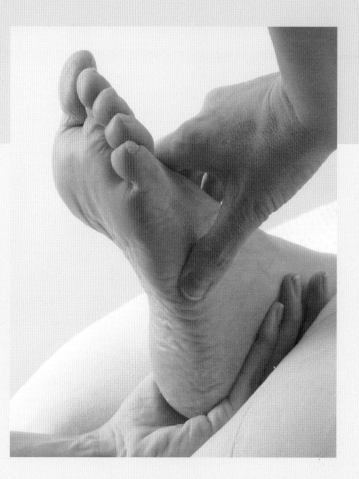

▼ Step 46

Continue to caterpillar walk along the outer edge of the foot until you reach the protrusion that is the knee reflex. Either perform several pressure circles, depending upon how much 'grittiness' you find, or caterpillar walk over the area, which is shaped like a half moon.

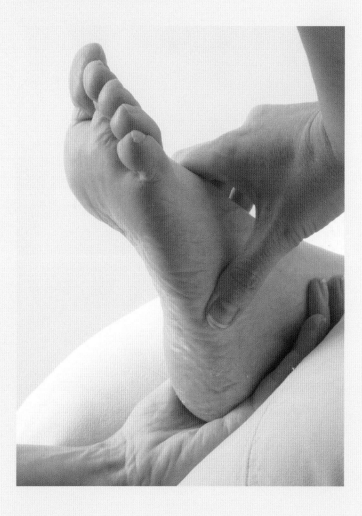

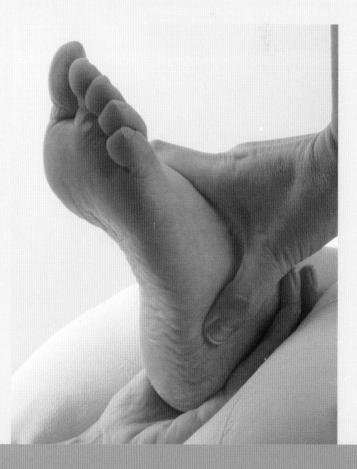

Step 47 ▶

Next to the knee reflex, you will find the hip reflex. Perform pressure circles on this, then use your thumb or fingers to caterpillar walk over this half moon-shaped reflex.

The reflexes of the sciatic nerve and pelvic muscles

Disorders eased by treating the reflexes of the sciatic nerve and pelvic muscles include:

- sciatica
- lower-back problems
- hip problems
- disc problems
- tightness in the muscles of the buttocks and pelvis

Step 48 ▼ ▶

To treat the muscles of the pelvis, cup the receiver's foot with your supporting hand. Make a loose fist with your working hand and then, moving in a circular direction, gently work your knuckles into the heel area below the pelvic girdle line.

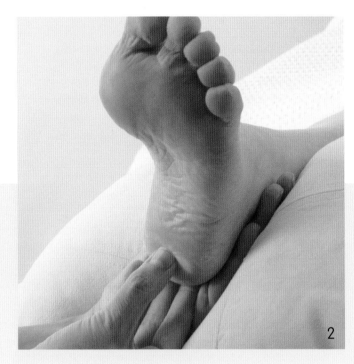

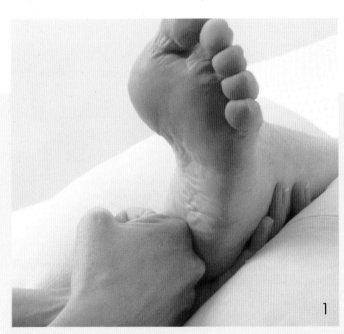

Alternatively, either caterpillar walk from the base of the heel up to the pelvic girdle line to cover the area completely or else caterpillar walk across the heel in horizontal rows.

Step 49 ▶

When treating the sciatic nerve reflex, first wrap your supporting hand around the receiver's foot and then use the palm of your working hand to stroke and squeeze the calf muscles at the back of the leg.

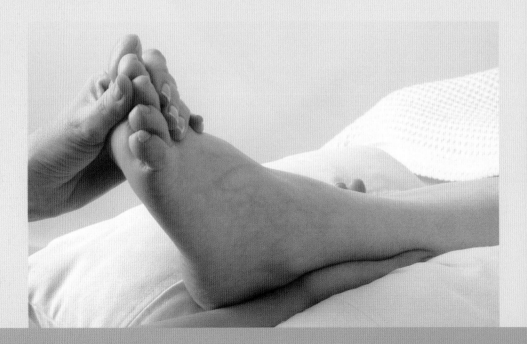

▼ **Step 50**

Now hold the ball of the receiver's left foot in your left hand and position your right thumb, tip pointing downwards, above the outer anklebone. Caterpillar walk down the side of the Achilles tendon, moving towards the heel.

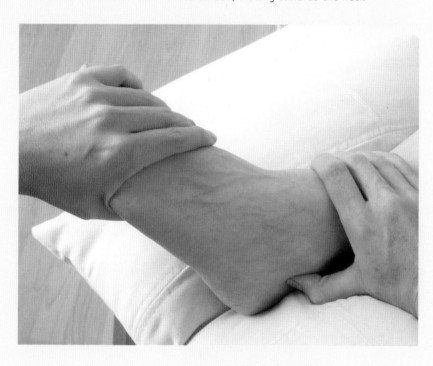

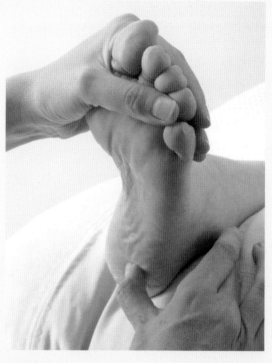

▲ **Step 51**

Continue to caterpillar walk across the sciatic nerve reflex on the heel pad.

▶ **Step 52**

Now change hands and use your left thumb to caterpillar walk up the other side of the Achilles tendon.

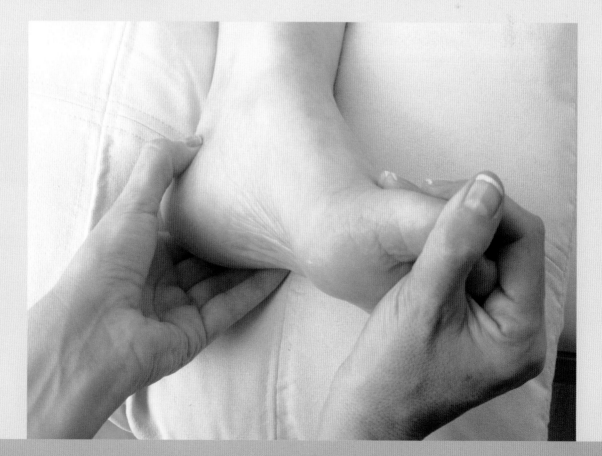

The reflexes of the reproductive organs

Areas treated by working on the reflexes of the reproductive organs and lymph nodes of the groin include:

- the right ovary or right testicle
- the right fallopian tube or the vas deferens
- the lymph nodes of the groin
- the uterus or prostate gland

Disorders eased by working on the reflexes of the reproductive organs and lymph nodes of the groin include:

- all menstrual problems
- premenstrual tension (PMT)
- the menopause
- infertility problems
- prostate problems

Step 53 ▶

To locate the left ovary reflex (in the case of a female receiver) or the left testicle reflex (if the receiver is male), first draw an imaginary, diagonal line running from the receiver's outer anklebone to the heel and then locate the midpoint.

Hold the top of the receiver's foot with your left hand, place your right thumb or index finger on the reflex and then perform gentle pressure circles over the area.

Caution

If the receiver is pregnant, then leave out these areas if there is a history of miscarriage. (A fully-qualified reflexologist may treat these reflexes, however.) If a female receiver has an intrauterine device (IUD) fitted, then gently stroke the uterus reflex area rather than pressing on it.

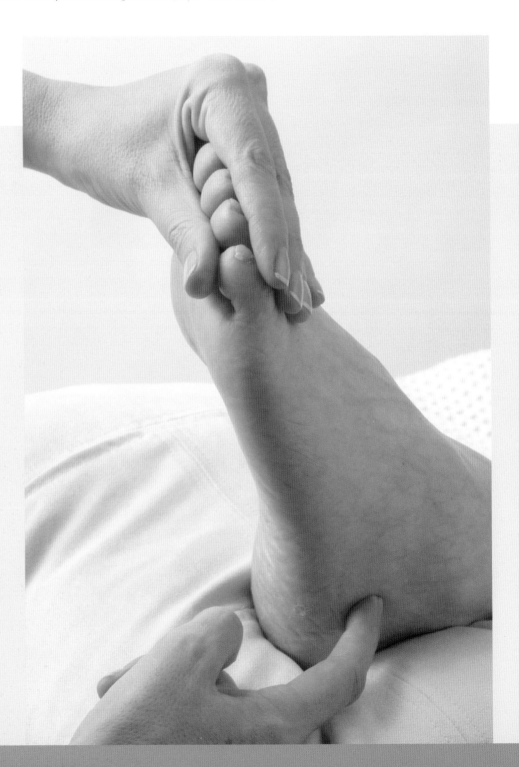

Step 54 ▶

Thumb walk or finger walk across the top of the foot to midway between the inner anklebone and the heel. This is the reflex for the left fallopian tube or the vas deferens. However, this is also the reflex for the lymphatics of the groin and since our lymphatics are often clogged up due to poor diet, lack of exercise and stress, a tender area will usually reveal a toxic lymphatic system. Caterpillar walk over this area several times if the lymphatics are congested which will be indicated by puffiness or 'grittiness'.

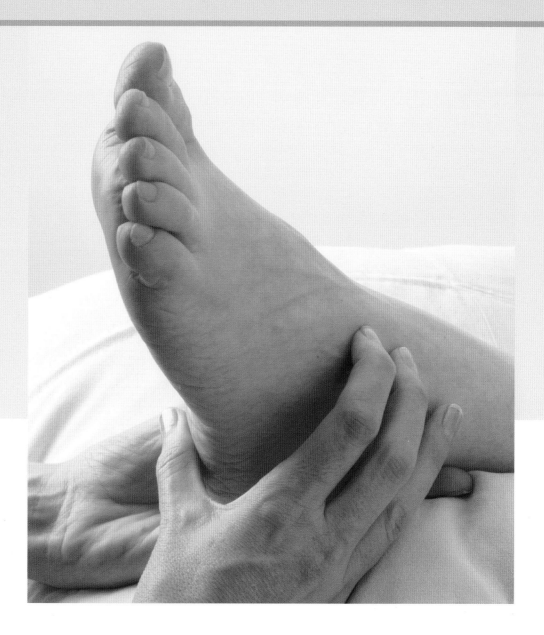

▼ Step 55

Place your left thumb or index finger on the uterus reflex (if the receiver is female) or the prostate reflex (if the receiver is male), which is located midway between the inner anklebone and the heel, and then perform gentle pressure circles over the area.

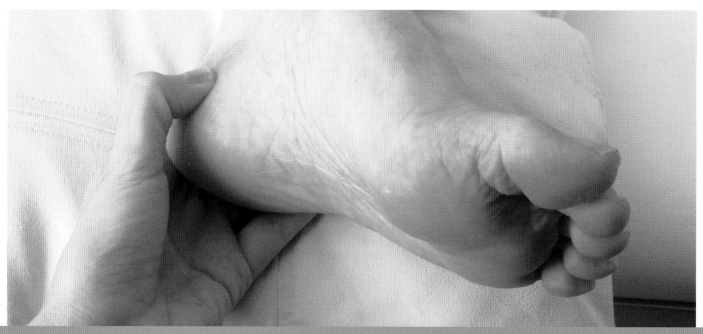

To finish

Step 1

To finish, stroke the receiver's left foot with both hands several times, both to ensure that all of the toxins have been dispersed and to relax the foot fully. Then gently clasp the receiver's foot between both hands and cover it up.

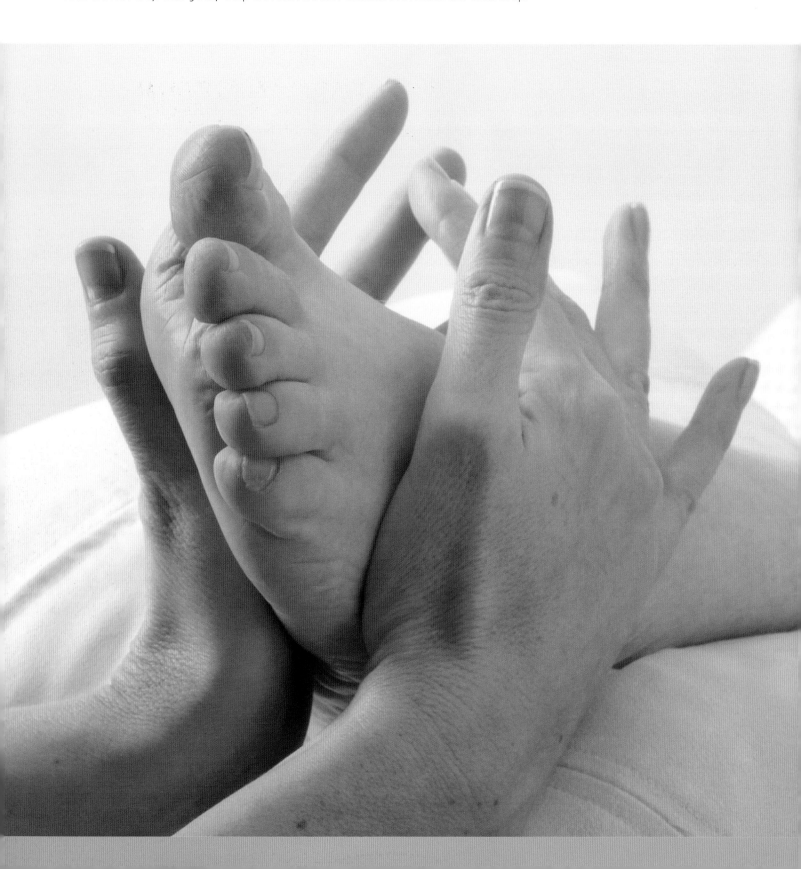

Step 2

Uncover both feet and return to any reflex areas that were tender during the initial treatment.

Step 3

Perform a few of your favourite relaxation techniques. If you wish to enhance your reflexology treatment, then massage the feet with your chosen blend of aromatherapy oils (see pages 236–41 for details).

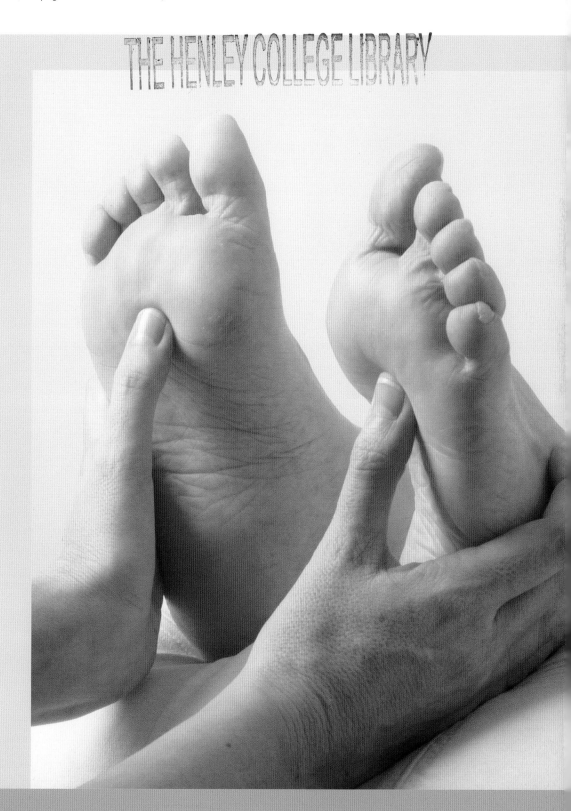

Step 4 ▶

Perform the solar plexus release on both feet to encourage a total state of relaxation. Hold the receiver's right foot with your left hand and his or her left foot in your right hand, with your fingers resting gently on the tops of the feet. Place both thumbs on the solar plexus reflexes and hold them gently for a few seconds. Ask the receiver to take a deep breath as you press gently, and slowly, into the solar plexus areas. As he or she breathes out, gradually release the pressure on the reflexes.

Step 5

Cover up the receiver's feet and allow him or her to relax for as long as necessary. When the receiver sits up, offer him or her a glass of water with which to flush away any toxins that may have been released during the treatment. Also encourage the receiver to drink at least six to eight glasses of water over the next 24 hours to encourage the detoxification process.

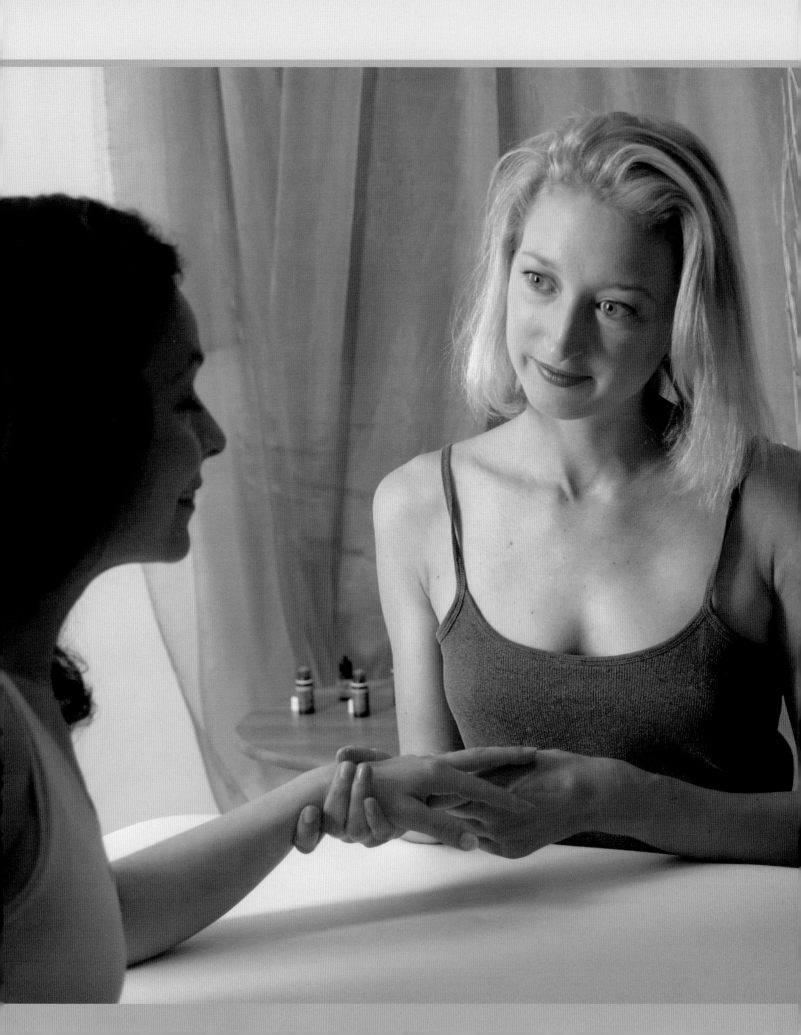

CHAPTER TWO

Hand reflexology

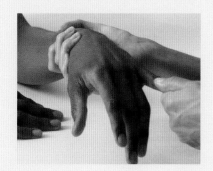 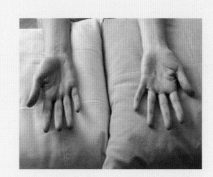 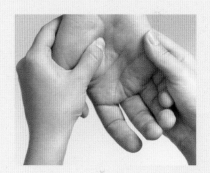

A hand reflexology treatment may be carried out anywhere and at any time. No special equipment is required – all you need is your own hands.

The bony structure of the hands

Twenty-seven bones make up each hand and wrist:

- 14 phalanges, phalanges being the finger and thumb bones. There are three phalanges in each finger and two in the thumb.
- 5 metacarpals. The metacarpals meet with the phalanges and form the palm of the hand. The heads of these bones make up the knuckles.
- 8 carpal bones, which make up the wrist. The carpals are small bones that are arranged in two rows of four and are bound closely together by ligaments. The row nearest the metacarpals comprises the trapezium, trapezoid, capitate and hamate. The second row, nearest the bones of the forearm, is made up of the scaphoid, lunate, triquetrum and pisiform.

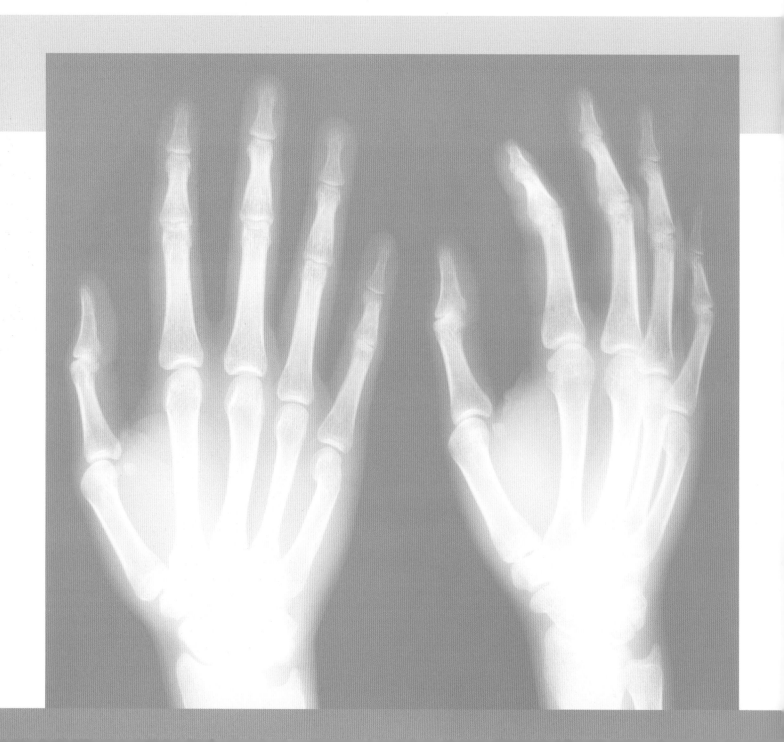

Preparing for a hand reflexology treatment

You do not need to buy any equipment in order to carry out a hand reflexology treatment – all you need is your own hands. The treatment can also be carried out anywhere, however, ideally, you should try to create the right ambience for the best possible results. Peaceful surroundings are essential for a successful treatment.

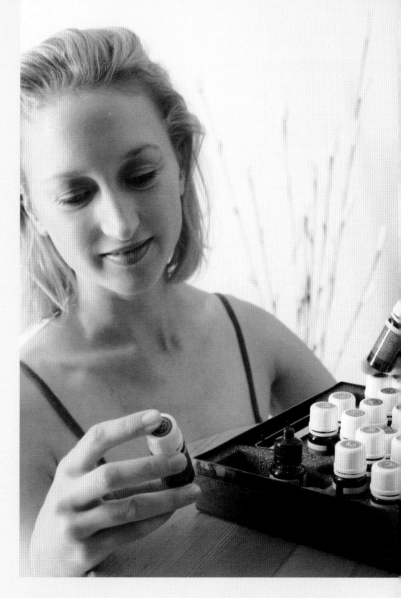

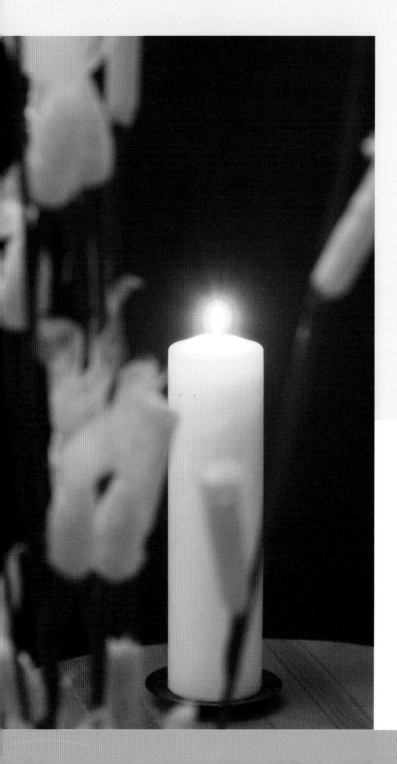

Firstly you will need a quiet room. You do not want to be disturbed during a treatment. Make sure the people around you know not to disturb you, and you are well away from the telephone. To enhance the soothing atmosphere you need subdued lighting. If you have a room with a dimmer switch this is ideal, or you can use small table lamps or even candles. Make sure the room temperature is comfortable before beginning the treatment, and have a blanket and pillows or cushions handy to ensure your partner is completely relaxed. It is up to you and your partner whether you have complete silence during the treatment – some people enjoy low music. It is best to keep conversation to a minimum however – not only will this help you focus, it will also enhance your partner's state of relaxation.

An atmosphere conducive to calm and healing can be enhanced by diffusing essential oils into the room. There are many types of oil burners available, and all you need do is fill the bowl with water, then add a few drops of your favourite oil or oils, depending on the mood you wish to create.

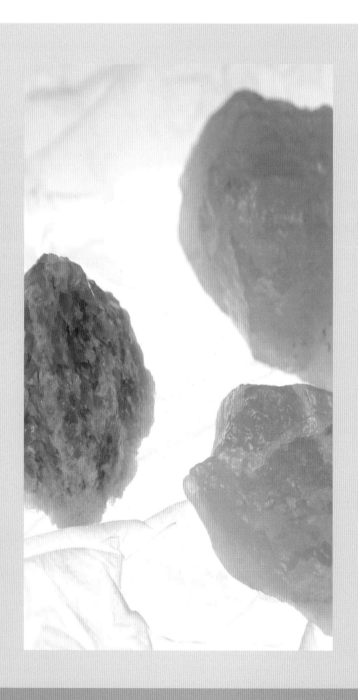

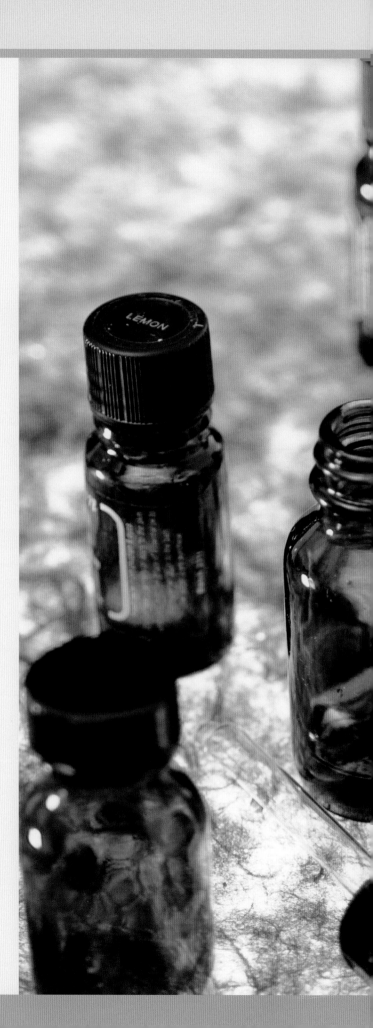

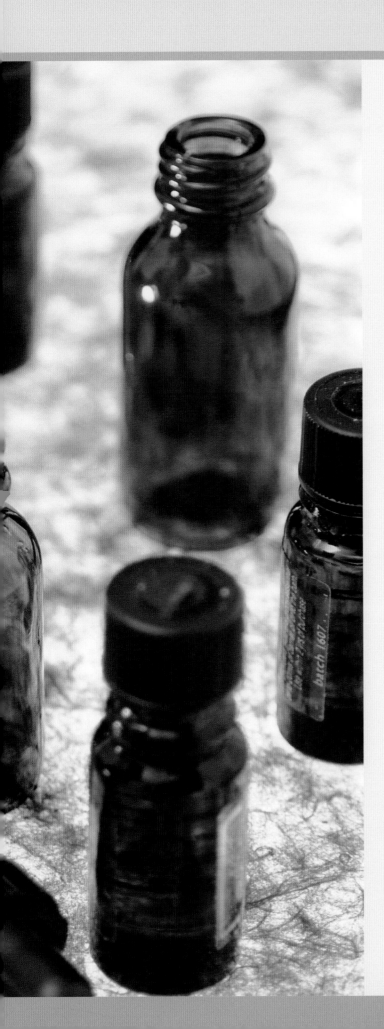

- For lifting depression, use grapefruit or bergamot.
- To calm a troubled mind, lavender is perfect.
- To enhance self-esteem, use either rosemary or black pepper.

Another way to create a soothing atmosphere is to place a few crystals around the room. As well as looking nice, they can also help aid the mood. Rose quartz will aid a feeling of contentment, while purple amethyst helps deflect feelings of negativity.

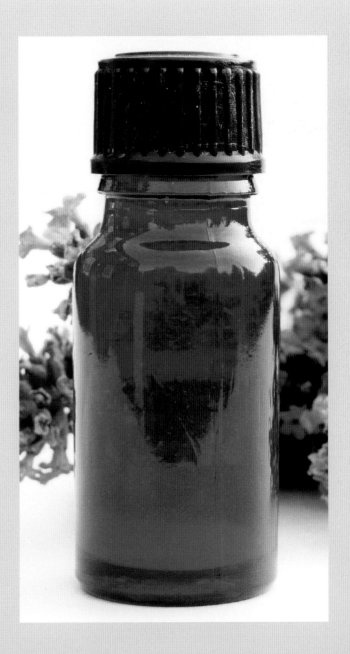

Positions for treatment

A hand reflexology treatment may be carried out with the receiver either lying or sitting down. Whichever position you opt for, it is essential that both of you are completely comfortable and relaxed.

The lying down option

If you would prefer the receiver to lie down, the following options are available to support him or her:

- a massage couch
- a bed
- a reclining chair or sun-lounger
- the floor (a thick duvet, some blankets or a sleeping bag can be used to create a firm, well-padded working surface)

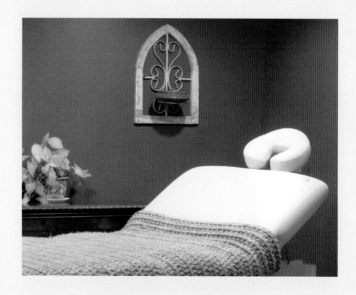

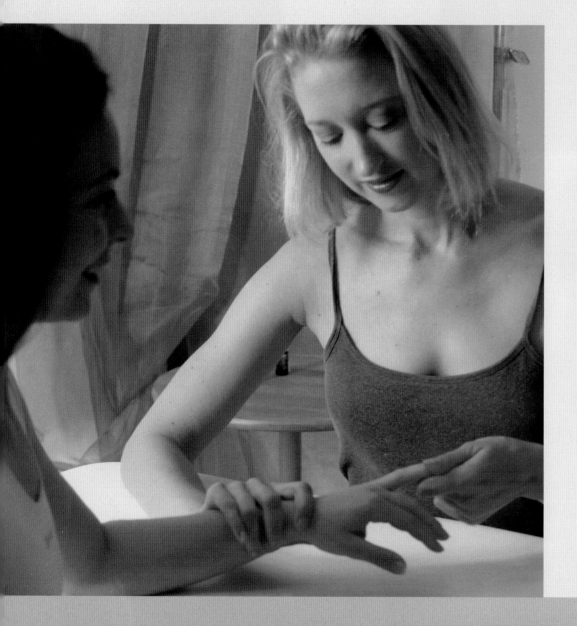

Remember to place some pillows or cushions under the receiver's head, both to support his or her neck comfortably and to enable you to observe his or her facial expressions. Also place a pillow or cushion under the receiver's knees in order to keep the lower back relaxed, as well as one under the hand that you are going to treat first.

Finally, cover the receiver with a towel, sheet or blanket, depending on the temperature, to enable him or her to relax completely.

You yourself will need a chair or stool on which to sit so that you can treat the receiver's hands without creating any tension in your own body.

The sitting down option

The receiver may prefer to sit down for a hand reflexology treatment. In this case, the receiver should sit facing you, with his or her hand resting on a cushion, table or stool. It is also possible to place the receiver's hand on one or two pillows or cushions resting on your lap.

You will again need to sit on a comfortable chair or stool so that the receiver's hands are easily accessible to you.

Other points

There are a few other points to remember before starting a reflexology session:

- trim your nails to prevent them from digging into the receiver's hands
- remove all of your jewellery to avoid scratching the receiver
- wash your hands before giving the treatment
- ask the receiver to remove his or her jewellery so that the treatment is not impeded

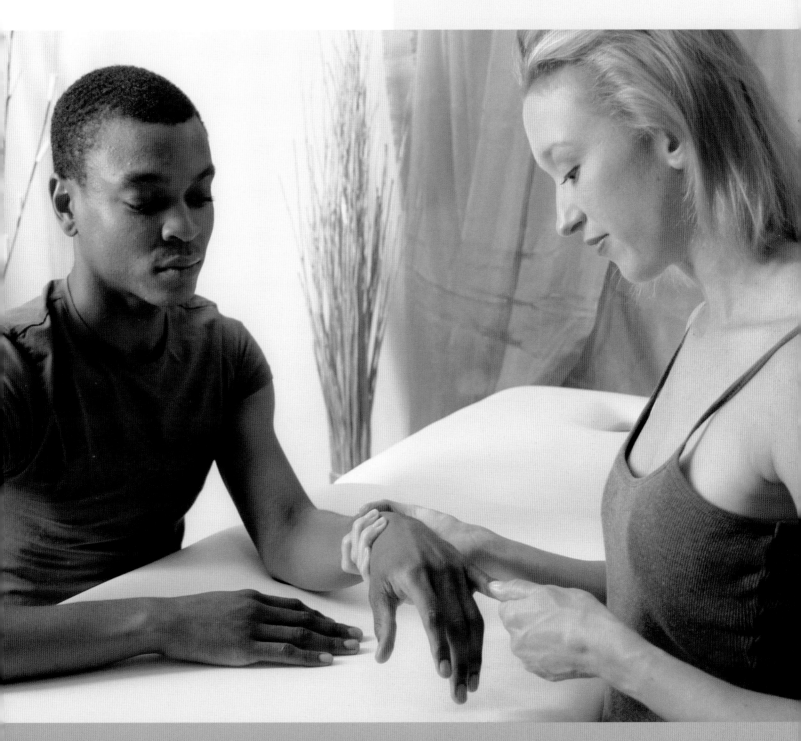

A physical examination of the hands
What the hands can tell you

Healthy hands should display an even colour, unblemished skin and good muscle tone. The hands should feel pleasantly warm, rather than moist or clammy, and they should also be supple and flexible, while the fingernails should be strong.

Any imbalances in the body will be reflected in the condition of the hands and nails, so it is important to consider the following aspects when examining the hands.

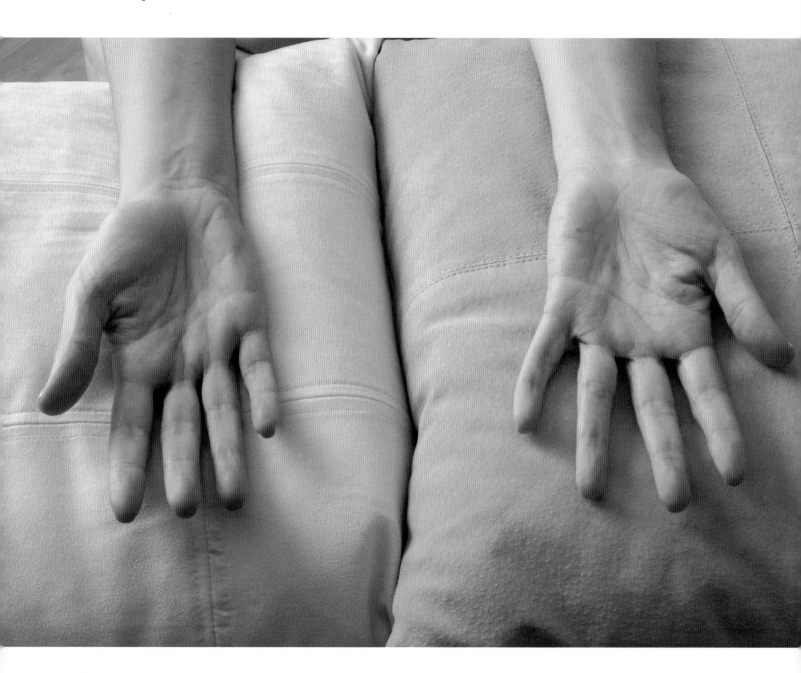

Skin colour

The hands' skin colour can send certain messages.

- White hands indicate that circulation is poor. Hands that are drained of colour usually suggest exhaustion and tiredness.
- Red hands indicate blockages of energy to the reflexes. Anger and frustration can also cause the hands to turn red.
- Yellow areas on the hands indicate toxins in the body. Smoking can cause an intense yellowing over the lung area. Chemicals, medications and poor diet can all turn the hands yellow.
- Brown spots on the hands also indicate toxicity. Is the receiver fed up, or 'browned off', with life?
- Blue hands indicate poor circulation, and the hands can even turn purple with congestion. Emotional trauma can also make the hands appear 'black and blue'.
- Green tinges on the hands not only indicate areas of toxicity, but can also reveal envy and dissatisfaction with life.
- Mottled hands reveal toxins in the body, as well as emotional hurts.

Skin condition

The condition of the skin of the hands can tell you more about the receiver's wellbeing.

- Dry or peeling skin indicates dehydration and the need to drink more water. During a period of change, areas of skin can peel off the hands as the body lets go of the past to make way for the future.
- Hard skin will impair the flow of energy to reflex areas. Areas of hard skin can also protect us from being hurt or suggest that we are hiding our true feelings.

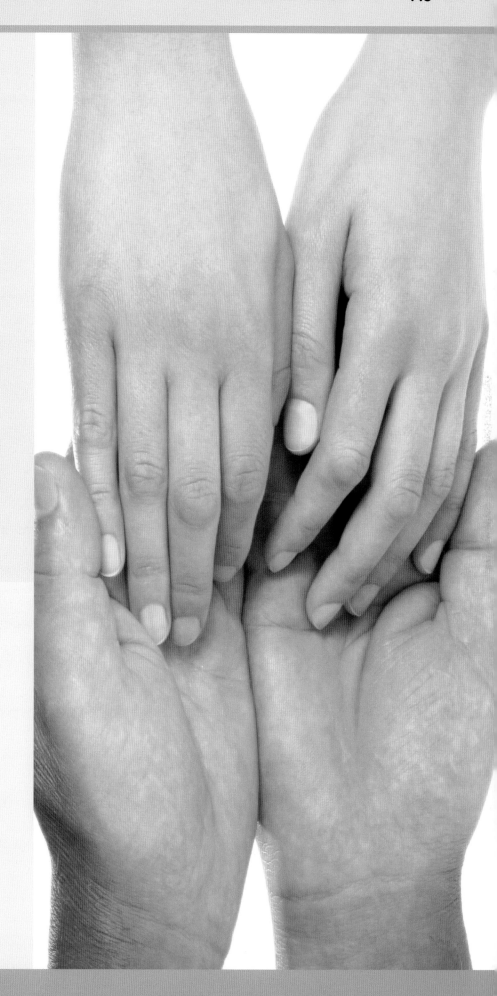

The nails

The nails can also give clues to the receiver's health.

- Pinkish nails reveal a good state of health.
- White, blue or purple nails indicate poor circulation.
- Soft or thin nails may reveal a nutritional imbalance. They can also indicate a weak constitution and are often seen in sensitive individuals with a delicate nervous system.
- Thicker nails reveal vitality and physical strength. However, if they become hard and discoloured, the reflex areas are blocked; such nails may also point to rigidity and stubbornness.
- Vertical ridges can indicate poor nutrition, tiredness and fatigue, as well as shock and trauma.
- Horizontal lines or indentations can also indicate trauma. They suggest changes in diet, too, and if there is more than one indentation, it is likely that more than one dietary change has taken place. (It takes over six months for a nail to grow.)
- White spots on the nails may indicate a weak constitution, trauma or a lack of zinc.
- Spoon-shaped nails can reveal an iron deficiency.
- Pitted nails can indicate a skin disorder, such as psoriasis.

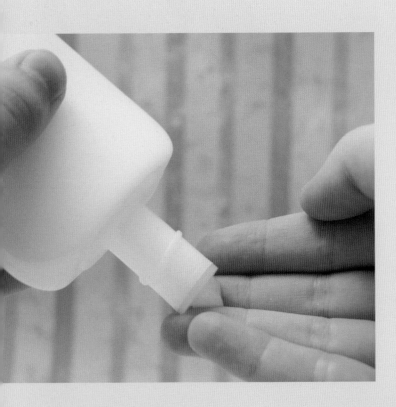

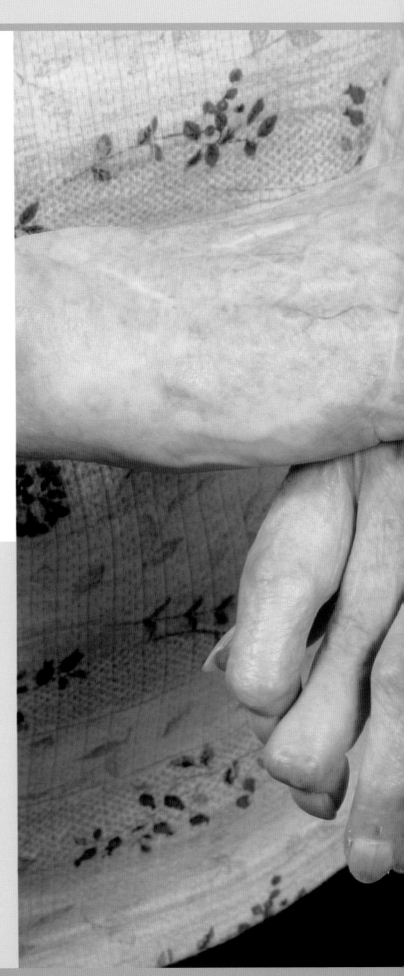

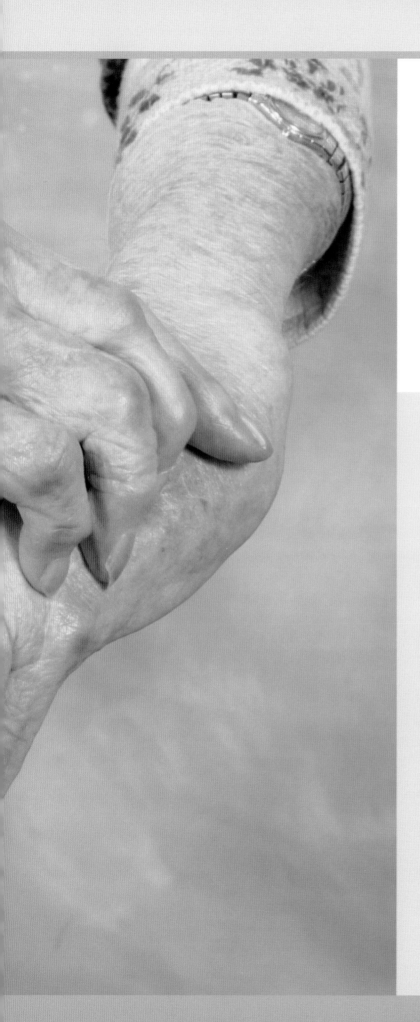

The hands' bony structure

Also observe the hands' bony structure for information.

- Distortions in the shape of the hands (caused by arthritis, for instance) will affect the reflex zones.
- Bent fingers may create an imbalance within the body.

Skin temperature

Note whether the receiver's hands feel clammy or cold. Clammy hands may indicate toxicity or excessive nervousness.

Cold hands reveal that the circulation is poor or may otherwise indicate an inability to express oneself.

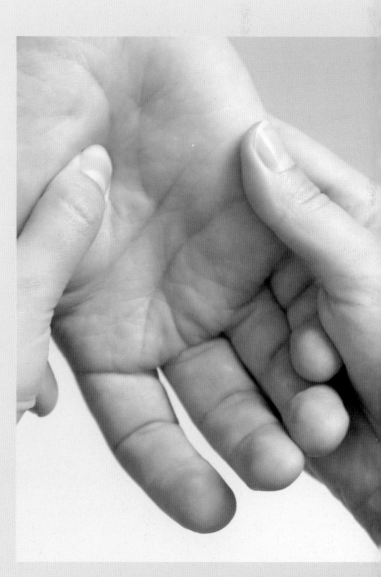

Other points to look out for

Look out for the following, too, any of which may create an imbalance in a reflex zone:

- swelling or puffiness around the wrists or fingers (indicating congestion)
- warts
- a ganglion , a (usually painless) lump, varying in size from that of a small pea to that of a golf ball
- scars, cuts, rashes, spots, blisters and calluses
- wrinkled and lined hands

The type of abnormality is irrelevant, what is important is the site of the abnormality. For example, a wart, or an area of hard skin, on the side of the thumb reflects a neck problem, for this is the neck's reflex area. And puffiness, or a scar, around the wrist indicates a clogged-up lymphatic system, for this is where the reflexes for the pelvic lymphatics are found. Remember! The type of abnormality is irrelevant – it is the site that counts!

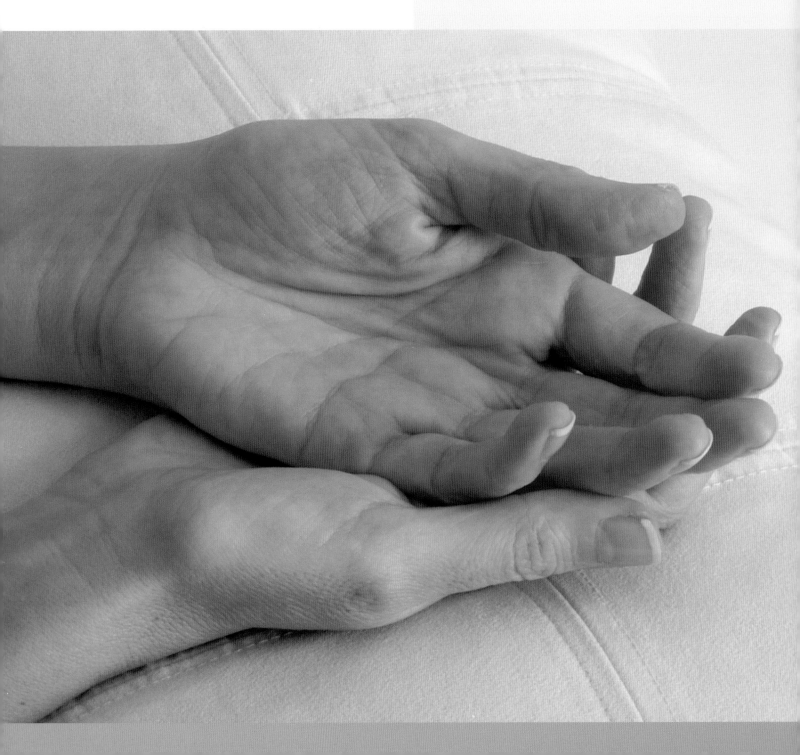

Hand reflexology – basic techniques

Many different treatment techniques are used for hand reflexology. The ones most widely used will be described in this section.

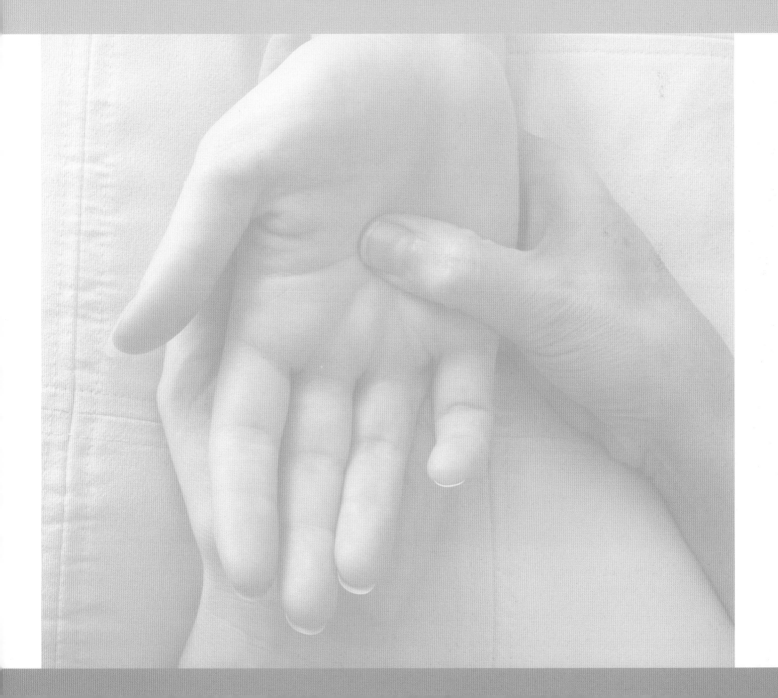

Supporting and holding techniques

It is essential to support and hold the receiver's hands properly during a reflexology session, so that you are able to:

- instil trust and confidence
- make the treatment comfortable for both you and the receiver
- pinpoint and reach the reflex points and zones accurately and effectively
- maintain control over the receiver's hands as you carry out the treatment

There are two standard holds for working on the hands: the first should be used when treating the palm, and the second, when treating the dorsal aspect (top) of the hand. Whichever hold you use, make sure, as you work, that you do not grip the receiver's hand too tightly and that you do not pull the skin taut. Also be aware of any painful joints or sensitive areas.

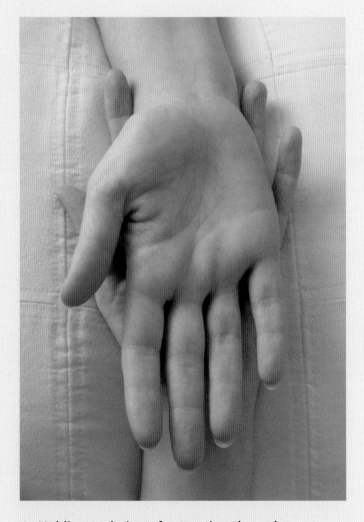

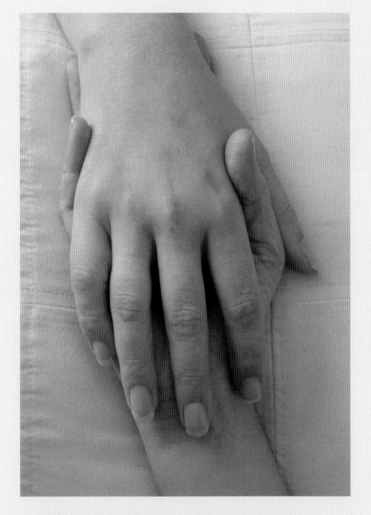

▲ **Holding technique for treating the palm**

Simply rest the receiver's hand, with the palm uppermost, in the palm of your own hand.

▲ **Holding technique for treating the dorsal aspect (top) of the hand**

Support the receiver's wrist from below, as if you were shaking hands.

Basic hand reflexology treatment techniques

Many different treatment techniques are used in reflexology, and I will describe some of the ones that are used the most frequently. Note that the area that you are working on will largely determine the technique that you should use.

How much pressure?

The amount of pressure that you should use depends on the individual that you are working on, and should be adjusted accordingly. Generally, your touch should be firm, yet gentle – not too light or it will tickle, and not too firm or the receiver will try to pull his or her hand away from you. If you are working on a strong, fit adult, then a firmer pressure will be required than you would use if you were working on a frail, older person or a child.

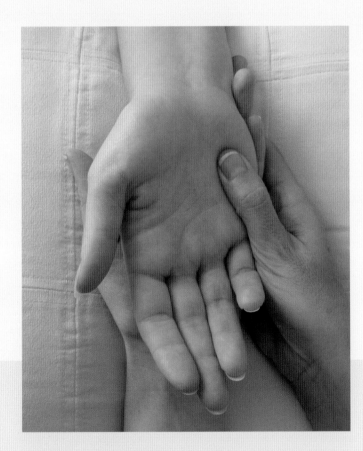

Although it is impossible to predict how much pressure it is best to use, I have noticed that stronger, earthier individuals like firmer pressure, whereas sensitive individuals prefer gentle pressure, although there will be times when they need a firmer touch.

◄ correct amount of pressure

▼ too much pressure

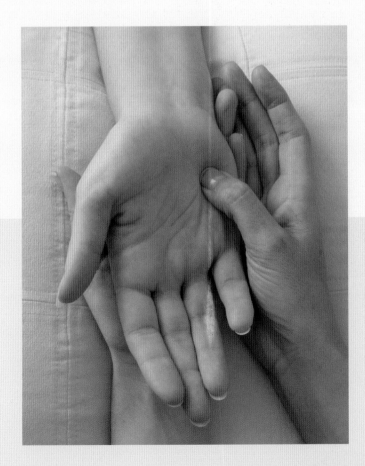

It is important to remember that reflexology should never be painful for the receiver, but a wonderfully relaxing, delightful experience. On most occasions, the receiver will drift off to sleep.

Always observe the receiver's facial expressions or reactions during the treatment, and do not be afraid to ask for feedback about the amount of pressure that you are applying. Try to tune in to the pressure that the receiver requires – trust your intuition!

The thumb walking or caterpillar walking technique

The thumb walking or caterpillar walking technique is the most widely used technique in reflexology, and is particularly suitable for working over large areas of the hand. The basis of the thumb walking technique is the bending of the first joint of the thumb to an angle of about 45°. The following exercise is excellent for beginners.

Let's practice

Step 1 ▶

Using your index finger and thumb, hold your other thumb just underneath the first joint. This will stabilise it and prevent the other joint from bending. Now bend and straighten the joint several times. Then swap hands and bend your other thumb repeatedly. If you are right-handed, you may well find that your right thumb bends more easily than your left one, but don't worry about this as it won't be long before both thumbs are equally proficient at performing the movement. Now practise bending the first joint of each thumb without providing stabilisation.

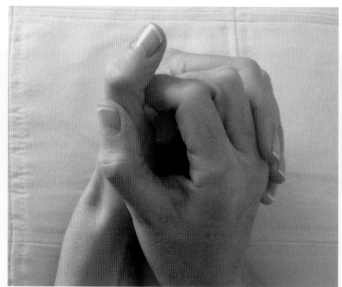

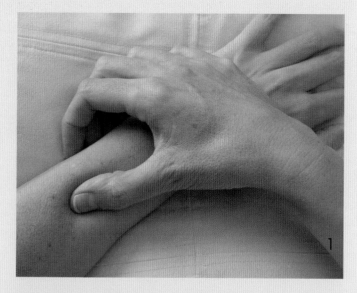

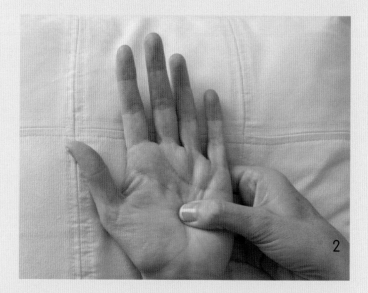

▲ **Step 2**

Once your thumbs are bending easily, place the outer edge of one of them on your forearm. (If you are unsure about which is the outer, and which is the inner edge of your thumb, place your hand, palm facing downwards, on a flat surface, such as a table. The outer edge is the one that is touching the flat surface. By using the outer edge of your thumb, you will prevent your nail from pressing into the receiver's hand.)

▲ Now try caterpillar walking along your arm towards the elbow; then swap hands and work on the other arm. Your thumb should bend at an angle of no more than 45°, and you should take small steps. Finally, try caterpillar walking on the palm of your own hand.

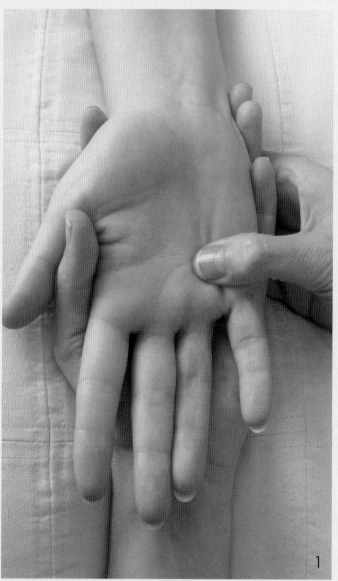

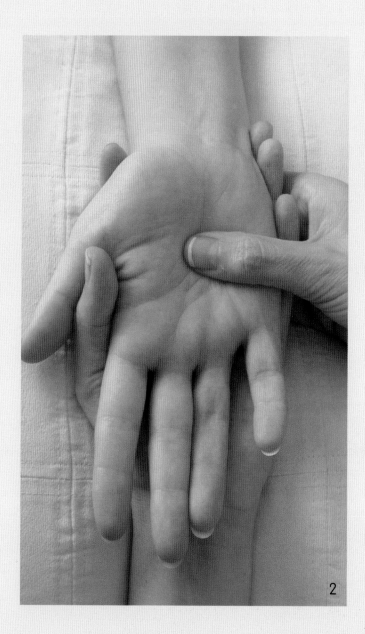

▲ Step 3

You are now ready to try caterpillar walking on your practice partner. Cup the receiver's hand, palm uppermost, in your left hand and use your right thumb to caterpillar walk across the palm of his or her hand.

Tips

You may find the following tips helpful.

1 Ensure that you are using the outer edge of your thumb.
2 Bend only the first joint of your thumb, to an angle of approximately 45°, and do not flex it completely.
3 Keep the pressure that you are applying steady and constant.
4 Only ever caterpillar walk forwards, not backwards or sideways.
5 Do not grip the receiver's hand too firmly.

Finger walking technique

The finger walking technique is similar to the thumb walking technique, except that it involves the bending of the first joint of one or more fingers. It is a gentler technique, and is applied mainly to the top of the hand, which is more bony and sensitive than the palm of the hand.

Let's practice

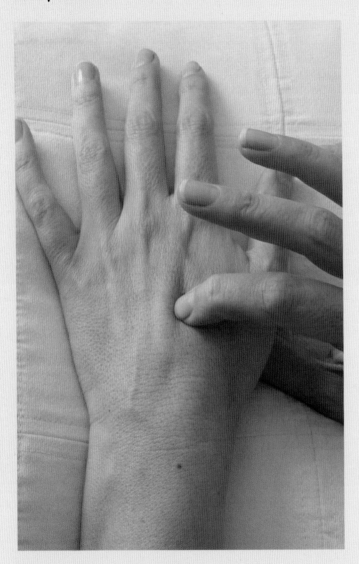

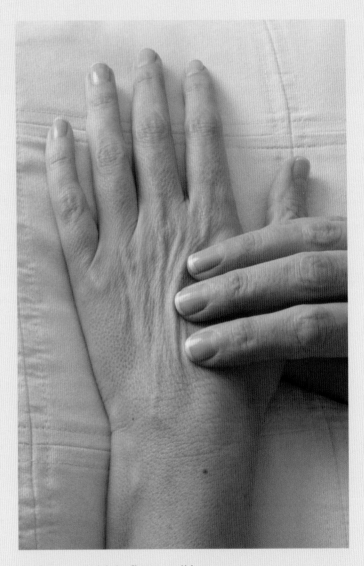

▲ **Step 1: single finger walking**

First of all, it is recommended that you practise finger walking on the top of your own hand. Try single finger walking across the top of your hand first. Gently position your thumb under the palm of your hand and then walk your index finger across the top of your hand. Do several rows of finger walking until you reach the wrist.

▲ **Step 2: multiple finger walking**

Now try finger walking using more than one finger. Try walking two fingers across the top of your hand first, then use three fingers and, finally, use all four fingers. (You may find this technique easier when you are using more than one finger.)

▶ **Step 3: time to practise on your partner!**
Now practise finger walking on your practice partner. Because this technique is designed for bony areas, we will practise it on the top of the hand. Gently rest the receiver's hand, palm facing downwards, on your palm. Place the pad of your index finger just below one of the knuckles and finger walk downwards, towards the wrist. Repeat several times until you have covered the whole of the top of the hand.

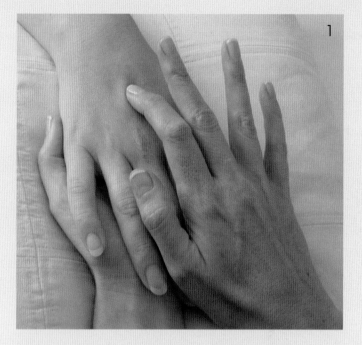

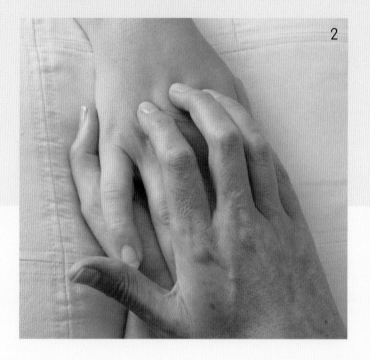

◀ Now for multiple finger walking. Try using two, three or four fingers to finger walk down the back of the receiver's hand. (You may find it easier to use more than one finger.) Either use the same hold that you used for single finger walking or, alternatively, provide support by placing your fist under the receiver's palm.

▶ Note that multiple finger walking is also useful for working across the top of the hand. Firstly, wrap your supporting hand around the receiver's wrist. Then place two or three fingers on the little-finger side of the top of the receiver's hand and walk right across the hand.

Tips
You may find the following tips helpful.

1 Apply gentle pressure.
2 Keep your movements constant and even.
3 Avoid digging your nails into the receiver's skin.
4 Keep your steps small.
5 Walk your fingers forwards.

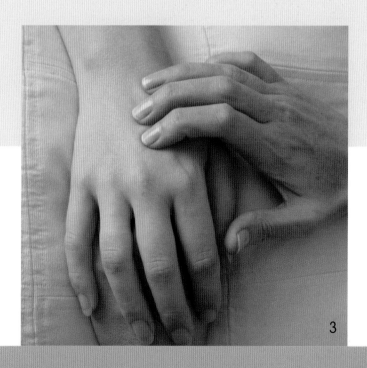

The hook in and back up technique

The hook in and back up technique is often compared to a bee inserting its sting. It is particularly useful for accurately pinpointing reflex points that are small, specific and deep. The hook in and back up technique would never be used over a large area. To perform this technique, place the outer edge of your flexed thumb on the reflex, push it in and then pull your thumb back, across the point.

Let's practice

Step 1 ▼

First of all, practise this technique on your own hand, on the pituitary gland reflex. Place your right thumb on the centre of the fleshy part of your other thumb, press it in firmly (hook in)

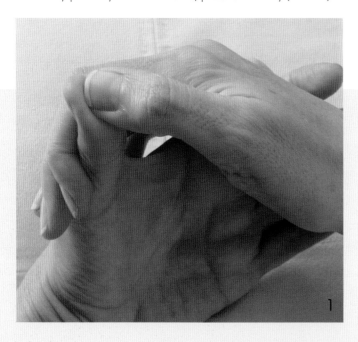

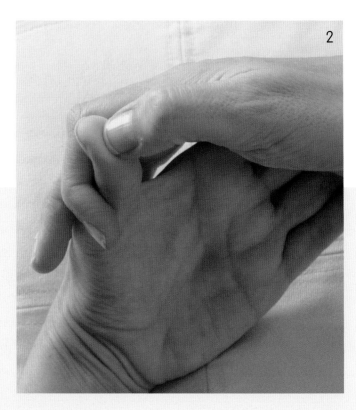

▲ and then pull it back, across the point (back up).

Step 2 ▶

Now practise this technique on your partner. Support the receiver's hand in your left hand and use your right thumb to hook in and back up over the pituitary gland reflex.

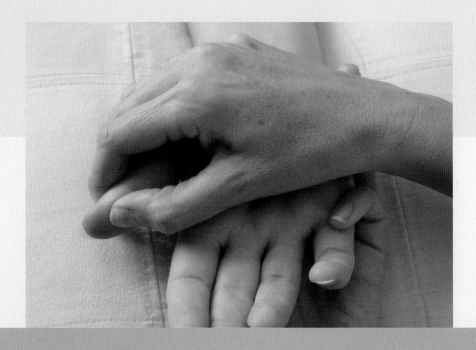

Tips

You may find the following tips helpful.

1 Avoid pressing in with your nail.
2 Do not grip the hand too tightly.

The pressure circle technique

Pressure circles are usually performed using the pad of the thumb, although the pad of a finger may be used if necessary. This technique is particularly useful for treating sensitive reflexes on the hand, enabling them to become unblocked and balanced; it is a soothing technique.

Tips

You may find the following tips helpful.

1 Keep your circling movement slow and even.
2 Do not dig into the receiver's hand with your thumb.

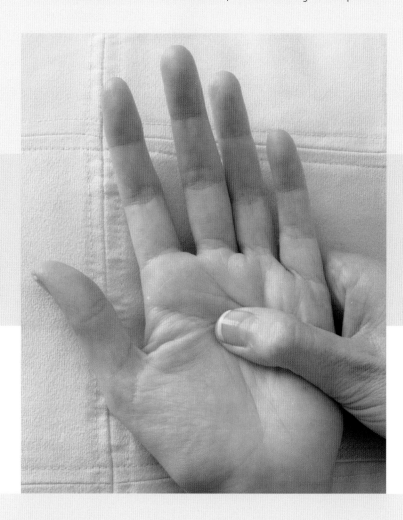

Let's practice

◀ **Step 1**

Select an area on your left hand, and then, using your right thumb, circle gently and slowly over the area, keeping your thumb in contact with the point.

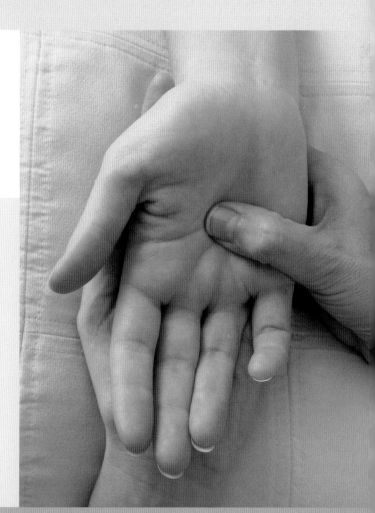

▶ **Step 2**

To practise on your partner, gently cup his or her right hand, palm uppermost, in the palm of your left hand. Place your right, working thumb on a reflex point on the palm of the receiver's hand and then slowly and gently circle over the area, keeping your thumb in contact with the point. Note that any initial tenderness will quickly subside after a few pressure circles have been performed.

The press and release technique

The press and release technique is particularly suitable for treating small reflex points. The palmar surface of the thumb pad is used, or, alternatively, sometimes the pad of a finger.

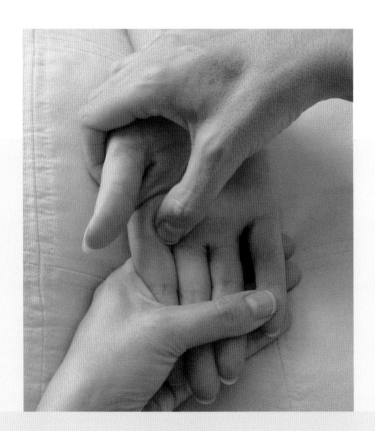

Let's practice ▶

Support the receiver's right hand, palm uppermost, with your left thumb positioned across his or her fingers, gently holding them back. Place your right thumb just below the base of fingers two and three and then press and release several times. In doing this, you are treating the right eye.

Tips

You may find the following tips helpful.

1 Do not press in with your nail.
2 Maintain a steady pressure.

The press and hold technique

The press and hold technique is highly effective for providing pain relief if, for instance, the receiver has a toothache or earache. The pads of the thumb and index finger are used together for this technique.

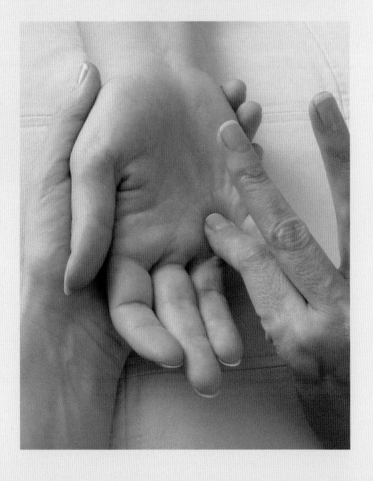

Let's practice ▶

Support the receiver's hand with your left hand. We will be working on the ear reflex point, which is located between the fourth and fifth fingers. Place your thumb just below the webbing on the palm and your index finger on the top of the hand and then gently squeeze your thumb and finger together, without pinching. Maintain the pressure for up to 20 seconds, until any tenderness subsides.

Tips

You may find the following tips helpful.

1 Do not pinch the area being worked on.
2 Try to apply equal pressure with both your thumb and index finger as you press and hold the reflex.

The rotation on a point technique

The rotation on a point technique is useful for treating a small reflex, and involves pinpointing an area and then rotating the receiver's hand around it. The pad of the thumb is usually employed in this technique, but you may use a finger if you prefer.

Let's practice ▶

Gently hold the fingers of your partner's left hand in your left hand. Place the pad of your thumb or one of your fingers on the uterus/prostate point, which is located on the thumb side of the wrist. Keep your thumb or finger stationary as you circle the wrist several times around the point with your supporting hand.

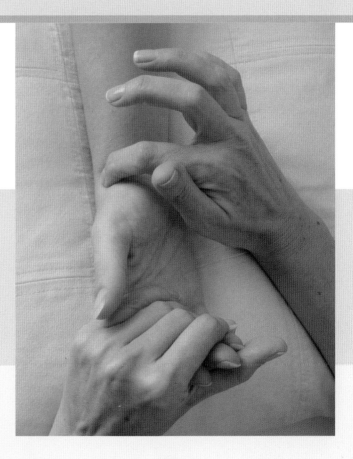

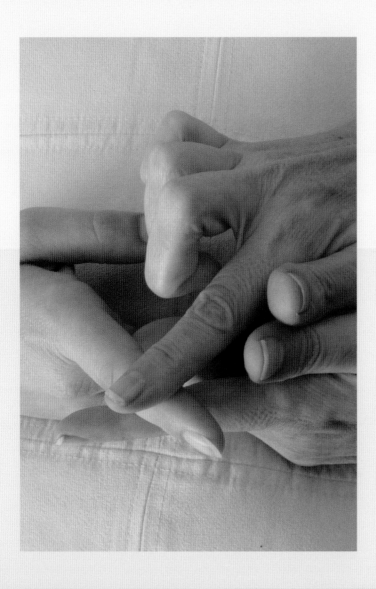

Tips

You may find the following tips helpful.

1 Do not grip the receiver's hand tightly with your holding hand.
2 Do not press your thumb or finger too firmly into the area.
3 For maximum comfort and effectiveness, always circle the hand slowly around the point.

The rubbing technique

The rubbing technique is useful when you wish to bring warmth to an area, to decongest a reflex or to de-stress and energise. Various parts of your hands may be employed for rubbing. For instance, the palms of both hands would be used when working on the inner and outer edges of the hand, whereas the index fingers would be used to rub the fingers. Rubbing creates friction, and therefore generates warmth.

◀ Let's practice

Select one of your partner's fingers and then simply place your index fingers or thumb and index finger on either side of your chosen finger and rub it gently, moving your working digits in opposite directions.

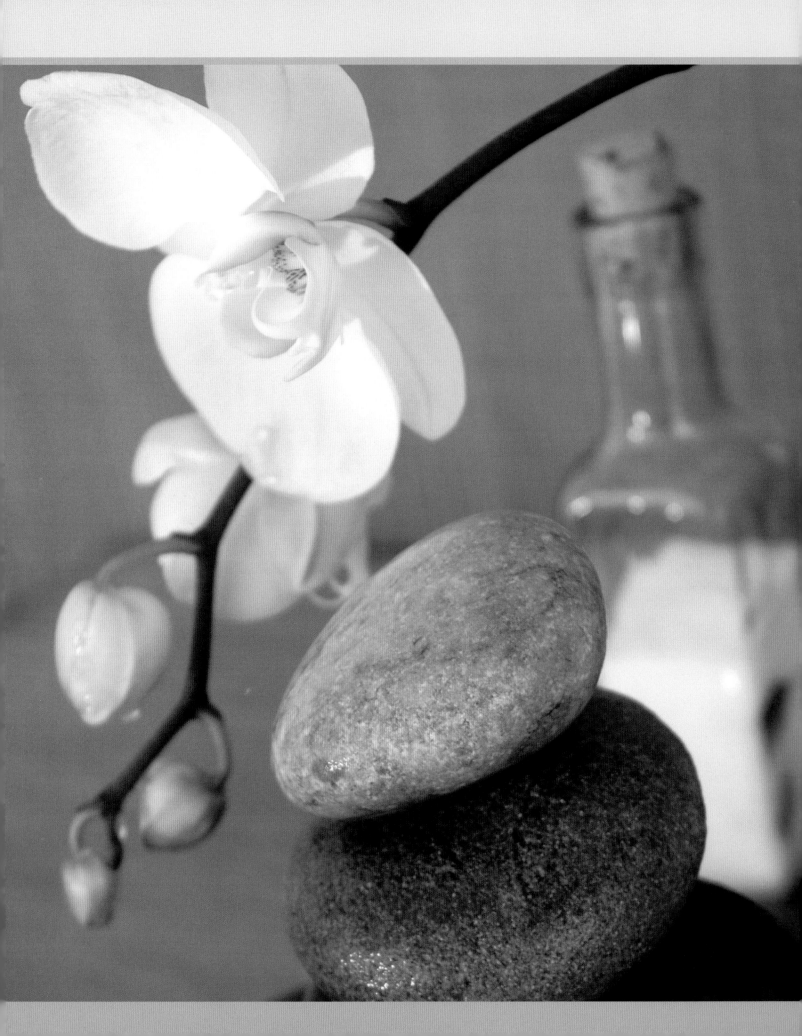

Hand reflexology – the sequence

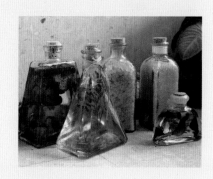 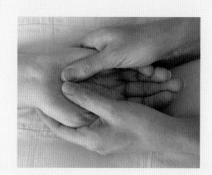 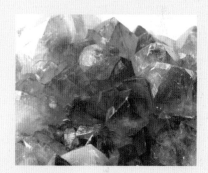

This section will enable you to carry out a complete reflexology routine. Detailed instructions and colour photographs will guide you through the treatment step by step. If you practise you may soon be able to carry out a complete treatment in less than thirty minutes! You may wish to familiarise yourself with the detailed colour hand charts at the back of the book prior to giving a treatment.

The sequence

How long should the treatment take?

With practice, a treatment should normally take about 30 minutes, and even less if you work on lots of hands. If you are working on an elderly or frail individual, then 15 minutes will be sufficient. A baby will need only a five-minute treatment, which should mostly consist of stroking movements combined with very gentle pressure applied to any reflex areas in need of attention. Do not think that a longer treatment will be more effective because it is possible to overstimulate a reflex and thereby induce excessive elimination, such as diarrhoea.

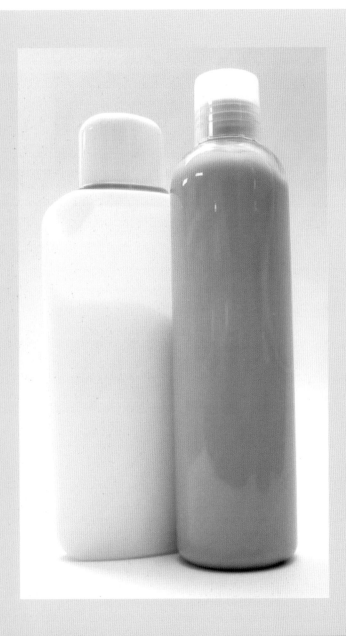

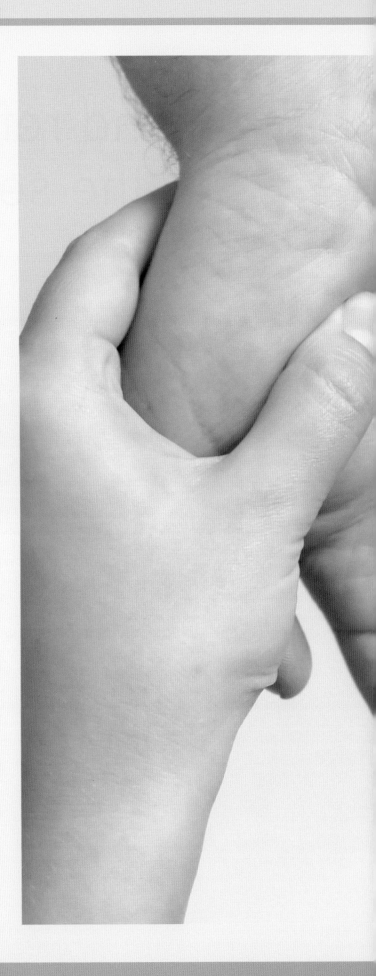

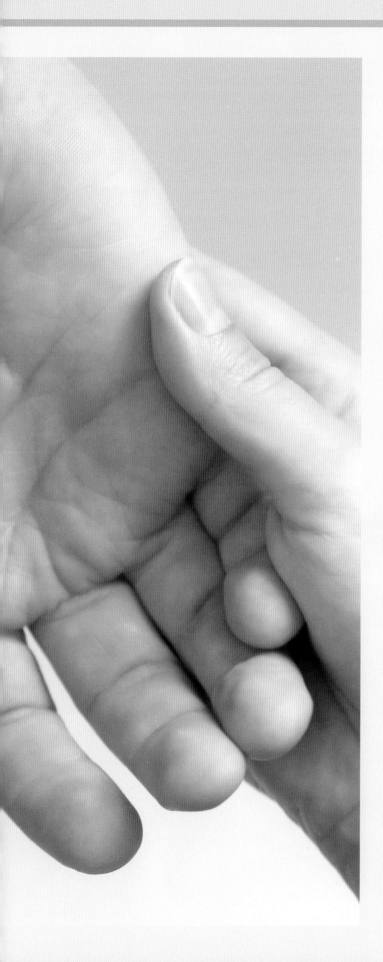

How often should I treat?

Providing treatment once a week to begin with would achieve excellent results. (It is necessary to leave time between treatments in order to allow healing to take place.)

How many sessions will be needed?

Just one session of reflexology is a wonderful experience for the receiver. You will be astounded by its effects, and the receiver will definitely want more! Providing approximately six sessions initially, and then one session per month in order to maintain health and prevent any problems from occurring, is ideal. This is not always possible, of course, in which case give or receive a treatment whenever you can.

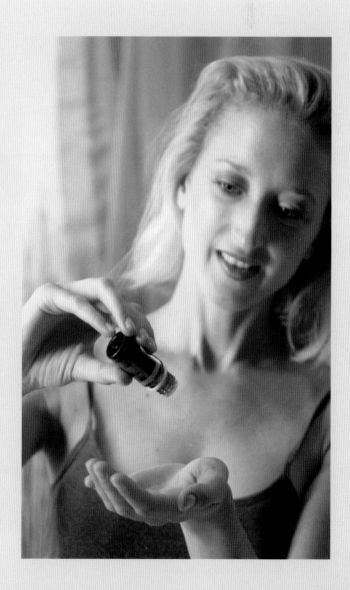

How quickly will I see results?

Remarkably, results are sometimes seen after just one session of reflexology, although it may take a few sessions before the full benefits become evident. Do not be discouraged if results are not immediately obvious, however, for this does not mean that the treatment is not working. Keep persevering, for you will eventually succeed!

Should I use oils or creams?

Do not use oils or creams either prior to or during the reflexology treatment, otherwise both the receiver's hands and your hands will become oily, causing your hands to slip and slide and making it difficult for you to find the reflex points.

You can use oils or creams for your final relaxation movements at the end of a treatment, however. You can make the most wonderful blended oils or creams tailored specially to the individual, and if this interests you, please refer to pages 236-41.

A reflexology checklist

Prior to the reflexology session, ensure the following.

1 Ensure that you have created the right ambience (see pages 139-41).
2 Ensure that you are positioned comfortably.
3 Ensure that both you and the receiver have removed any jewellery.
4 Ensure that your nails are short and your hands are clean.
5 Ensure that you have checked for any contraindications.
6 Ensure that you have carried out a physical examination of the receiver's hands.
7 Ensure that you have washed your hands.
8 Ensure that you feel relaxed and full of positivity. Consciously try to clear your mind and take a few deep breaths to release any tension. Try to be serene, peaceful and loving.

Relaxation techniques are recommended for use prior to a specific reflexology treatment as they:

• encourage initial relaxation
• build up a relationship of trust between giver and receiver
• put both of you at ease
• increase flexibility in the hands
• provide the perfect opportunity for you to judge how much pressure is needed

Relaxation techniques may also be used during the reflexology routine gently to disperse any toxins released during treatment. And when used at the end of a session, they provide a wonderful 'dessert'.

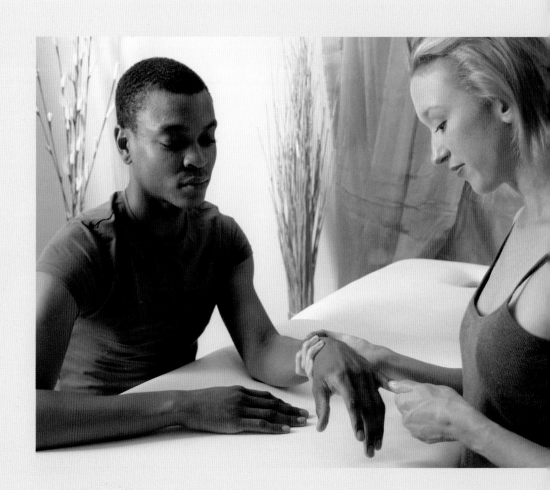

Relaxation sequence – right hand

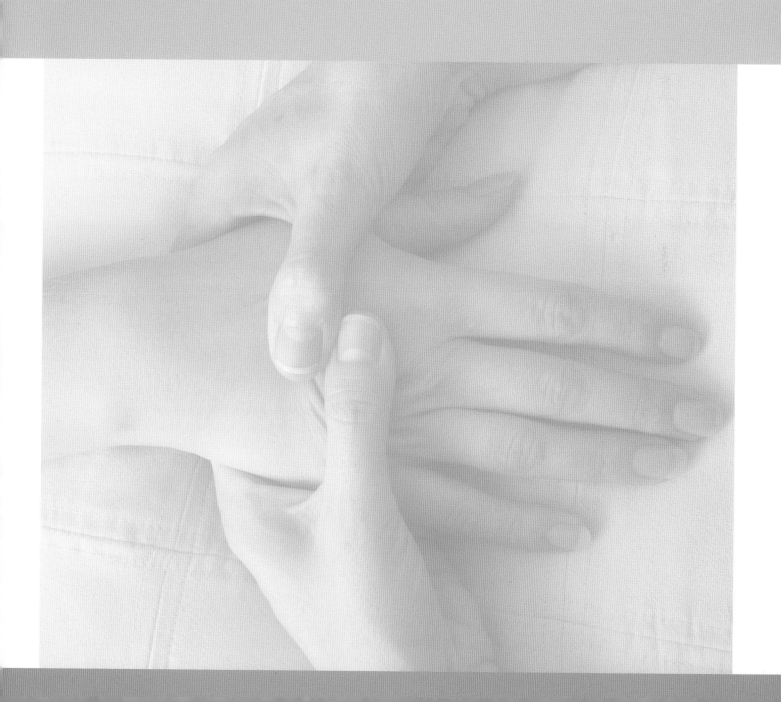

It is not necessary to use all of the relaxation techniques described here, just as many as you wish. These techniques are very flexible, and it is not essential to use them in a set order.

Opening moves

Relaxation movement 1: greeting the hand ▶
Take hold of the receiver's hand and clasp it gently between both of your hands. Hold it for about 30 seconds and notice how relaxed you both become. This initial contact will enable you to tune in to the receiver.

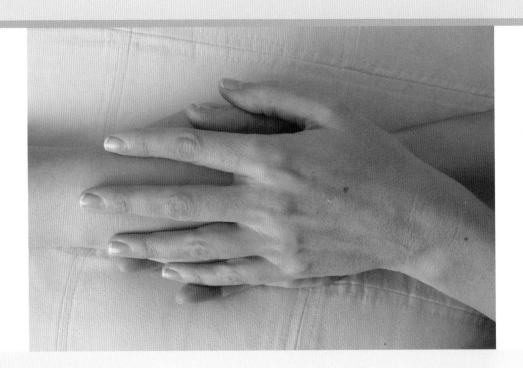

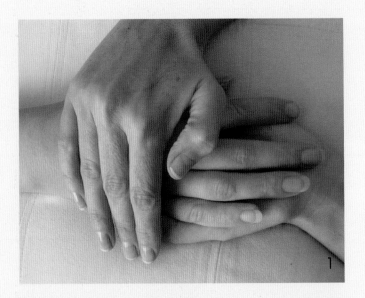

1

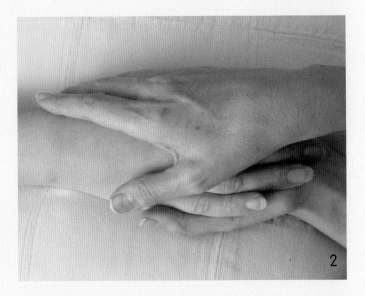

2

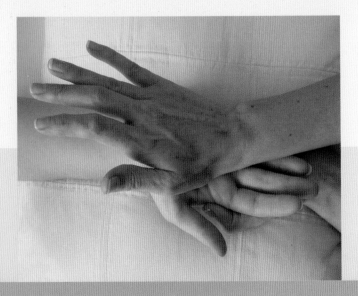

▲ **Relaxation movement 2: stroking the hand**
Supporting the receiver's right hand, palm facing downwards, with your left hand, gently stroke up to the top of his or her hand with your right hand. Glide lightly back, applying no pressure. Repeat this movement several times and then turn the receiver's hand over and repeat it on the palm of his or her hand.

◀ **Relaxation movement 3: deep hand stroking**
Supporting the receiver's right hand with your left hand, use the heel of your right hand to stroke deeply into the palm of the receiver's hand.

Working the palm of the hand

Relaxation movement 4: opening the palm of the hand ▶
Take the receiver's right hand, palm uppermost, in both of your
hands. Position your thumbs so that they are parallel and
touching in the centre of the receiver's palm, then slide your
thumbs gently outwards, to the sides.

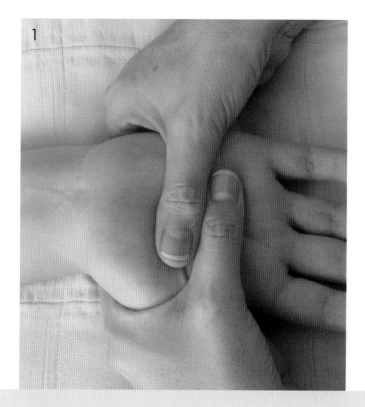

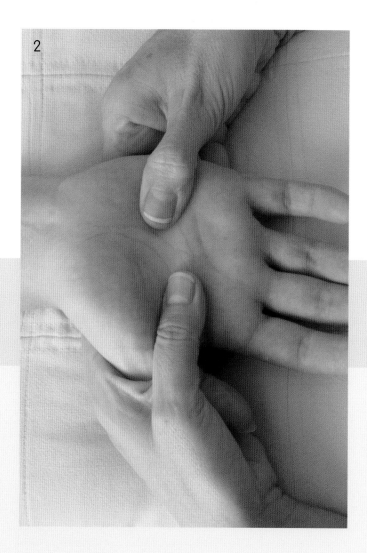

◀ Repeat this movement several times in rows to open up
the palm gradually.

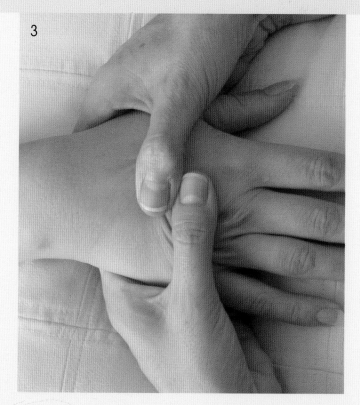

You may then turn the receiver's hand over in order to ▶
repeat these movements on the dorsum (top) of the hand.

▼ **Relaxation movement 5: stretching the palm**
Place your thumbs at the bottom of the palm of the
receiver's hand, with your fingers on top. Push your thumbs
upwards, towards the fingers, several times to stretch the
palm gently.

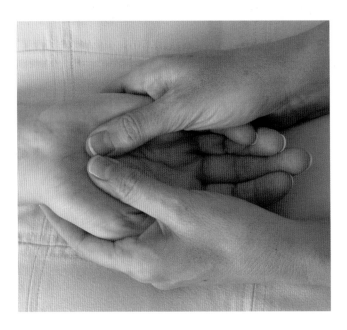

▼ **Relaxation movement 6: knuckling the palm
(metacarpal kneading)**
Make a loose fist with your right hand while supporting the
receiver's hand, palm uppermost, with your left hand. Place
your fist on the receiver's palm and then make gentle, circular
movements to loosen up the muscles, joints and tendons and
to open the hand further.

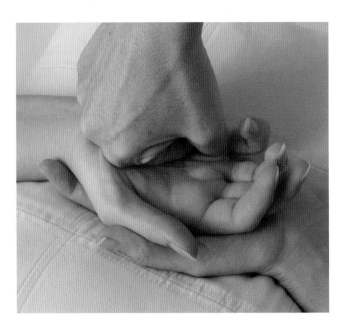

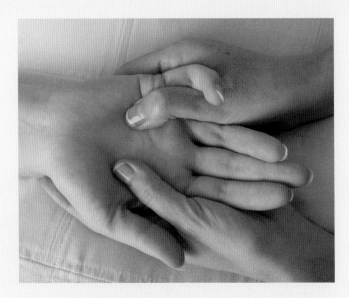

▲ **Relaxation movement 7: thumb circling on the palm**
With the palm of the receiver's hand uppermost, interlock
both of your thumbs with the receiver's hand. Place both
thumbs on the palm and then work the whole of the palm,
using small, circular movements directed outwards.

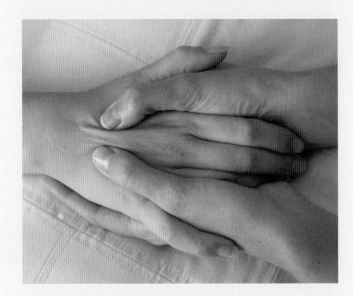

Working the top of the hand

▲ **Relaxation movement 8: finger circling on the
top of the hand**
With the receiver's hand positioned with the palm facing
downwards, place your right thumb between his or her thumb
and index finger and your left thumb between fingers four
and five. Using the pads of your fingers, make tiny, circular
movements as you move from the fingers up towards the
wrist. Gently glide your fingers back to their starting position
and repeat several times.

▼ **Relaxation movement 9: thumb sliding on the top of the hand**
Supporting the receiver's hand, with the palm facing downwards, between both of your hands, gently slide your thumbs down the hand, towards the wrist, and then glide back again. Repeat several times to loosen the top of the hand.

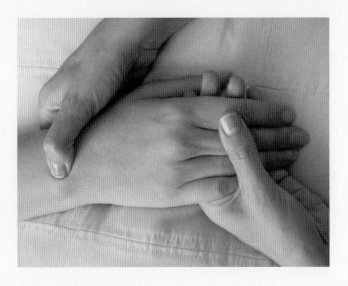

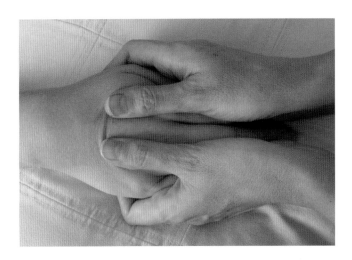

Loosening the joints

▲ **Relaxation movement 10: loosening the wrist**
Gently holding the receiver's hand between your fingers, gently use your thumbs to work in small circles all around the wrist.

▼ **Relaxation movement 11: moving the wrist**
Interlock your fingers with the receiver's fingers. Working gently and slowly, move the wrist backwards and forwards, from side to side, and then in both a clockwise and an anti-clockwise direction. (This movement is marvellous for keeping the wrists supple and mobile.)

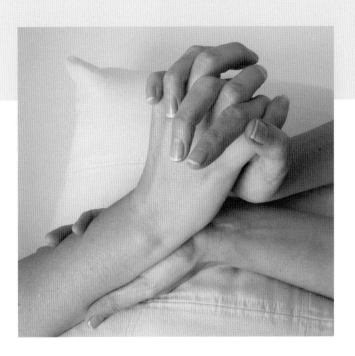

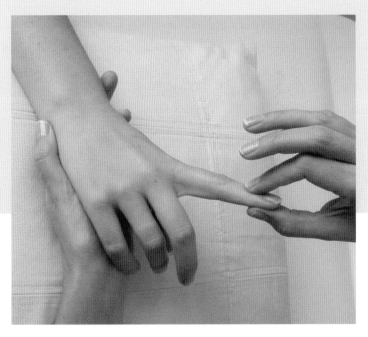

▲ **Relaxation movement 12: loosening and moving the fingers and thumb**
Gently grasp the receiver's wrist to provide support. Using your thumb and index finger, gently stretch and circle each digit in turn. You may also flex and extend each of the finger joints to encourage extra flexibility.

Final moves

Relaxation movement 13: the solar plexus release ▶ Support the receiver's right hand, palm uppermost, in the palm of your left hand. Place your right thumb on the solar plexus reflex, which is located almost in the centre of the palm. Now move your thumb very gently in a circular direction three times. As you do this, you may notice the receiver's breathing start to deepen as he or she completely lets go of any residual tension.

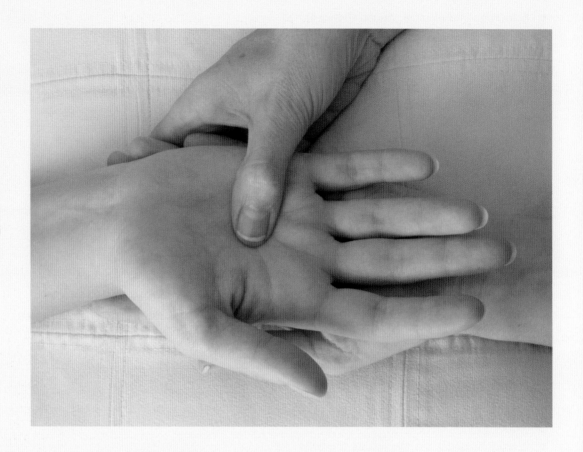

◀ Relaxation movement 14: To complete your relaxation sequence, gently stroke the receiver's right hand with the tips of your fingers, using a featherlight touch.

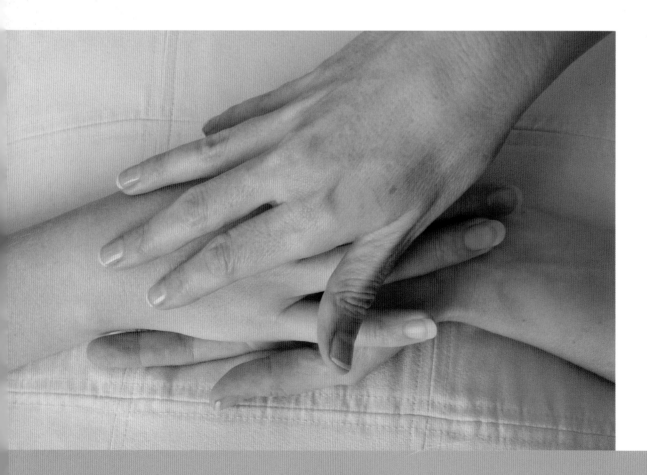

The reflexes of the right hand

The head and neck reflexes

Areas treated when working on the head and neck reflexes include:

- the head and brain
- the teeth and gums
- the pituitary gland, pineal gland and hypothalamus
- the face
- the right eye
- the neck
- the sinuses
- the thyroid gland and throat
- the upper lymphatics
- the vocal cords
- the right ear and Eustachian tube

The thumb

The head and brain reflex

Disorders eased by treating the head and brain reflex include:

- headaches and migraines
- lack of concentration
- the inability to think clearly
- mental congestion
- memory defects
- Alzheimer's disease
- amnesia
- neuralgia
- loss of balance
- fainting
- Bell's palsy (facial paralysis)
- Parkinson's disease
- multiple sclerosis
- stroke and paralysis
- epilepsy
- poor co-ordination
- the aftereffects of anaesthetics
- baldness
- scalp problems
- learning difficulties, e.g., dyslexia
- Attention Deficit Disorder (ADD)
- lack of confidence and low self-esteem
- depression
- a lack of intuition and a closed mind.

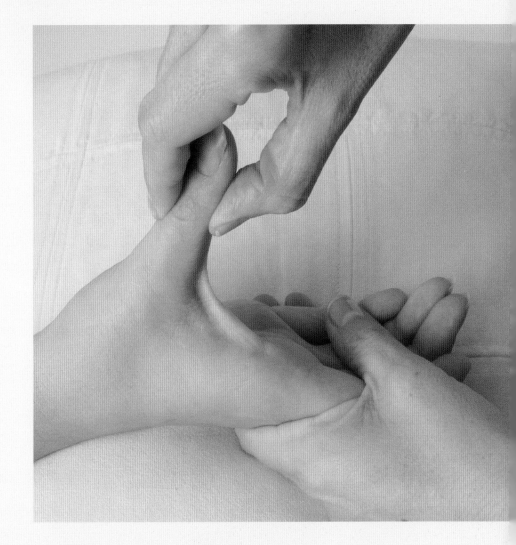

Step 1 ▶

Rest the receiver's right hand, palm uppermost, on a cushion and use your left hand to gently support it. Remember not to grip the receiver's hand too tightly and to take tiny, little steps. Place the pad of your right thumb on the tip of the receiver's right thumb and caterpillar walk down it to the base several times. Make sure that you cover the outside, back and inside of the thumb. Note that you will need to caterpillar walk for several rows to cover the area completely.

The pituitary gland reflex

Disorders eased by treating the pituitary gland reflex include:

- hormonal imbalances
- premenstrual syndrome (PMS)
- scanty, heavy or painful menstruation
- difficulties conceiving
- the menopause

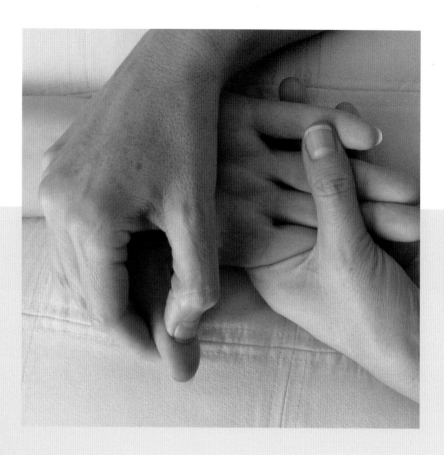

Step 2 ▶

Be prepared to have to search to pinpoint the pituitary gland reflex. It is often positioned off-centre on the thumb pad, be it slightly higher, lower, to the right or to the left. If you are very lucky, a small lump may be visible or palpable, indicating the exact location.

Supporting the receiver's hand in your left hand, use your right thumb to press in firmly (hook in) and then pull back, across the pituitary gland reflex (back up). Note that this is often a sensitive point.

The pineal gland and hypothalamus reflexes

Disorders eased by treating the pineal gland and hypothalamus reflexes include:

- Seasonal Affective Disorder (SAD)
- sleep problems
- mood swings
- hormonal imbalances
- a lack of insight, intuition or vision

◀ Step 3

The pineal gland and hypothalamus reflexes are situated very close to the pituitary gland reflex. Move your thumb up very slightly, towards the tip of the receiver's thumb, and then rock your thumb onto its outer edge to circle over the pineal gland reflex. Then rock your thumb onto its inner edge and treat the hypothalamus reflex with pressure circles.

The face reflex

Disorders eased by treating the face reflex include:

- eye problems, e.g., conjunctivitis
- teeth and gum problems
- nasal problems
- sinusitis
- jaw problems
- facial acne
- Bell's palsy (facial paralysis)
- facial neuralgia

Step 4 ▶

Gently turn over the receiver's hand and support it with your left hand. Using your thumb, caterpillar walk down the front of the thumb, moving from the tip to the base. You may need to caterpillar walk down the thumb three or four times, depending on its size. Depending on the size of the receiver's thumb and your fingers, you may find it easier to use your index finger instead (1). You may prefer to finger walk across the face reflex. With your thumb positioned on the back of the receiver's thumb for support, use two fingers to walk across the front of the thumb (2).

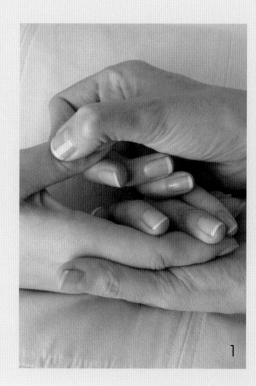
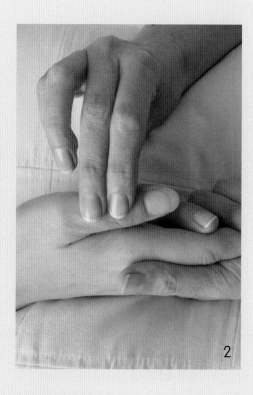

The neck reflex

Disorders eased by treating the neck reflex include:

- aches and pains in the neck
- a lack of mobility in the neck
- whiplash injuries   • arthritis in the neck
- throat problems, such as tonsillitis and problems with the adenoids, pharynx and larynx, when working across the front of the neck reflex.

Step 5 ▶

Support the receiver's hand with your left hand. Gently hold the receiver's thumb between your index finger and thumb and then rotate it both clockwise and anti-clockwise. This movement is excellent for alleviating a stiff neck. If a thumb joint grates, or does not move very well, gently encourage it, but never force it.

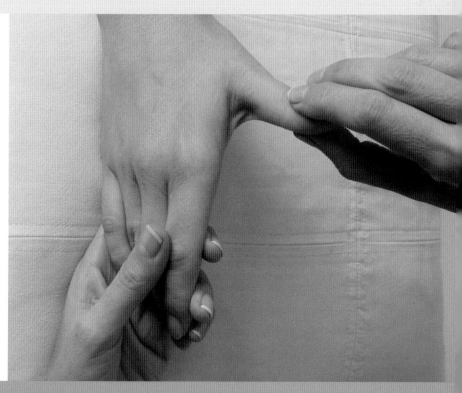

The neck, thyroid gland and throat reflex

Disorders eased by treating the neck, thyroid gland and throat reflex include:

- all neck and throat problems as outlined for step 5
- parathyroid disorders
- osteoporosis
- thyroid problems
- muscle-twitching
- weight problems
- arthritis

Step 6 ▶

Supporting the receiver's hand, palm uppermost, caterpillar walk your right thumb across the back of the base of the thumb several times (1).

Turn the receiver's hand over and grasp the thumb between your left thumb and index finger. Then caterpillar walk your right thumb across the front of the base of the thumb (2).

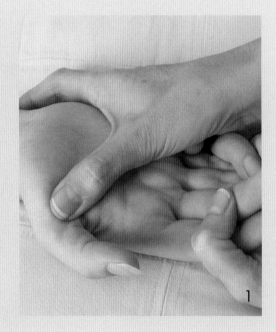

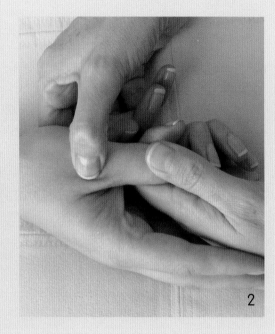

The vocal cords reflex

Disorders eased by treating the vocal cords reflex include:

- vocal cord problems
- laryngitis
- pharyngitis
- tracheitis
- difficulty expressing oneself
- a 'lump' in the throat
- an inability to say what one thinks
- speech problems
- an overuse of the voice.

Step 7 ▶

To locate the reflex for the vocal cords, place the thumb of your working hand at the bottom of the webbing between the receiver's thumb and index finger. Now gently circle over this reflex.

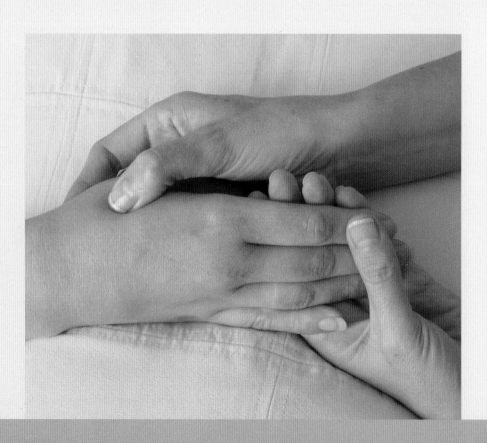

The fingers

The sinus reflexes

Disorders eased by treating the sinus reflexes include:

- sinus problems
- allergies
- catarrh
- hay fever
- rhinitis
- colds
- a loss of the sense of smell
- nasal polyps

Step 8 ▶
Support the receiver's hand, palm uppermost, in the palm of your left hand. Use your right thumb to caterpillar walk from the tip of the little finger to its base. You will need to caterpillar walk for about three rows to cover the area thoroughly. Repeat on the ring, middle and index fingers (1).

To treat the sides of the fingers, you may use your thumb and index finger to caterpillar walk down both sides of each finger at the same time (2).

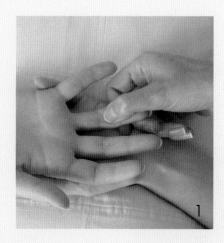
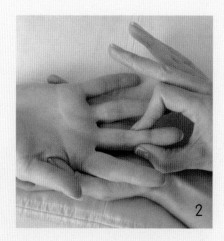

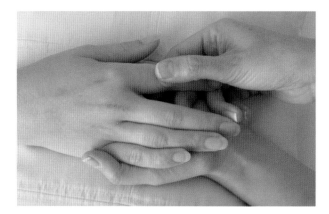

The teeth and gum reflexes

Disorders eased by treating the teeth and gum reflexes include:

- toothache
- gum problems
- painful or sensitive teeth
- abscesses
- teething
- pain after dental procedures

◀ **Step 9**
The reflexes for the teeth and gums are found on the top of all of the fingers. Turn the receiver's hand over and support the fingers with your left hand. Commencing at the top of the index finger, perform about three or four rows of thumb walking to cover the dorsal (top) side of the finger. Repeat on the middle, ring and little fingers.

The upper lymphatic reflexes

Disorders eased by treating the upper lymphatic reflexes include:

- a poor immune function, e.g., if a person suffers from recurrent infections
- myalgic encephalomyelitis (ME)
- ear, nose and throat problems
- a toxic lymphatic system (which is often due to poor diet and a lack of exercise)
- acne (this technique will help to drain the head and neck area)

Step 10 ▶
Supporting the receiver's hand with your left hand, gently squeeze the webbing between each of the fingers with your right thumb and index finger. Repeat several times.

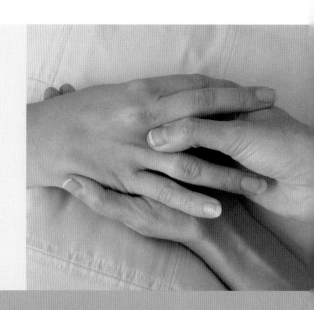

Reflexes for the right ear and Eustachian tube, and the right eye

Disorders eased by treating the reflexes for the right ear and Eustachian tube, and the right eye include:

- earache
- ear infections
- glue ear
- hearing problems
- balance problems
- vertigo or dizziness
- hay fever
- tinnitus
- watery eyes
- sore eyes
- itchy eyes
- blocked tear ducts
- conjunctivitis
- glaucoma

▼ **Step 11**

Support the receiver's right hand, palm uppermost, with your left thumb positioned across the fingers, gently holding them back. Now use your right thumb to caterpillar walk across the ridge at the base of the fingers, working from the little finger to the index finger.

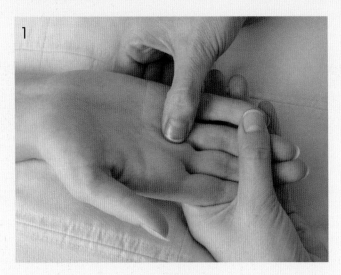

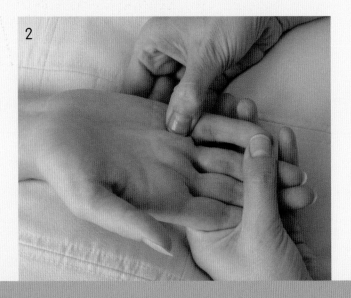

▼ To pinpoint the right ear reflex, slowly caterpillar walk across the area again and stop between the fourth and fifth fingers (the ring and little finger). Then either press and release the right ear reflex point or perform pressure circles over the area if it is sensitive.

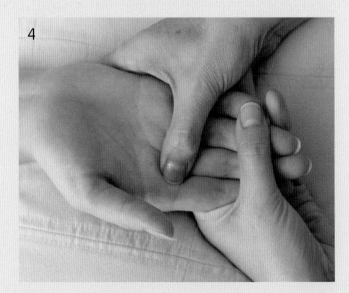

▲ To treat the Eustachian tube, take just a few more tiny steps and stop between fingers three and four (the middle and ring fingers). Now either perform pressure circles or press and release the Eustachian tube reflex point.

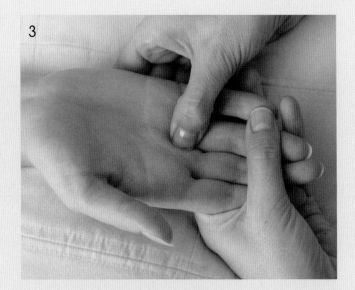

▲ Continue to caterpillar walk and stop between fingers two and three (the index and middle fingers) to treat the right eye reflex point. Again, either press and release it or perform pressure circles over it in order to treat the right eye.

The spinal and sciatic reflexes

Disorders eased by treating the spinal and sciatic reflexes include:

- backache
- muscle spasm
- arthritis of the spine
- stiffness and lack of mobility
- disc problems;
- sciatica

▼ **Step 12**

With the receiver's hand positioned with the palm uppermost, place your right hand, palm facing downwards, on his or her hand to steady and support it. Now place your left thumb on the edge of the receiver's thumb, just below the nail bed, and begin to caterpillar walk down the side of the thumb. In your initial steps, you are covering the neck area of the spine (the cervical vertebrae), before continuing down the middle of the back (the thoracic vertebrae) and into the lumbar area.

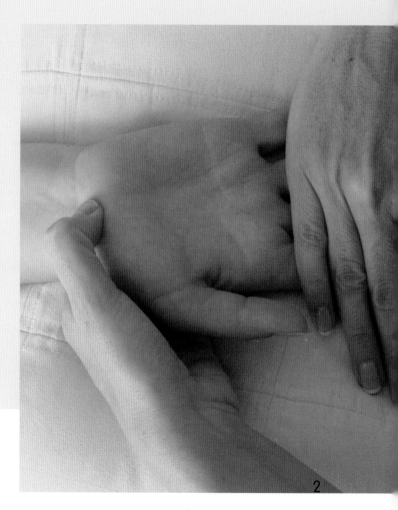

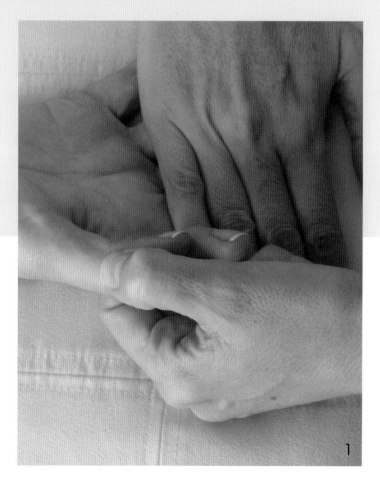

▲ Continue to caterpillar walk right across the wrist in order to treat the sciatic nerve.

You may also use your other thumb to repeat this thumb walking exercise in the opposite direction, working across the wrist and then upwards, towards the thumbnail.

The palm of the hand

The chest, shoulder and abdomen reflexes

Areas treated by working on the chest, shoulder and abdomen reflexes include:

- the right lung
- the right shoulder
- the liver
- the right adrenal gland
- the appendix

- the right breast
- the diaphragm
- the gallbladder
- the right kidney, ureter and bladder
- the ileocaecal valve

- the ribs and sternum
- the solar plexus
- the stomach, pancreas and duodenum
- the small intestine
- the large intestine (ascending and transverse colon)

The right lung, right breast, ribs and sternum reflexes

Disorders eased by treating the right lung, right breast, ribs and sternum reflexes include:

- lung problems
- asthma
- hyperventilation
- shallow breathing
- difficulty in expressing emotions
- a lack of self-esteem;
- overwhelming emotions (it helps to get them off the receiver's chest)
- tension and anxiety

- coughs and colds
- emphysema
- panic attacks
- the effects of smoking
- fear and anxiety
- harmless breast lumps

- chest infections
- bronchitis
- hysteria
- emotional dependence
- exhaustion from nurturing others
- mastitis
- breast problems; e.g., tenderness prior to menstruation
- palpitations and hyperventilation

Step 13

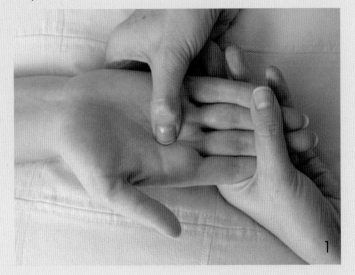

1

▲ Clasp the receiver's hand, palm uppermost, with your fingers positioned underneath and your thumb gently pressing back the fingers. Starting just below the ridge at the base of the fingers, use your right thumb to caterpillar walk in horizontal strips across the hand. Continue until you reach the diaphragm line.

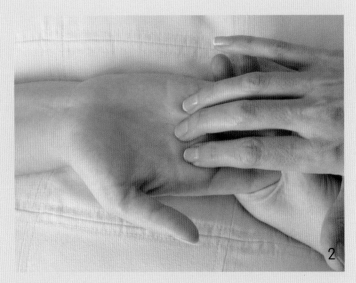

2

▲ You may also work on the same area in vertical, instead of horizontal, strips. Try finger walking with one or more fingers.

Step 14 ▶

Turn the receiver's hand over and rest it on your palm, gently pressing down the fingers with your left thumb. Now finger walk in vertical strips down the troughs on top of the hand, moving from the base of the fingers to the diaphragm line.

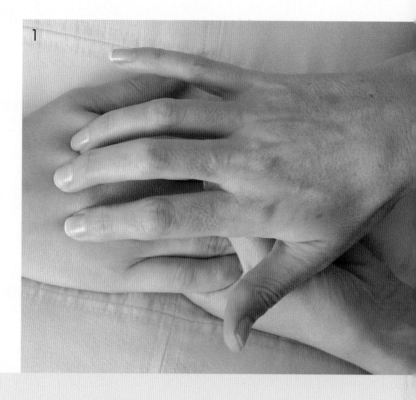

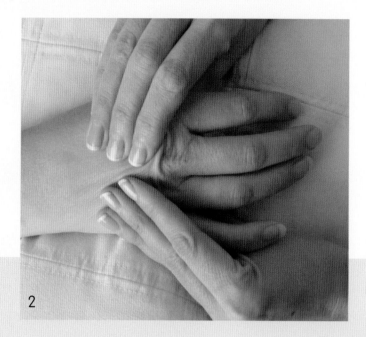

◀ You may prefer to walk across the hand in horizontal strips instead,

or, alternatively, to place the thumb of your working hand on the receiver's palm and your fingers on the top of the hand and then perform large, circular movements over the top of the hand. ▶

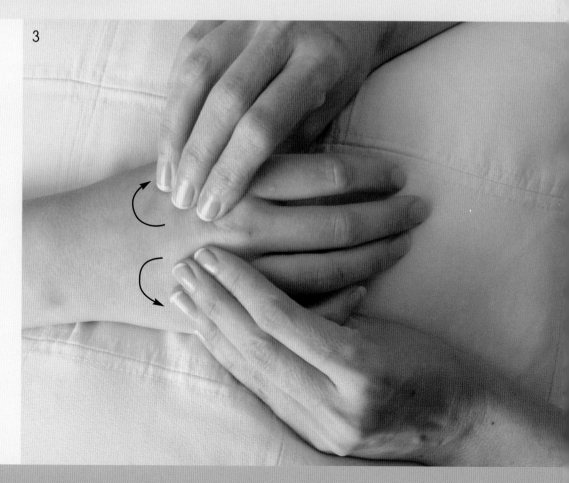

The right shoulder reflex

Disorders eased by treating the right shoulder reflex include:

- tension and pain in the shoulder
- a frozen shoulder
- arthritis
- a lack of mobility
- shouldering too much responsibility

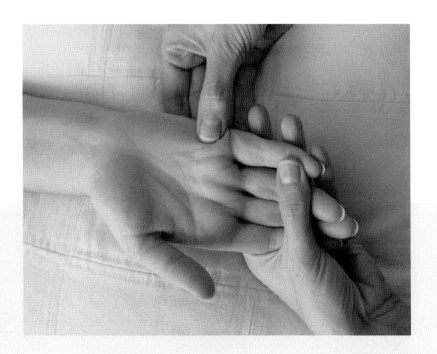

Step 15 ▶
Supporting the receiver's hand, place your right thumb just below the little finger and perform pressure circles there to treat the right shoulder. This area usually feels very 'gritty' and hard because most people suffer from tension in their shoulders.

The diaphragm and solar plexus reflex

Disorders eased by treating the diaphragm and solar plexus reflex include:

- respiratory problems
- panic attacks
- stress and tension
- hysteria
- fear
- hyperventilation
- shallow breathing

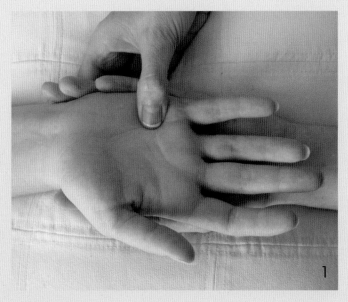

1

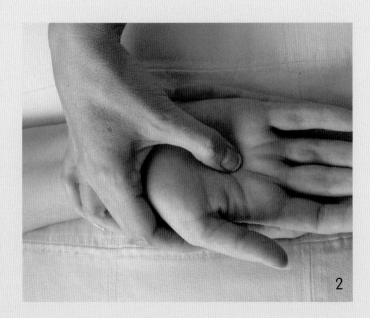

2

▲ **Step 16**
Rest the receiver's right hand, palm uppermost, in the palm of your left hand. Caterpillar walk across the diaphragm line with your right thumb, and as you reach the centre, perform gentle pressure circles over the solar plexus reflex.

The liver and gallbladder reflexes (the right hand only)

Disorders eased by treating the liver and gallbladder reflexes include:

- liver problems
- gallbladder problems
- digestive disturbances
- toxicity
- overindulgence in drink or food
- difficulties in breaking down fats

Step 17 ▶

Support the receiver's hand, palm uppermost, with your left thumb positioned over the top of the receiver's fingers to open up the liver reflex area. Use your right thumb to work from zone 5, which is the little-finger side of the hand, to zone 3.

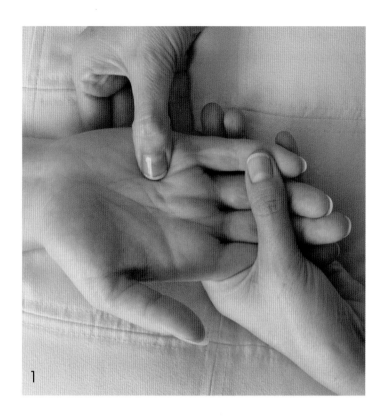

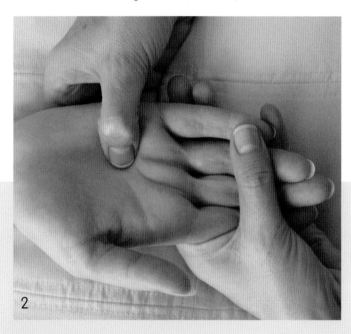

◀ Pinpoint the gallbladder reflex, which is located roughly in line with the third and fourth fingers. This is often a tender area that may feel like a small indentation or a slight swelling. Use pressure circles to treat this area or else the rotation on a point technique by placing the pad of your right thumb on the gallbladder reflex and rotating the receiver's hand in a circular motion around your thumb.

The stomach, pancreas and duodenum reflexes

Disorders eased by treating the stomach, pancreas and duodenum reflexes include:

- general digestive problems
- ulcers
- indigestion and heartburn
- diabetes
- stomach cramps
- low blood sugar

Step 18 ▶

Using your right hand to provide support, caterpillar walk with your left thumb in horizontal rows, moving from the diaphragm line to the waist line and covering zones 1 and 2. (If you wish, you may walk in the opposite direction.)

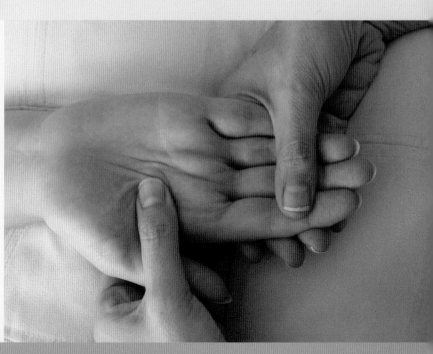

The right adrenal gland reflex

Disorders eased by treating the right adrenal gland reflex include:

- nervous conditions
- inflammatory disorders, such as irritable bowel syndrome and rheumatoid arthritis
- allergies
- pain
- a lack of energy

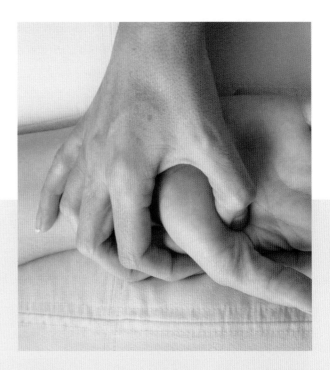

Step 19 ▶

The adrenal glands are easily pinpointed because they are usually tender (this is because most of us have stress in our lives!). Cup the receiver's hand, palm uppermost, in your left hand and either use your right thumb to perform pressure circles on the right adrenal gland reflex (which is found beneath the index finger, just below the webbing of the thumb and index finger) or else press and release it. If it is not tender, try the hook in and back up technique.

The right kidney, ureter and bladder reflexes

Disorders eased by treating the right kidney, ureter and bladder reflexes include:

- kidney problems
- bladder infections
- cystitis
- fluid retention
- incontinence

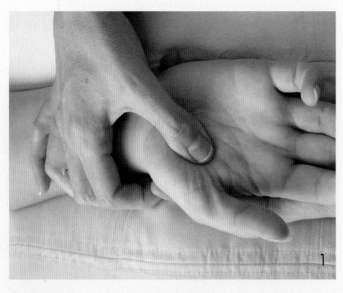

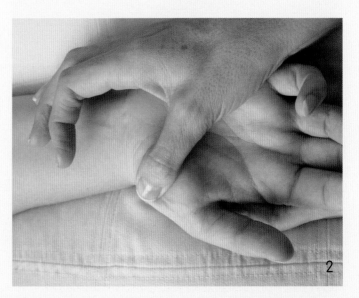

▲ Step 20
Place the pad of your thumb on the right kidney reflex, which is located on the waist line between zones 2 and 3, and perform gentle pressure circles.

▲ Then caterpillar walk towards zone 1, on the inside of the hand, just above the wrist, and use pressure circles to massage the bladder reflex.

The small intestine reflex

Disorders eased by treating the small intestine reflex include:

- all digestive disorders
- abdominal cramps
- bloating
- allergies

Step 21 ▼

The reflex area for the small intestine is found covering zones 1 and 4, between the waist line and the pelvic girdle line. Support the receiver's hand, palm uppermost, with your right hand. Place your left thumb slightly below the waist line, on the thumb side of the receiver's hand, and caterpillar walk in horizontal rows until you are slightly above the pelvic girdle line. Note that you will need to caterpillar walk for several rows, and that you may wish to change hands and caterpillar walk in the opposite direction.

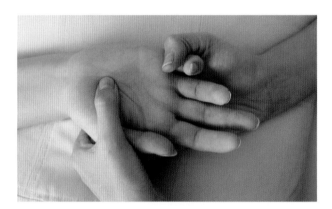

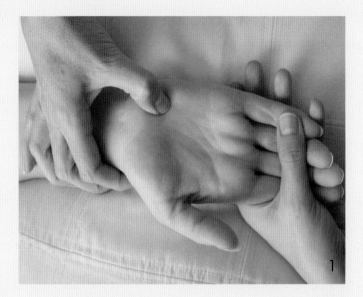

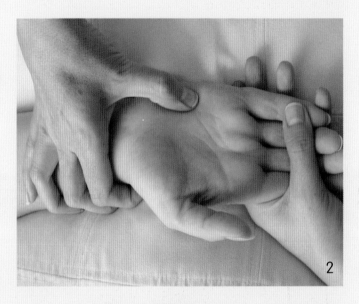

The appendix, ileocaecal valve and large intestine (ascending and transverse colon) reflexes

Disorders eased by treating the appendix, ileocaecal valve and large intestine (ascending and transverse colon) reflexes include:

- all digestive problems
- irritable bowel syndrome
- constipation
- diarrhoea

Step 22 ▶

The ileocaecal valve and appendix reflexes are located in the right hand only. Place the pad of your right thumb between zones 4 and 5 (between the little finger and ring finger), slightly above the wrist. Perform pressure circles on the appendix reflex, where you may feel a small hollow. Move your thumb up very slightly to circle over the ileocaecal valve reflex. Then caterpillar walk upwards, towards the waist line (the ascending colon reflex), before turning 90° and walking across the hand, just below the waist line, until you reach the inside of the hand. (Note that you may need to practise this step several times.)

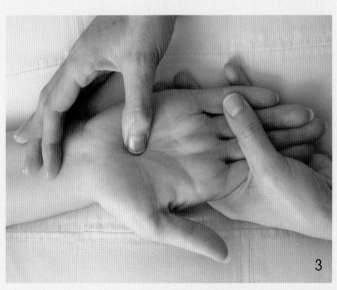

The reflexes of the joints

Areas treated by working on the reflexes of the joints include:

- the right shoulder
- the right elbow
- the right knee
- the right hip

Disorders eased by treating the reflexes of the joints include:

- all joint problems
- tennis elbow
- arthritis
- housemaid's knee
- sports injuries
- sprains and strains
- hip disorders
- cartilage and ligament problems
- a frozen shoulder

Step 23 ▼

The reflexes for the joints are located along the outer edge of the hand. Hold the receiver's hand, palm uppermost, with your left hand, gently holding the fingers back. Place your right thumb at the base of the little finger (the shoulder joint reflex) and ensure that you cover all of the joints thoroughly by caterpillar walking down the outer edge of the hand until you reach the wrist.

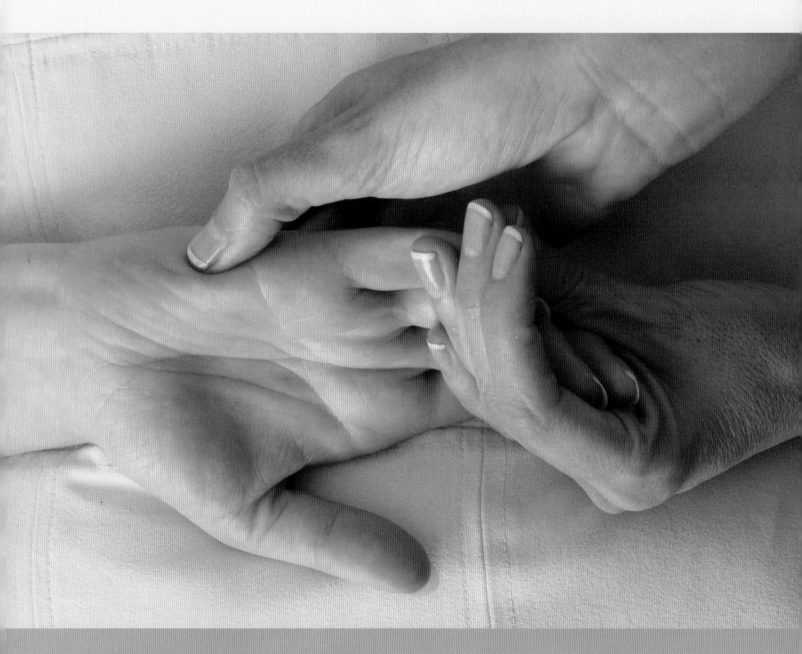

The reflexes of the reproductive organs and lymph nodes of the groin

Areas treated by working on the reflexes of the reproductive organs and lymph nodes of the groin include:

- the right ovary or right testicle
- the uterus or prostate gland;
- the right fallopian tube or the vas deferens
- the lymph nodes of the groin

Disorders eased by working on the reflexes of the reproductive organs and lymph nodes of the groin include:

- all menstrual problems
- the menopause
- prostate problems
- premenstrual tension (PMT)
- infertility problems
- an accumulation of toxins

Caution

If the receiver is pregnant, then leave out these areas if there is a history of miscarriage. (A fully qualified reflexologist may treat these reflexes, however.) If a female receiver has an intrauterine device (IUD) fitted, then gently stroke the uterus reflex area rather than pressing on it.

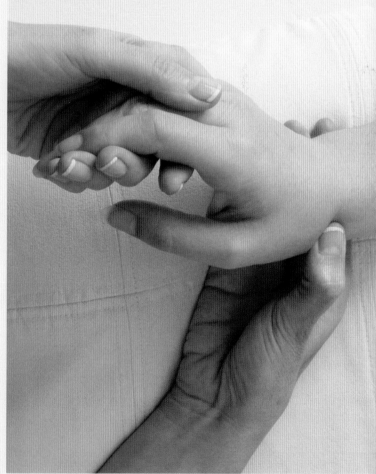

2

▼ Step 24
The reflexes for the reproductive organs are all to be found around the wrist. Grasp the receiver's fingers with your right hand and place the pad of your left thumb on the right ovary (if the receiver is female) or right testicle (if he is male) reflex on the outer edge of the wrist. Either use the rotation on a point technique to treat the ovary or testicle or, alternatively, use the press and release technique or perform gentle pressure circles.

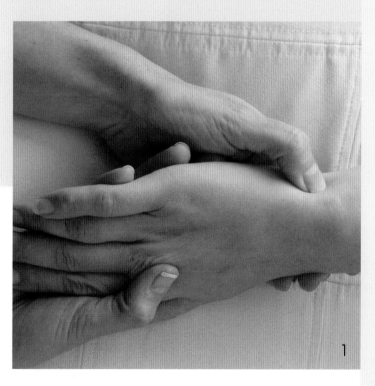

1

▲ Step 25
Grasp the receiver's fingers with your left hand and place your right thumb on the prostate (if the receiver is male) or uterus (if she is female) reflex. Treat this reflex using either the rotation on a point technique or the press and release technique or by performing pressure circles on it.

Step 26 ▶

The area that circles the wrist relates to the right fallopian tube (if the receiver is female) or the vas deferens (if he is male) and the lymph nodes of the groin. Rest the receiver's hand, palm facing downwards, on the palm of your hand. Now thumb or finger walk right across the wrist on the back of the hand.

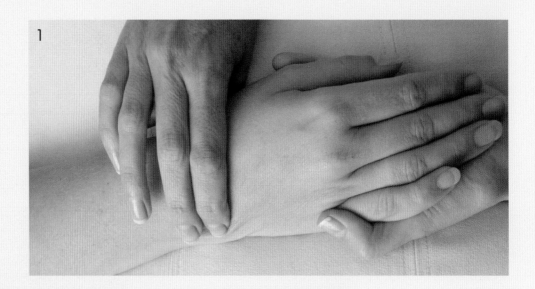

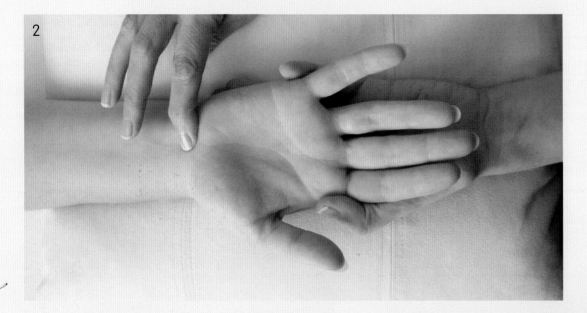

◀ Then turn the hand over and continue thumb or finger walking across the wrist. Note that if this area feels congested, it usually indicates a sluggish lymphatic system due to poor diet, a lack of exercise and stress.

To finish ▶

To finish, gently stroke the receiver's hand to ensure that any toxins that have been released are dispersed. Place the receiver's hand between both of your hands, rest it there for a few moments and then cover it up.

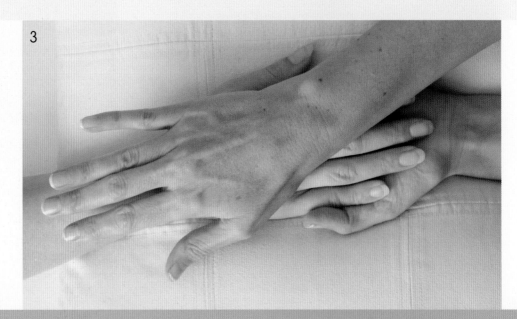

Relaxation sequence – left hand

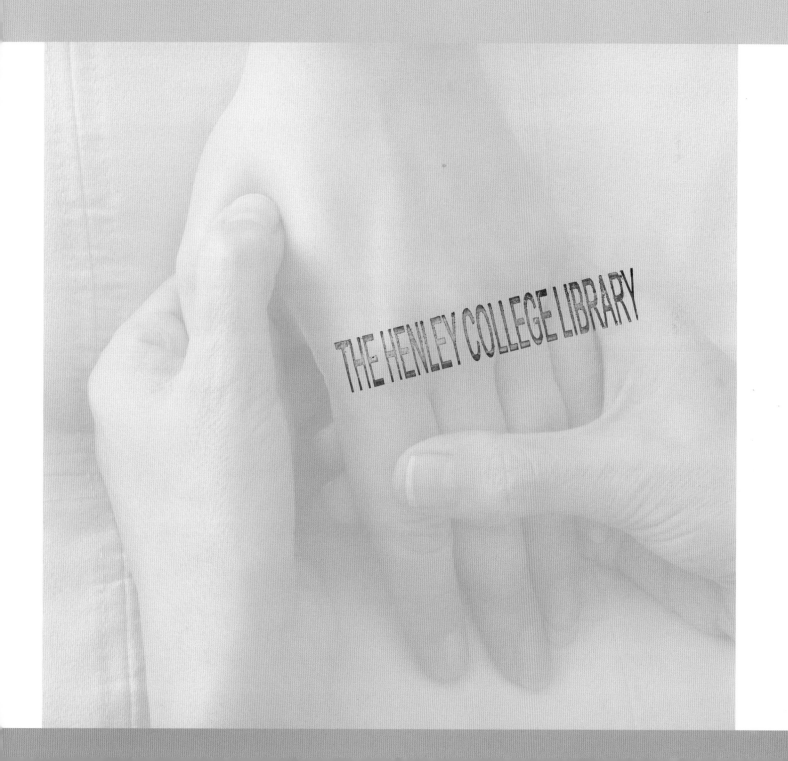

Uncover the receiver's left hand and then perform some of your favourite relaxation techniques on it.

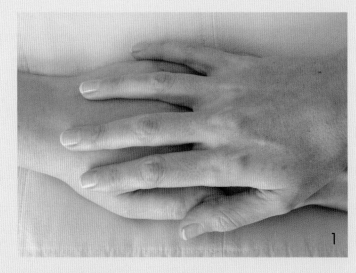

▲ Greeting the hand

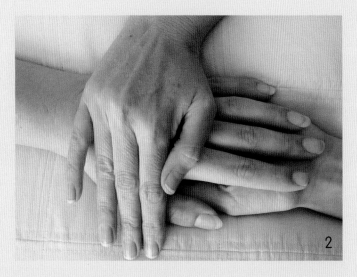

▲ Stroking the hand

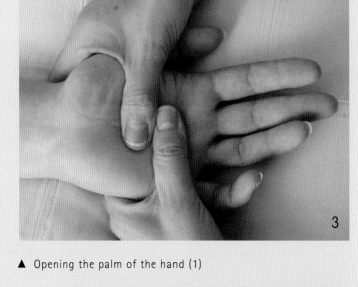

▲ Opening the palm of the hand (1)

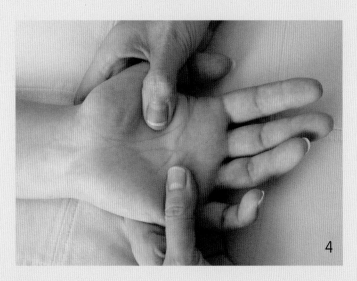

▲ Opening the palm of the hand (2)

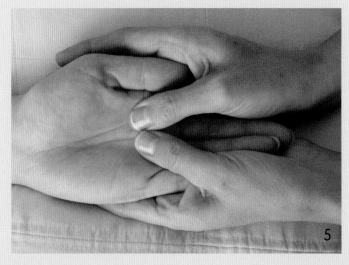

▲ Stretching the palm

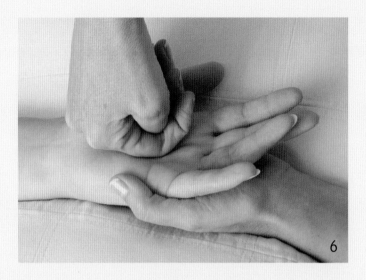

▲ Knuckling the palm (metacarpal kneading)

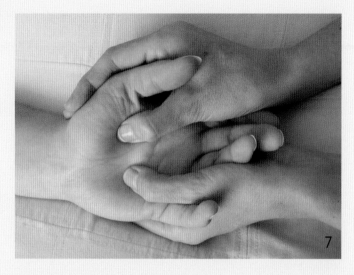

▲ Thumb circling on the palm

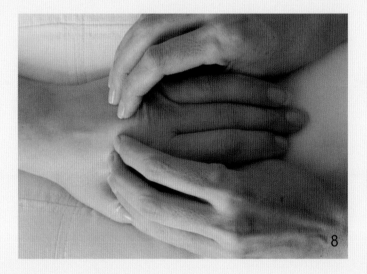

▲ Finger circling on the top of the hand

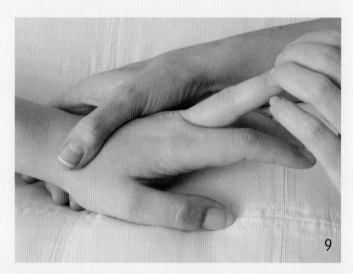

▲ Loosening the joints

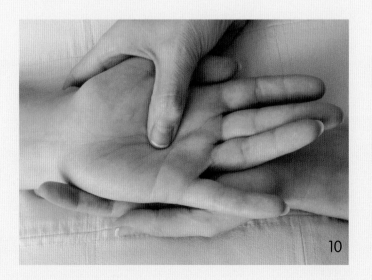

▲ Solar plexus release

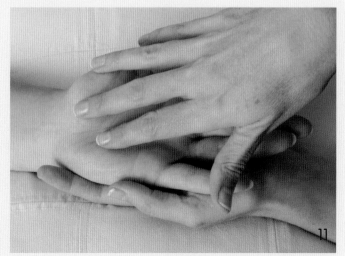

▲ Featherlight stroking of the hand

The reflexes of the left hand

The head and neck reflexes

Areas treated when working on the head and neck reflexes include:

- the head and brain
- the pituitary gland, pineal gland and hypothalamus
- the face
- the neck
- the thyroid gland and throat
- the vocal cords
- the sinuses
- the teeth and gums
- the upper lymphatics
- the left ear and Eustachian tube
- the left eye

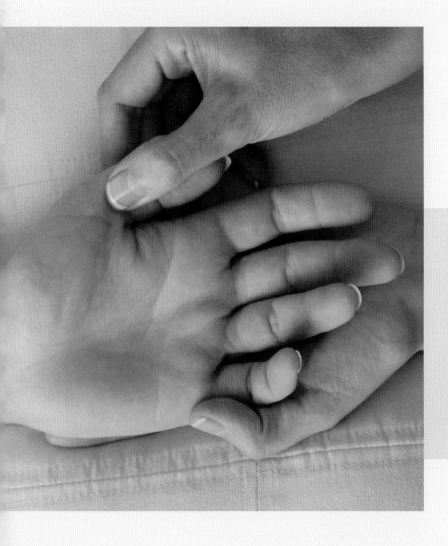

The thumb

The head and brain reflex

Disorders eased by treating the head and brain reflex include:

- headaches and migraines
- lack of concentration
- the inability to think clearly
- mental congestion
- memory defects
- Alzheimer's disease
- amnesia
- neuralgia
- loss of balance
- fainting
- Bell's palsy (facial paralysis)
- Parkinson's disease
- multiple sclerosis
- stroke and paralysis
- epilepsy
- poor co-ordination
- the aftereffects of anaesthetics
- baldness
- scalp problems
- learning difficulties, e.g., dyslexia
- Attention Deficit Disorder (ADD)
- lack of confidence and low self-esteem
- depression
- a lack of intuition and a closed mind

◄ **Step 1**

Rest the receiver's left hand, palm uppermost, on a cushion and place your right hand on top of the receiver's palm. Remember not to grip the receiver's hand too tightly and to take tiny, little steps. Place the pad of your right thumb on the tip of the receiver's left thumb and caterpillar walk down it to the base several times. Make sure that you cover the outside, back and inside of the thumb. Note that you will need to caterpillar walk for several rows to cover the area completely.

The pituitary gland reflex

Disorders eased by treating the pituitary gland reflex include:

- hormonal imbalances
- premenstrual syndrome (PMS)
- scanty, heavy or painful menstruation
- difficulties conceiving;
- the menopause

▶ **Step 2**

Be prepared to have to search to pinpoint the pituitary gland reflex. It is often positioned off-centre on the thumb pad, be it slightly higher, lower, to the right or to the left. If you are very lucky, a small lump may be visible or palpable, indicating the exact location.

Supporting the receiver's hand in your left hand, use your right thumb to press in firmly (hook in) and then pull back, across the pituitary gland reflex (back up). Note that this is often a sensitive point.

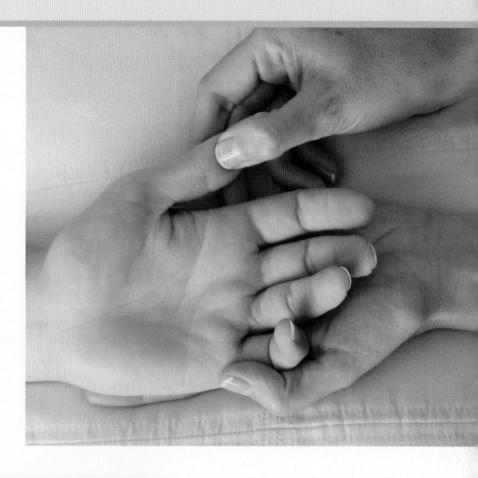

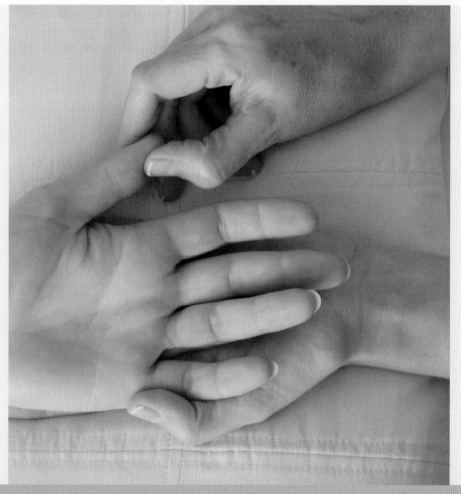

The pineal gland and hypothalamus reflexes

Disorders eased by treating the pineal gland and hypothalamus reflexes include:

- seasonal affective disorder (SAD)
- sleep problems
- mood swings
- hormonal imbalances
- a lack of insight, intuition or vision

◀ **Step 3**

The pineal gland and hypothalamus reflexes are situated very close to the pituitary gland reflex. Move your thumb up very slightly, towards the tip of the receiver's thumb, and then rock your thumb onto its outer edge to circle over the pineal gland reflex. Then rock your thumb onto its inner edge and treat the hypothalamus reflex with pressure circles.

The face reflex

Disorders eased by treating the face reflex include:

- eye problems, e.g., conjunctivitis
- Bell's palsy (facial paralysis)
- sinusitis
- nasal problems
- facial neuralgia
- facial acne
- jaw problems
- teeth and gum problems

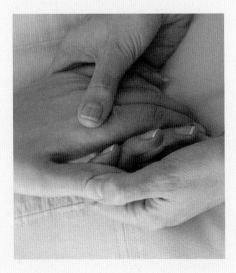

▲ **Step 4**
Gently turn over the receiver's hand and support it with your right hand. Using your left thumb, caterpillar walk down the front of the thumb, moving from the tip to the base.

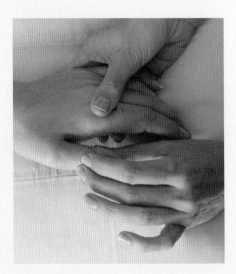

▲ You may need to caterpillar walk down the thumb three or four times, depending on its size. (Depending on the size of the receiver's thumb and your fingers, you may find it easier to use your index finger instead.)

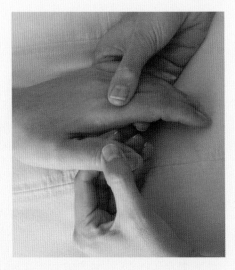

▲ You may prefer to caterpillar walk across the face reflex. With your thumb positioned on the back of the receiver's thumb for support, use two fingers to walk across the front of the thumb.

The neck reflex

Disorders eased by treating the neck reflex include:

- aches and pains in the neck
- a lack of mobility in the neck
- whiplash injuries
- arthritis in the neck
- throat problems, such as tonsillitis and problems with the adenoids, pharynx and larynx, when working across the front of the neck reflex

Step 5 ▶
Support the receiver's hand with your right hand. Gently hold the receiver's thumb between your index finger and thumb and then rotate it both clockwise and anti-clockwise. This movement is excellent for alleviating a stiff neck. If a thumb joint grates, or does not move very well, gently encourage it, but never force it.

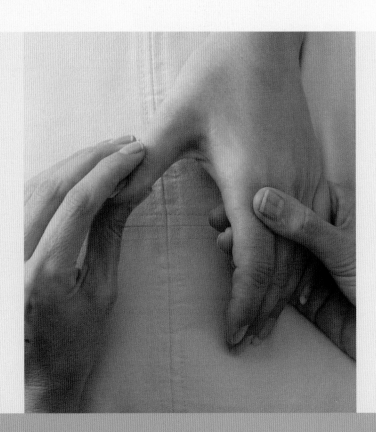

The neck, thyroid gland and throat reflex

Disorders eased by treating the neck, thyroid gland and throat reflex include:

- all neck and throat problems as outlined for step 5
- parathyroid disorders
- osteoporosis
- thyroid problems
- muscle-twitching
- weight problems
- arthritis

Step 6 ▼ ▶

Supporting the receiver's hand, palm uppermost, caterpillar walk your right thumb across the back of the base of the thumb several times.

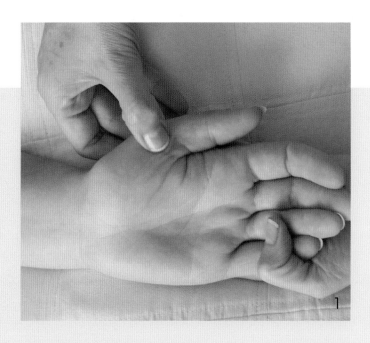

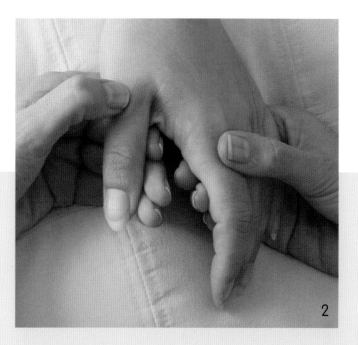

Turn the receiver's hand over and support it with your right hand. Now use your left thumb to caterpillar walk across the front of the base of the thumb.

The vocal cords reflex

Disorders eased by treating the vocal cords reflex include:

- vocal cord problems
- speech problems
- a 'lump' in the throat
- difficulty expressing oneself
- an inability to say what one thinks
- an over-use of the voice
- laryngitis
- pharyngitis
- tracheitis

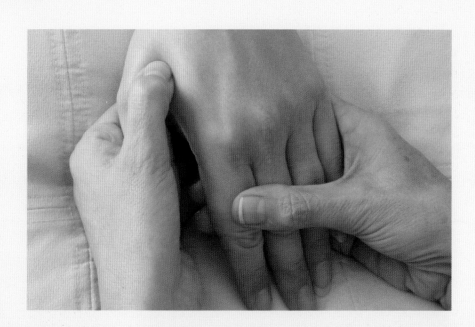

Step 7 ▶

To locate the reflex for the vocal cords, place the thumb of your working hand at the bottom of the webbing between the receiver's thumb and index finger. Now gently circle over this reflex.

The fingers

The sinus reflexes

Disorders eased by treating the sinus reflexes include:

- sinus problems
- allergies
- catarrh
- hay fever
- rhinitis
- colds
- a loss of the sense of smell
- nasal polyps

▼ **Step 8**

Support the receiver's hand, palm uppermost, in the palm of your right hand. Use your left thumb to caterpillar walk from the tip of the little finger to its base. You will need to caterpillar walk for about three rows to cover the area thoroughly. Repeat on the ring, middle and index fingers.

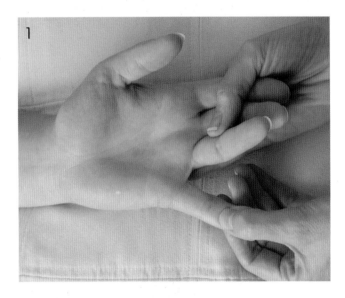

▼ To treat the sides of the fingers, you may use your thumb and index finger to caterpillar walk down both sides of each finger at the same time.

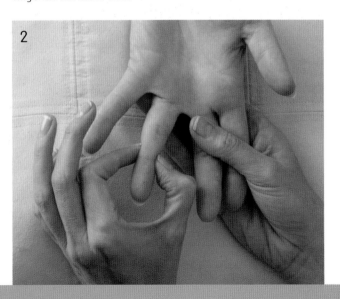

The teeth and gum reflexes

Disorders eased by treating the teeth and gum reflexes include:

- toothache
- painful or sensitive teeth
- gum problems
- abscesses
- pain after dental procedures
- teething

▼ **Step 9**

The reflexes for the teeth and gums are found on the top of all of the fingers. Turn the receiver's hand over and support the fingers with your left hand. Commencing at the top of the index finger, perform about three or four rows of thumb walking to cover the dorsal (top) side of the finger. Repeat on the middle, ring and little fingers.

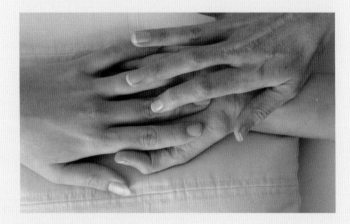

The upper lymphatic reflexes

Disorders eased by treating the upper lymphatic reflexes include:

- a poor immune function
- ear, nose and throat problems
- myalgic encephalomyelitis (ME)
- a toxic lymphatic system (which is often due to poor diet and a lack of exercise)
- acne (this technique will help drain the head and neck area)

Step 10

Supporting the receiver's hand with your right hand, gently squeeze the webbing between each of the fingers with your left thumb and index finger. Repeat several times.

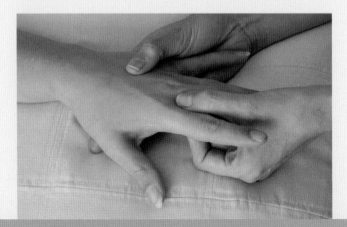

Reflexes for the left ear and Eustachian tube, and the left eye

Disorders eased by treating the reflexes for the left ear and Eustachian tube, and the left eye include:

- earache
- tinnitus
- ear infections
- watery eyes
- glue ear
- sore eyes
- glaucoma
- itchy eyes
- conjunctivitis
- hay fever
- balance problems
- blocked tear duct
- vertigo or dizziness
- hearing problems

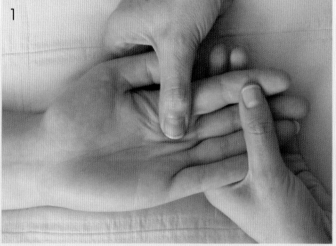

▲ **Step 11**
Support the receiver's left hand, palm uppermost, with your right thumb positioned across the fingers, gently holding them back. Now use your left thumb to caterpillar walk across the ridge at the base of the fingers, working from the little finger to the index finger.

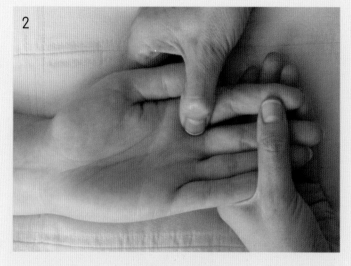

▲ To pinpoint the left ear reflex, slowly caterpillar walk across the area again and stop between the index and middle fingers. Then either press and release the reflex point or perform pressure circles over the area if it is sensitive.

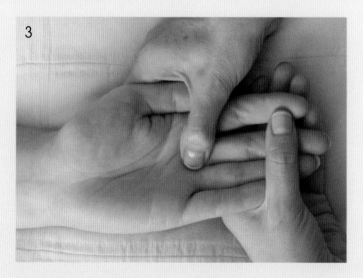

▲ To treat the Eustachian tube, take just a few more tiny steps and stop between fingers three and four (the middle and ring fingers). Now either perform pressure circles or press and release the Eustachian tube reflex point.

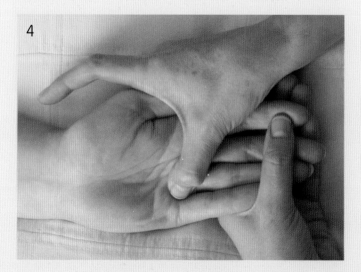

▲ Continue to caterpillar walk and stop between fingers four and five (the ring and little fingers) to treat the left eye reflex point. Again, either press and release it or perform pressure circles over it in order to treat the left eye.

The spinal and sciatic reflexes

Disorders eased by treating the spinal and sciatic reflexes include:

- backache
- disc problems
- muscle spasm
- sciatica
- arthritis of the spine
- stiffness and lack of mobility

Step 12 ▼

Support the receiver's hand, palm uppermost, with your left hand. Place your right thumb on the edge of the receiver's thumb, just below the nail bed, and caterpillar walk down the side of the thumb.

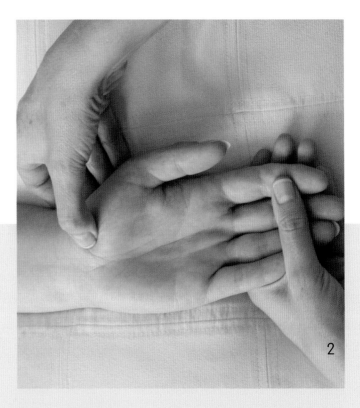

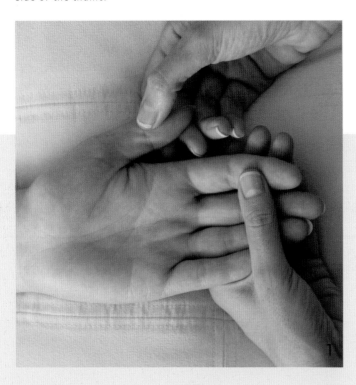

▲ Continue to caterpillar walk right across the wrist in order to treat the sciatic nerve.

The palm of the hand

The chest, shoulder and abdomen reflexes

Areas treated by working on the chest, shoulder and abdomen reflexes include:

- the left lung
- the heart
- the pancreas
- the small intestine
- the left kidney, ureter and bladder
- the large intestine (transverse and descending colon)
- the left breast
- the diaphragm
- the duodenum
- the rectum and anus
- the ribs and sternum
- the solar plexus
- the spleen
- the left shoulder
- the stomach
- the left adrenal gland

The left lung, left breast, ribs and sternum reflexes

Disorders eased by treating the left lung, left breast, ribs and sternum reflexes include:

- lung problems
- coughs and colds
- chest infections
- asthma
- emphysema
- hyperventilation
- panic attacks
- hysteria
- shallow breathing
- bronchitis
- the effects of smoking
- emotional dependence
- fear and anxiety
- difficulty in expressing emotions
- a lack of self-esteem
- exhaustion from nurturing others
- harmless breast lumps
- mastitis
- tension and anxiety
- palpitations and hyperventilation
- breast problems; e.g., tenderness prior to menstruation
- overwhelming emotions (it helps to get them off the receiver's chest)

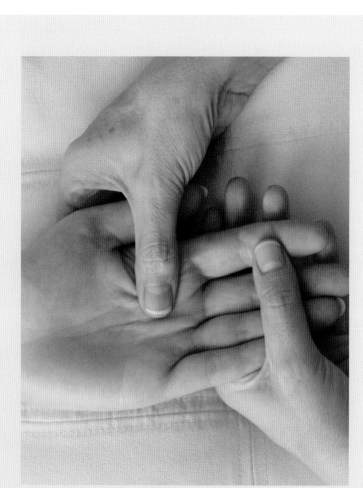

You may also work on the same area in vertical, instead ▶
of horizontal, strips. Try finger walking with one or more fingers.

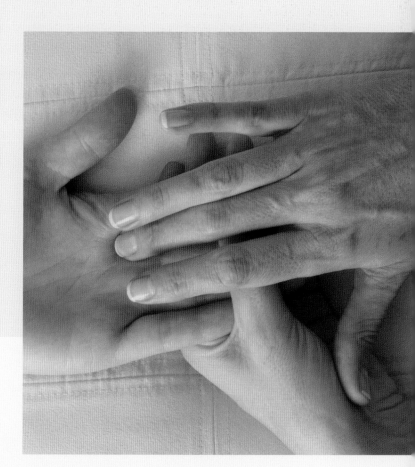

◀ **Step 13**

Clasp the receiver's hand, palm uppermost, with your fingers positioned underneath and your thumb gently pressing back his or her fingers. Starting just below the ridge at the base of the fingers, use your left thumb to caterpillar walk in horizontal strips across the hand. Continue until you reach the diaphragm line.

Step 14 ▶

Turn the receiver's hand over and rest it on your palm. Now finger walk in vertical strips down the troughs on top of the hand, moving from the base of the fingers to the diaphragm line.

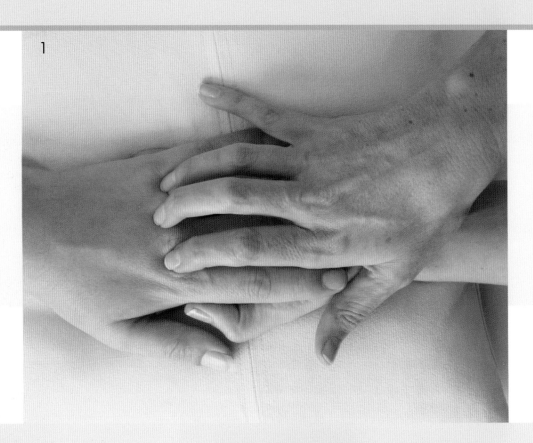

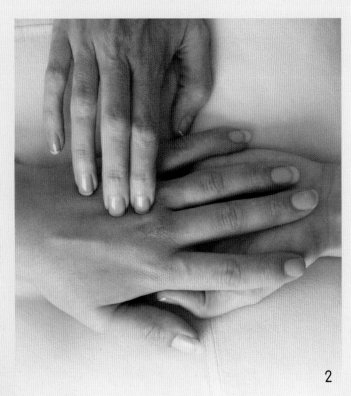

▲ You may prefer to walk across the hand in horizontal strips instead.

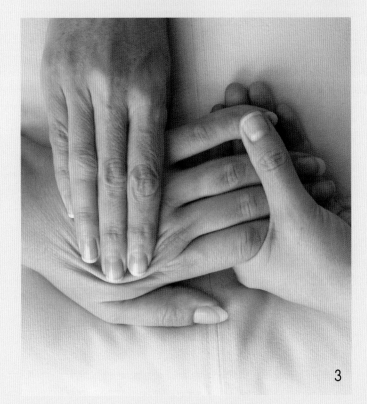

▲ Alternatively, place the thumb of your working hand on the receiver's palm and your fingers on the top of the hand and perform large, circular movements over the top of the hand.

The left shoulder reflex

Disorders eased by treating the left shoulder reflex include:

* tension and pain in the shoulder
* a frozen shoulder • arthritis • a lack of mobility
* shouldering too much responsibility

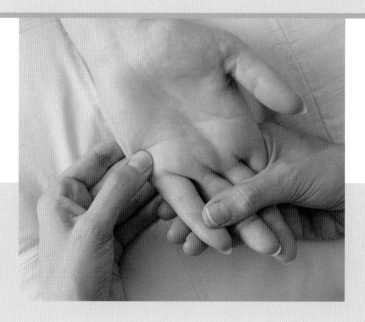

Step 15 ▶
Supporting the receiver's hand, place your left thumb just below the little finger and perform pressure circles there to treat the left shoulder. This area usually feels very 'gritty' and hard because most people suffer from tension in their shoulders.

The heart reflex (the left hand only)

Disorders eased by treating the heart reflex include:

* palpitations • heart problems
* blood pressure problems

> **Caution**
>
> Leave out the heart reflex if the receiver has severe heart problems or a pacemaker.

▲ Step 16
To treat the heart reflex, support the receiver's hand, palm uppermost, with your left hand and use your right thumb to massage the upper third of the receiver's palm, using a circular action.

Now turn the receiver's hand over and use your right index finger or index and middle finger to massage the upper third of the top of the receiver's hand, using a circular motion. ▶

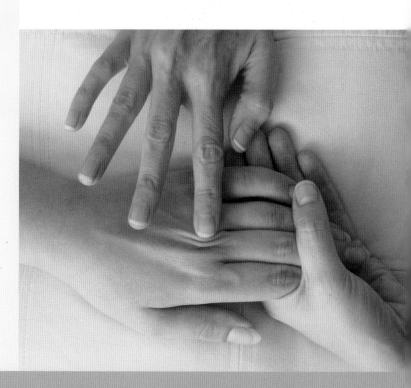

The diaphragm and solar plexus reflex

Disorders eased by treating the diaphragm and solar plexus reflex include:

- respiratory problems
- stress and tension
- fear
- shallow breathing
- panic attacks
- hysteria
- hyperventilation

The stomach, pancreas and duodenum reflexes

Disorders eased by treating the stomach, pancreas and duodenum reflexes include:

- general digestive problems
- stomach cramps
- diabetes
- indigestion and heartburn
- stomach ulcers
- low blood sugar

▼ Step 18

Using your left hand to support the receiver's hand, thumb walk in horizontal rows from the diaphragm line to the waist line, covering zones 1 and 2. (If you wish, you may thumb walk in the opposite direction.)

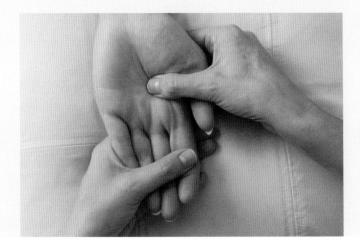

▼ Step 17

Rest the receiver's left hand, palm uppermost, in the palm of your right hand. Caterpillar walk across the diaphragm line with your left thumb.

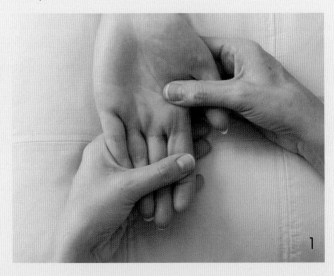

1

▼ As you reach the centre, perform gentle pressure circles over the solar plexus reflex.

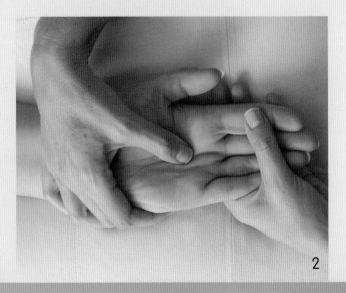

2

The spleen reflex (the left hand only)

Disorders eased by treating the spleen reflex include:

- a poorly functioning immune system

▼ Step 19

Support the receiver's left hand with your right, fingers underneath and thumb on top. Use the pad of your left thumb to caterpillar walk from zone five to four working in horizontal rows from the diaphragm line to the waist line.

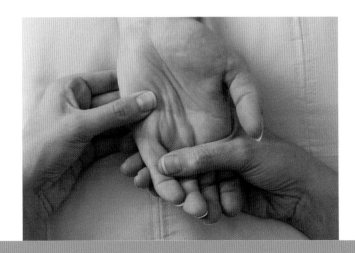

The left adrenal gland reflex

Disorders eased by treating the left adrenal gland reflex include:

- nervous conditions • allergies • pain • a lack of energy
- inflammatory disorders, such as irritable bowel syndrome and rheumatoid arthritis

Step 20 ▶

The adrenal glands are easily pinpointed because they are usually tender (this is because most of us have stress in our lives!). Cup the receiver's hand, palm uppermost, in your left hand and either use your right thumb to perform pressure circles on the left adrenal gland reflex (which is found beneath the index finger, just below the webbing of the thumb and index finger) or else press and release it. If it is not tender, try the hook in and back up technique.

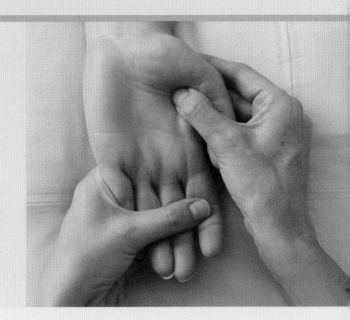

The left kidney, ureter and bladder reflexes

Disorders eased by treating the left kidney, ureter and bladder reflexes include:

- kidney problems • bladder infections • cystitis • fluid retention • incontinence

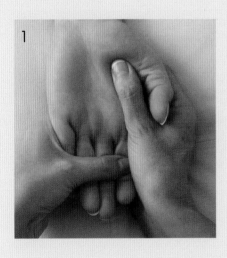
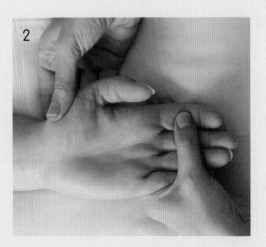

◀ Step 21

Place the pad of your thumb on the left kidney reflex, which is located on the waist line between zones 2 and 3, and perform gentle pressure circles (1).

Then caterpillar walk towards zone 1, on the inside of the hand, just above the wrist, and use pressure circles to massage the bladder reflex (2).

The small intestine reflex

Disorders eased by treating the small intestine reflex include:

- all digestive disorders • abdominal cramps • bloating • allergies

▶ Step 22

The reflex area for the small intestine is found covering zones 1 and 4, between the waist line and the pelvic girdle line. Support the receiver's hand, palm uppermost, with your left hand. Place your right thumb slightly below the waist line, on the thumb side of the receiver's hand, and caterpillar walk in horizontal rows until you are slightly above the pelvic girdle line. Note that you will need to caterpillar walk for several rows, and that you may wish to change hands and caterpillar walk in the opposite direction.

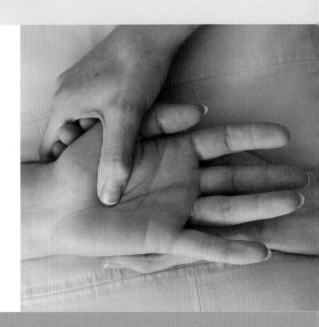

The large intestine (transverse and descending colon), rectum and anus reflexes

Disorders eased by treating the large intestine (transverse and descending colon), rectum and anus reflexes include:

- all digestive problems
- irritable bowel syndrome
- constipation
- diarrhoea
- flatulence
- diverticulitis
- Crohn's disease
- abdominal bloating
- allergies
- haemorrhoids

Step 23 ▶
Support the receiver's hand, with the palm facing upwards, with your left hand. Place your right thumb just below the waist line in zone 1 and then thumb walk across the palm (transverse colon) to between zone 4 and zone 5, where the splenic flexure is located. Perform several pressure circles on this reflex.

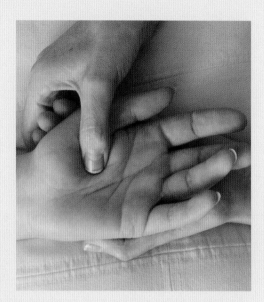

Step 24 ▶
Change hands and then thumb walk down the receiver's hand with your left thumb (over the descending colon reflex) (1).

Just before you reach the wrist, turn your left thumb 90° and thumb walk across the palm of the hand (over the sigmoid colon reflex) to the rectum and anus reflex point, which is just underneath the bladder (2).

Perform several pressure circles over this reflex (3).

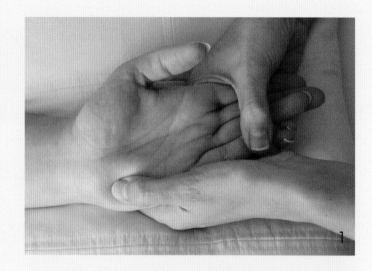

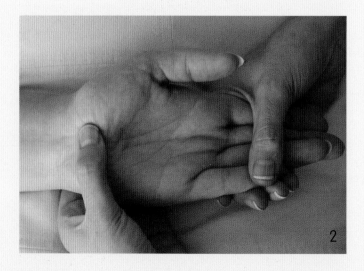

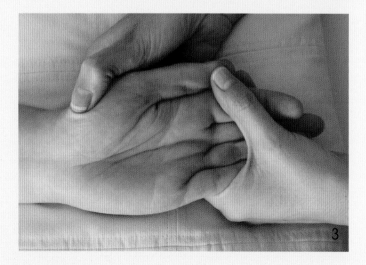

The reflexes of the joints

Areas treated by working on the reflexes of the joints include:

- the left shoulder
- the left elbow
- the left knee
- the left hip

Disorders eased by treating the reflexes of the joints include:

- all joint problems
- arthritis
- sports injuries
- hip disorders
- a frozen shoulder
- tennis elbow
- housemaid's knee
- sprains and strains
- cartilage and ligament problems

Step 25 ▶
The reflexes for the joints are located along the outer edge of the hand. Hold the receiver's hand, palm uppermost, with your right hand, with your thumb positioned on top and gently holding the fingers back. Place your left thumb at the base of the little finger (the shoulder joint reflex)

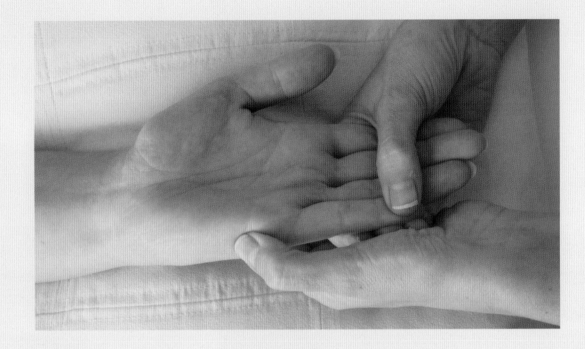

and ensure that you cover all of the joints thoroughly by caterpillar walking down the outer edge of the hand until you reach the wrist. ▶

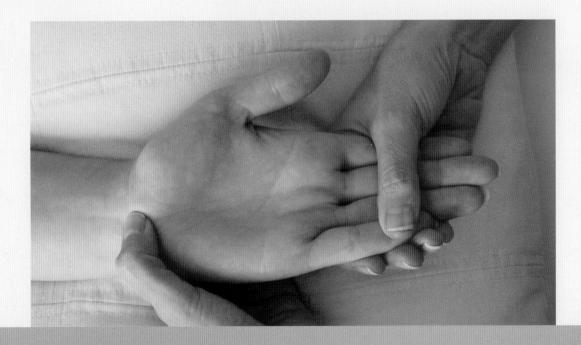

The reflexes of the reproductive organs and lymph nodes of the groin

Areas treated by working on the reflexes of the reproductive organs and lymph nodes of the groin include:

- the left ovary or left testicle
- the uterus or prostate gland
- the left fallopian tube or the vas deferens
- the lymph nodes of the groin

Disorders eased by working on the reflexes of the reproductive organs and lymph nodes of the groin include:

- all menstrual problems
- premenstrual tension (PMT)
- the menopause
- infertility problems
- prostate problems
- an accumulation of toxins

Caution

If the receiver is pregnant, then leave out these areas if there is a history of miscarriage. (A fully qualified reflexologist may treat these reflexes, however.) If a female receiver has an intrauterine device (IUD) fitted, then gently stroke the uterus reflex area rather than pressing on it.

▼ Step 26

The reflexes for the reproductive organs are all to be found around the wrist. Grasp the receiver's fingers with your right hand and place the pad of your left thumb on the left ovary (if the receiver is female) or left testicle (if he is male) reflex on the outer edge (the little finger side) of the wrist. Either use the rotation on a point technique to treat the ovary or testicle or, alternatively, use the press and release technique or perform gentle pressure circles.

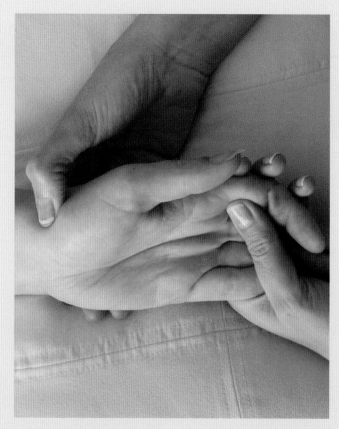

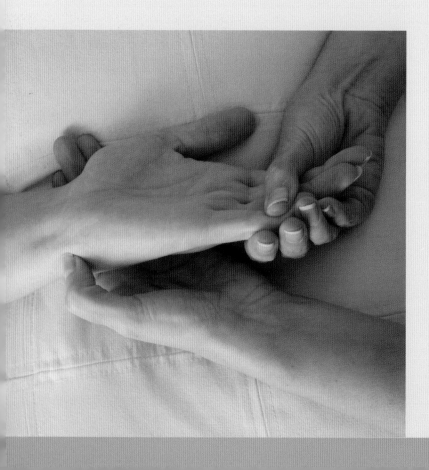

▲ Step 27

Grasp the receiver's fingers with your left hand and place your right thumb on the prostate (if the receiver is male) or uterus (if she is female) reflex. Treat this reflex using either the rotation on a point technique or the press and release technique or by performing pressure circles on it.

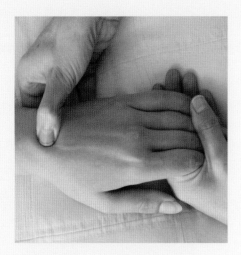

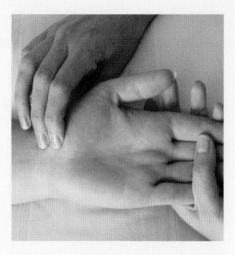

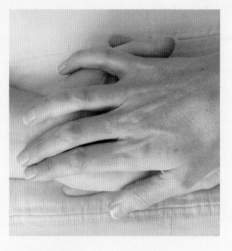

▲ **Step 28**
The area that circles the wrist relates to the left fallopian tube (if the receiver is female) or the vas deferens (if he is male) and the lymph nodes of the groin. Hold the receiver's hand, palm facing downwards, with your thumb across the top of the fingers and fingers underneath. Now thumb or finger walk right across the wrist on the back of the hand.

▲ Then turn the hand over and continue thumb or finger walking across the wrist. Note that if this area feels congested, it usually indicates a sluggish lymphatic system due to poor diet, a lack of exercise and stress.

▲ **To finish**
To finish, gently stroke the receiver's hand to ensure that any toxins that have been released are dispersed. Place the receiver's hand between both of your hands, rest it there for a few moments.

Completing the hands

Complete your treatment of the receiver's hands as follows.

Step 1
Return to any reflex areas that were tender during the initial treatment.

Step 2 ▶
Perform a few of your favourite relaxation techniques. If you wish to enhance your reflexology treatment, then massage the receiver's hands with your chosen blend of aromatherapy oils (see pages 237-41 for details).

Step 3
Allow the receiver to relax for as long as necessary. Offer him or her a glass of water with which to flush away any toxins that may have been released during the treatment. Also encourage the receiver to drink at least six to eight glasses of water over the next 24 hours to encourage the detoxification process.

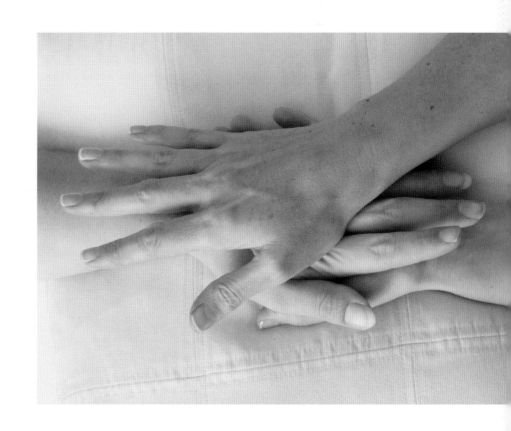

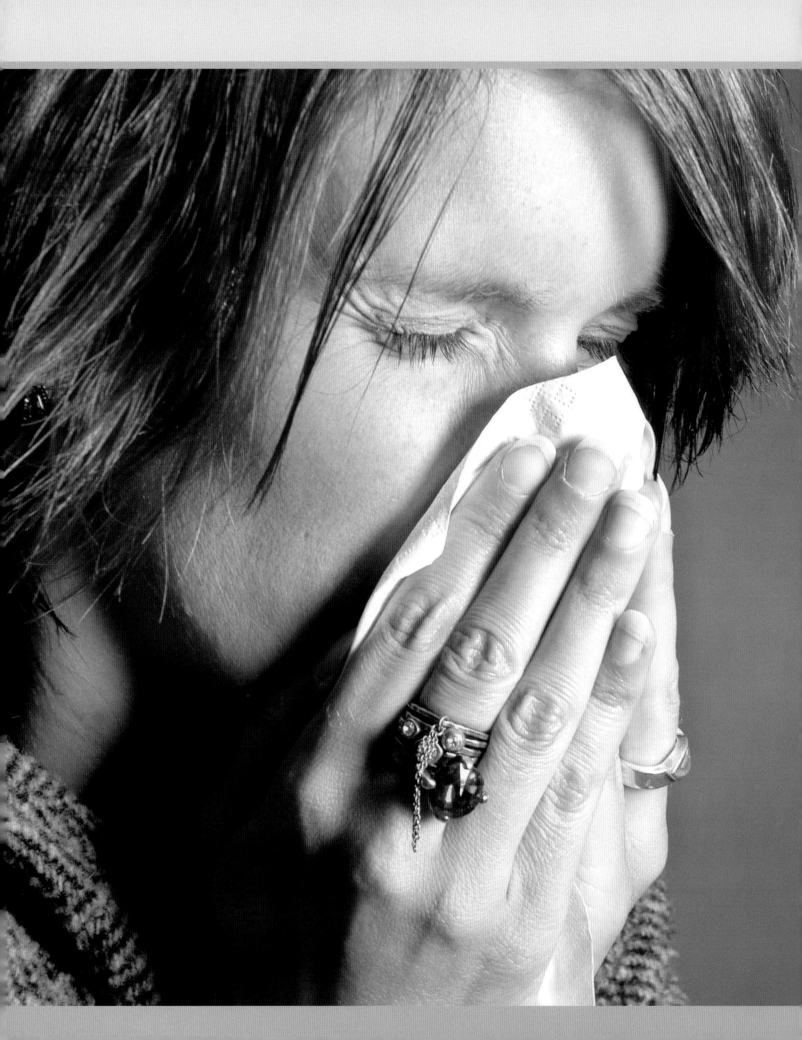

CHAPTER THREE

Treating common ailments and conditions

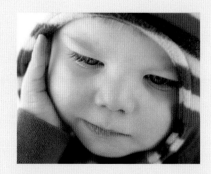 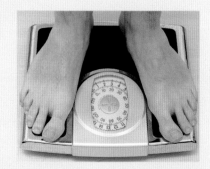 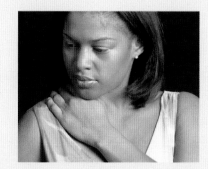

In this section a wide variety of common ailments and conditions will be described with the reflex points that are particularly important to treat.

Common ailments and conditions

Regardless of the disorder or condition from which the receiver may be suffering, all of the reflex areas in the hands or the feet should be treated in order to bring the body back to a state of balance. Some areas will benefit from additional treatment, however.

Many of the most common ailments and conditions are briefly described in this section of the book, together with the reflex points on the hands or feet that are particularly important when it comes to treating them.

Remember, however, that if the receiver's health problems are persistent or serious, it is always vital to consult a medically qualified doctor. Reflexology and orthodox medicine can work remarkably well together!

Acne

Acne is most prevalent in adolescence, but may affect adults. In this condition, the skin's sebaceous glands (oil-secreting glands) become overactive, resulting in blocked pores, blackheads, spots and, in some cases, scarring. Hormonal factors, diet and stress can all cause, or exacerbate, acne.

It is important to focus on the following reflex points when treating acne:

- the face (and other affected areas, such as the neck and back)
- the pituitary gland
- the thyroid and parathyroid glands
- the adrenal glands
- the thymus
- the lymphatic system
- all areas of the digestive system, including the large and small intestines, the liver, stomach and pancreas
- the kidneys
- the lungs
- the solar plexus
- the reproductive organs (the ovaries and uterus or the testes and prostate gland)

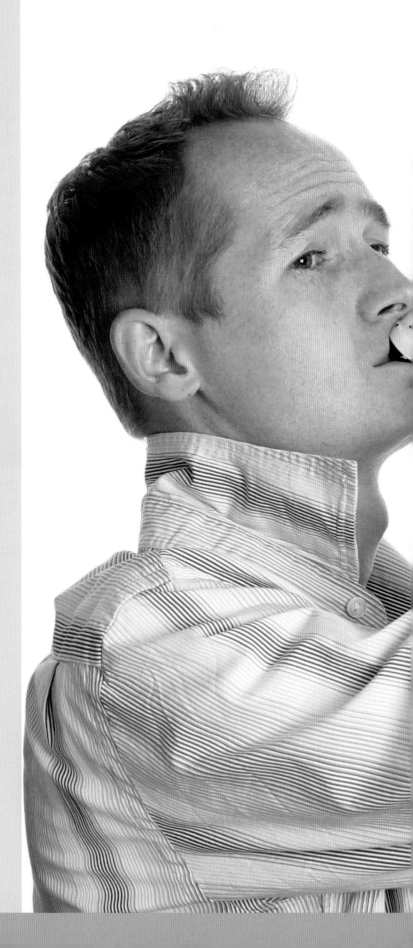

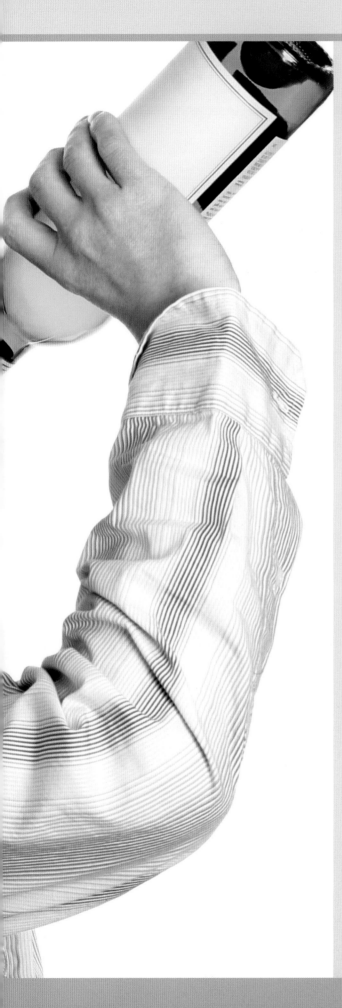

Alcohol and drug abuse

◄ The stresses of modern living are causing an increasing number of people to become addicted to drugs and alcohol. Addictions are self-destructive behavioural patterns that result from self-hatred, and addicts will often direct their abusive behaviour towards others. When trying to overcome alcohol and drug abuse, the intention to break an addiction is a most important factor.

It is important to focus on the following reflex points when treating alcohol or drug abuse:

- the head and brain
- the pineal gland
- the solar plexus
- the diaphragm
- the liver
- the pancreas
- the intestines
- the kidneys and bladder
- the pituitary gland
- the hypothalamus
- the adrenal glands
- the lungs

Caution

Note that you should not treat anyone who is under the influence of alcohol or drugs.

Allergies

Allergies are an overreaction of the body's immune system to such substances as certain foods (e.g., wheat or dairy products), dust, animal hair, pollen, medications and chemicals. Symptoms include itching, weals, bowel problems, wheezing, sneezing, runny eyes and headaches.

It is important to focus on the following reflex points when treating allergies:

- the pituitary gland
- the adrenal glands
- the solar plexus
- the diaphragm
- the lungs
- the lymphatic system
- the ears
- the eyes
- the throat
- all areas of the digestive system

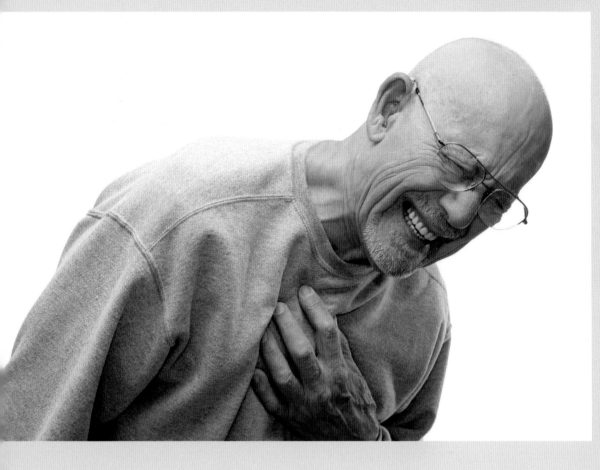

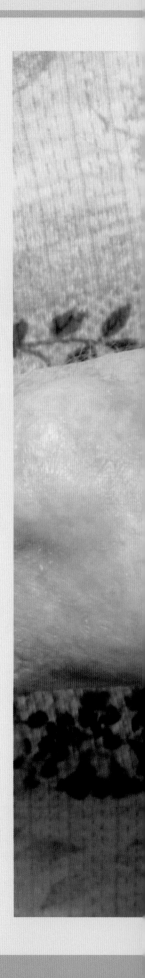

Anaemia

Anaemia is a disorder caused by a deficiency of the haemoglobin (iron-containing) components of the red blood cells. The main symptoms are fatigue, dizziness, palpitations, a rapid pulse, loss of appetite and paleness. Loss of blood (e.g., during menstruation) is a common anaemia-causing factor, and anaemia is also prevalent among pregnant women.

It is important to focus on the following reflex points when treating anaemia:

- the pituitary gland
- the solar plexus
- the adrenal glands
- the spleen
- the heart
- the thyroid gland

Angina

▲ Caused by insufficient oxygen reaching the heart muscle, angina is pain in the chest area that may radiate down the left arm.

It is important to focus on the following reflex points when treating angina:

- the solar plexus
- the heart (but note the caution)
- the adrenal glands
- the shoulder and arm
- the spine

Caution

If the angina is severe, then do not treat the heart reflex.

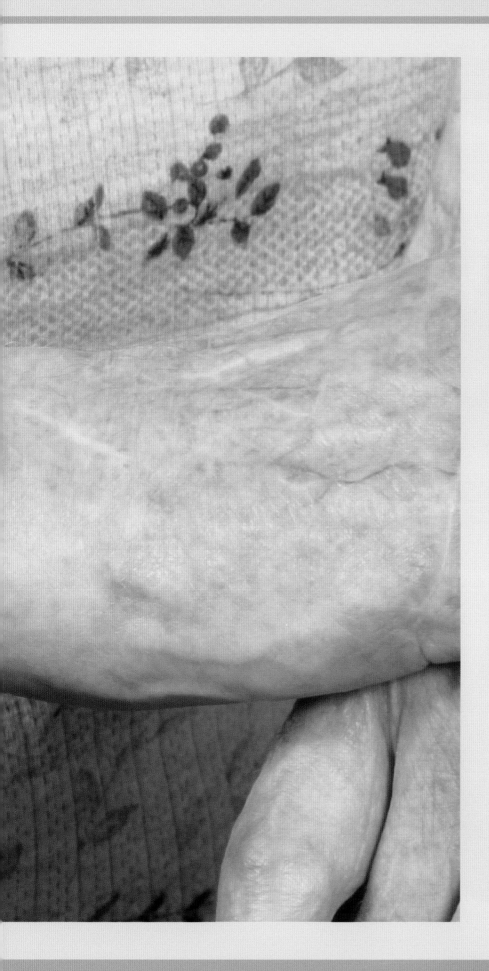

Anorexia nervosa and bulimia

Anorexia nervosa is a disorder that is most common among teenage girls who have become obsessed with their weight. Symptoms include a refusal to eat, self-induced vomiting, laxative abuse, the loss of menstruation, a decrease in body temperature, digestive problems and depressive, obsessional thoughts. Bulimia is another eating disorder whereby the sufferer binges on food and then induces vomiting and/or abuses laxatives.

It is important to focus on the following reflex points when treating anorexia nervosa or bulimia:

- the solar plexus
- the adrenal glands
- the pituitary gland
- the thyroid and parathyroid glands
- all areas of the reproductive system
- all areas of the digestive system
- the head and brain

Arthritis

◄ There are many different types of arthritis, but the most common are osteoarthritis and rheumatoid arthritis. Any joint may be involved, and the major symptoms include pain, stiffness, loss of movement and inflammation.

It is important to focus on the following reflex points when treating arthritis:

- all affected joints
- the spine
- the pituitary gland
- the parathyroid glands
- the solar plexus
- the adrenal glands
- the kidneys
- the lymphatic system
- all areas of the digestive system

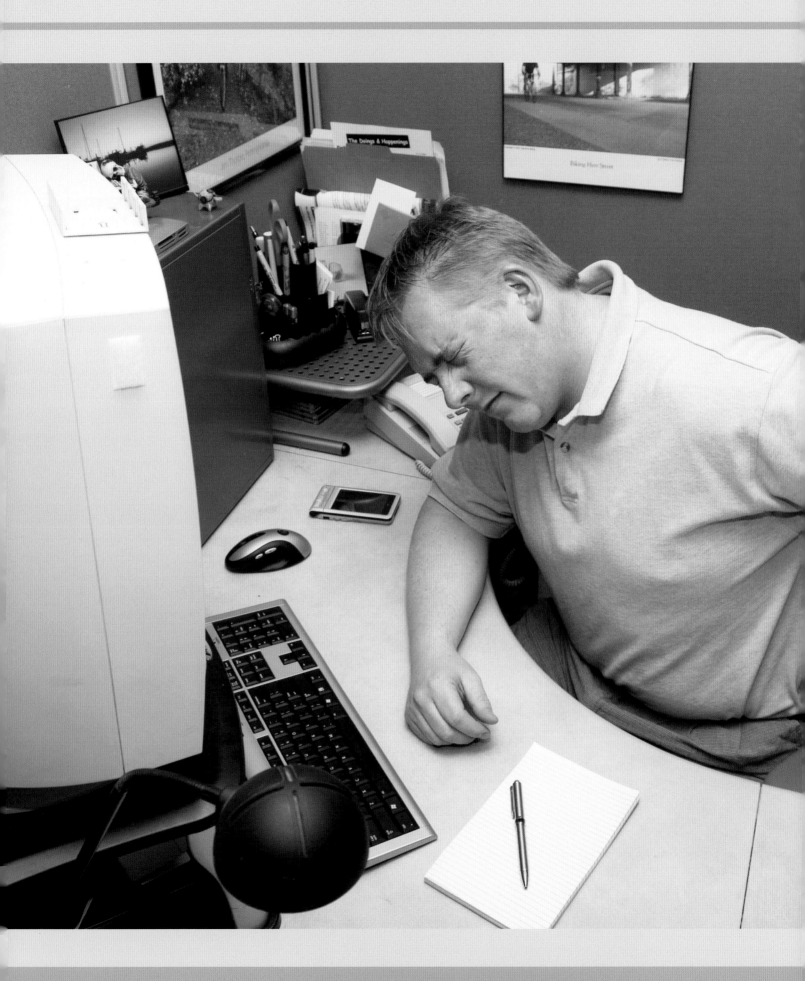

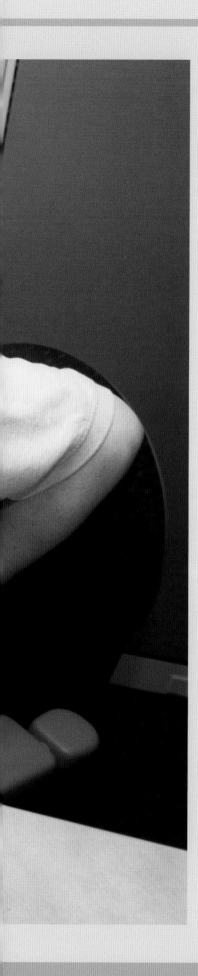

Asthma

Asthma can be caused by allergies, such as to pollen, house dust, foods, fur and pollutants, as well as by stress. Its symptoms include such breathing difficulties as wheezing and coughing.

It is important to focus on the following reflex points when treating asthma:

- the lungs
- the diaphragm
- the solar plexus
- the adrenal glands
- the spine
- the pituitary gland
- the heart
- the lymphatic system
- all areas of the digestive system

Bell's palsy

Bell's palsy usually comes on suddenly and affects only one side of the face, which becomes distorted due to the inflammation of, or damage to, the facial nerves. It is normally a temporary condition.

It is important to focus on the following reflex points when treating Bell's palsy:

- the face
- the head and brain
- the eye of the affected side
- the ear of the affected side
- the solar plexus
- the adrenal glands
- the neck

Back problems

◄ Most of us will suffer from pain in an area of our backs at some time in our lives, whether it be in the cervical area (that of the neck) or in the lumbar area (that of the lower back).

It is important to focus on the following reflex points when treating back problems:

- the spine
- the sciatic nerve
- the joints
- the adrenal glands
- the solar plexus

Bladder problems

Bladder conditions include cystitis, incontinence and bedwetting in children.

It is important to focus on the following reflex points when treating bladder problems:

- the bladder
- the kidneys
- the ureter
- the lymphatic system
- the adrenal glands
- the lower back
- the solar plexus

Breast lumps

If a woman detects a lump in her breast, then she should always seek medical advice in case it is cancerous. However, many lumps in the breasts, such as cysts, are not serious. Prior to menstruation, some women notice that their breasts become tender and lumpy; these lumps will shrink once menstruation is over.

It is important to focus on the following reflex points when treating breast lumps:

- the breasts
- the pituitary gland
- the thyroid gland
- the reproductive organs
- the lymphatic system
- the solar plexus
- the spine

Bronchitis

Bronchitis is an inflammatory disease of the respiratory system that may be caused by bacteria, viruses, smoke or chemicals. Symptoms include fever, coughing and mucus.

It is important to focus on the following reflex points when treating bronchitis:

- the lungs
- the diaphragm
- the lymphatic system
- the ears
- the eyes
- the solar plexus
- the adrenal glands
- the heart
- all areas of the digestive system

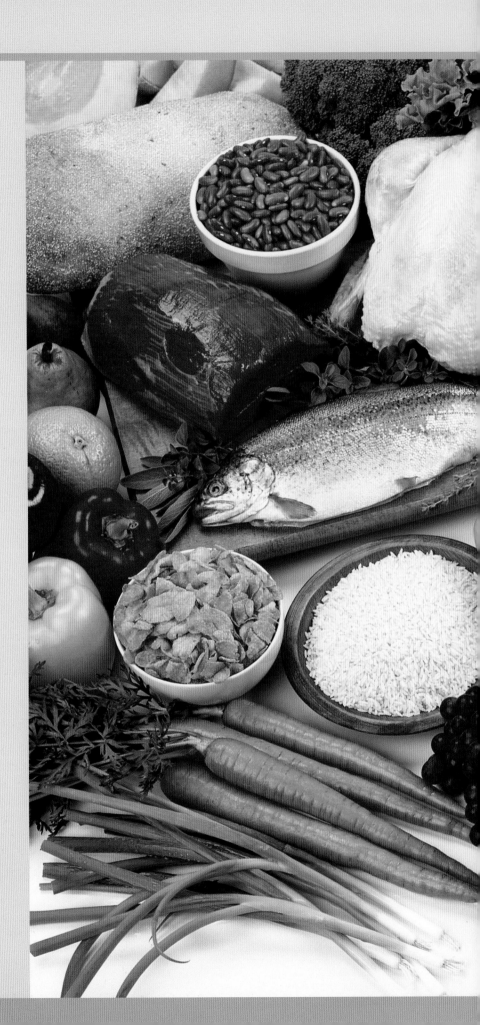

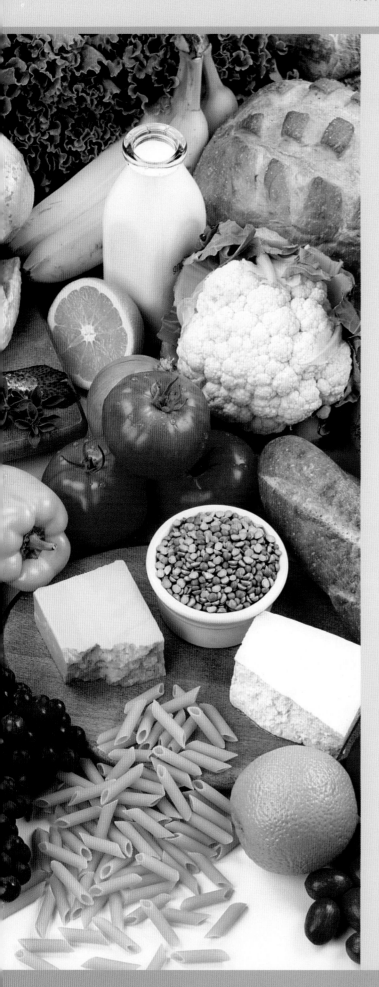

Candida

Candida albicans (thrush) is a type of yeast that is present in all of us, and is usually harmless. However, if the yeast multiplies and grows too much, it can cause a multitude of symptoms. Bloating, flatulence, itching, bowel problems, heartburn, fatigue, headaches, poor concentration, depression, mood swings, allergies, menstrual disorders and skin problems can all be caused by candida.

It is important to focus on the following reflex points when treating candida:

- the pituitary gland
- the small and large intestines
- the stomach
- the duodenum
- the gallbladder
- the rectum and anus
- the reproductive organs
- the adrenal glands
- the diaphragm
- the kidneys and bladder
- the head and brain
- the thymus
- the ileocaecal valve
- the pancreas
- the liver
- the spleen
- the spine
- the solar plexus

Constipation

Poor diet, an inadequate intake of water, stress, a lack of exercise, the regular use of laxatives and certain drugs (e.g., painkillers) are all contributory factors when it comes to constipation. Most of us suffer from it at some point in our lives.

It is important to focus on the following reflex points when treating constipation:

- the small and large intestines
- the rectum and anus
- the pancreas
- the liver
- the spleen
- the spine
- the solar plexus
- the adrenal glands
- the ileocaecal valve
- the stomach
- the duodenum
- the gallbladder
- the diaphragm
- the lungs
- the pituitary gland
- the kidneys and bladder

◀ **A healthy diet is vital for the prevention of constipation and other digestive disorders.**

Coughs and colds

▼ A few of the many symptoms of the common cold include a sore throat, sneezing, coughing, watery eyes, swollen lymph glands, tiredness, aching muscles and fever .

It is important to focus on the following reflex points when treating coughs and colds:

- the lungs
- the throat
- the Eustachian tubes
- the face
- the head and brain
- the spleen
- the pituitary gland
- the solar plexus
- the kidneys and bladder
- the diaphragm
- the ears
- the eyes
- the sinuses
- the thymus
- the adrenal glands
- the neck
- the lymphatic system

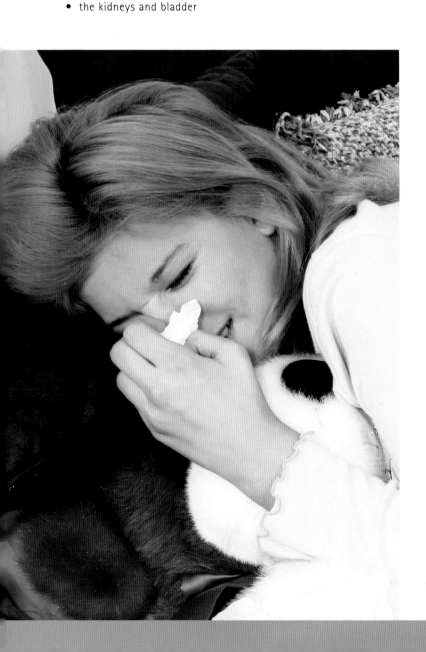

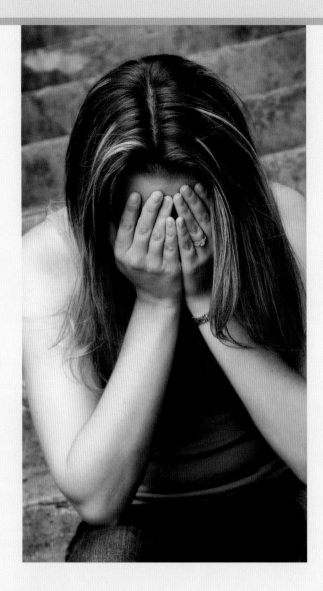

Depression

▲ There are various forms of depression, ranging from mild, temporary depression to severe cases in which suicide may be attempted and admission to a psychiatric unit is necessary.

It is important to focus on the following reflex points when treating depression:

- the head and brain
- the solar plexus
- the adrenal glands
- the heart
- the lungs
- the diaphragm
- the pituitary gland
- the pineal gland
- the thyroid gland
- all areas of the reproductive system

Diabetes

Diabetes is caused by insufficient, or absent, production of the hormone insulin by the pancreas. This lack of insulin results in an increase in the blood sugar level, causing such problems as excessive thirst, the frequent passing of urine, increased appetite and loss of weight. Long-term complications include damage to the retina at the back of the eye, cataracts, kidney damage, nerve damage, ulcers, high blood pressure and heart disorders.

It is important to focus on the following reflex points when treating diabetes:

- the pancreas
- the adrenal glands
- the kidneys and bladder
- the pituitary gland
- the thyroid gland
- the intestines
- the eyes
- the heart
- the liver

Caution

Use gentle pressure when treating a diabetic because the skin of people who suffer from diabetes is thinner, bruises more easily, is less sensitive, has a slower healing rate and can be more prone to ulceration than the skin of non-diabetics. Be sure either to use particularly gentle pressure over the pancreas reflex or to avoid it altogether.

Earache

▼ Earache may occur due to an infection, and symptoms typically include pain, fever, secretions from the ear, dizziness, impaired hearing or even deafness.

It is important to focus on the following reflex points when treating earache:

- the adrenal glands
- the neck
- the Eustachian tubes
- the throat
- the lymphatic system
- the thymus
- the solar plexus
- the ears

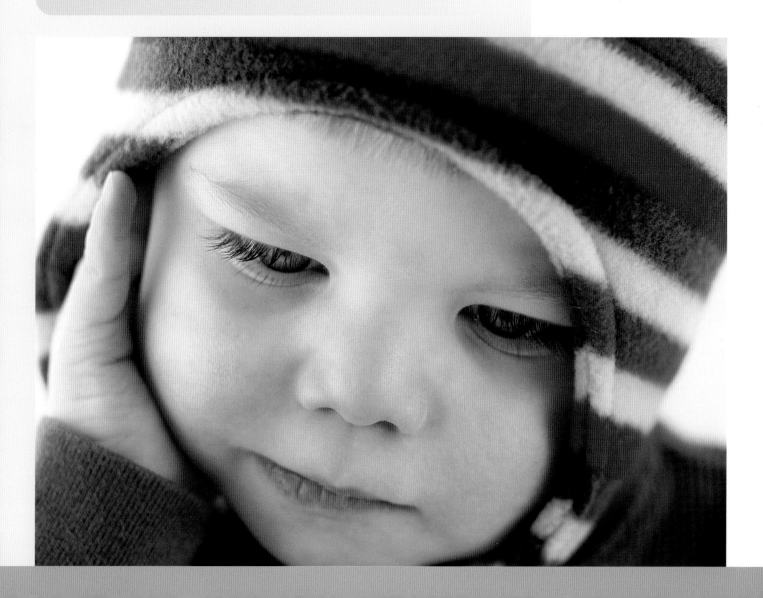

Eczema

Eczema is characterised by inflamed skin accompanied by itching, and sometimes by scaling skin or blisters. This skin condition may be related to allergies, and is aggravated by stress, but can also appear for no known reason.

It is important to focus on the following reflex points when treating eczema:

- all areas of the affected skin
- the solar plexus
- the adrenal glands
- the pituitary gland
- all areas of the digestive system
- the kidneys and bladder
- the liver
- the lymphatic system
- the lungs
- the diaphragm
- the thyroid gland

Eye problems

Eye problems include impaired vision, ▶ conjunctivitis, tired eyes, watery eyes, squints, cataracts, glaucoma, burning eyes and blocked tear ducts.

It is important to focus on the following reflex points when treating eye problems:

- the eyes
- the head and brain
- the face
- the neck
- the spine
- the solar plexus
- the adrenal glands
- the lymphatic system

Epilepsy

Epilepsy is a disorder of the nervous system that is characterised by seizures due to abnormal electrical activity in the brain. This disorder usually appears in childhood or adolescence, and there are different types of seizures, including grand mal and absence (or petit mal) seizures.

It is important to focus on the following reflex points when treating epilepsy:

- the head and brain (but see the caution)
- the solar plexus
- the adrenal glands
- the pituitary gland
- the thyroid gland
- all areas of the digestive system
- the diaphragm
- the neck
- the spine

Caution

Do not overstimulate the head and brain reflex point.

Fibroids

Fibroids are common, harmless tumours that grow within the uterus. They may be small or may grow to the size of a grapefruit. A larger fibroid can cause such symptoms as heavy or prolonged menstruation, leading to anaemia. Other problems include back pain, constipation and frequent urination.

It is important to focus on the following reflex points when treating fibroids:

- the uterus
- the ovaries
- the Fallopian tubes
- the pituitary gland
- the lymphatic system
- the spine
- all areas of the digestive system
- the kidneys and bladder

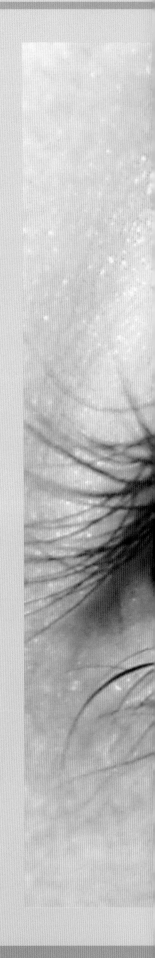

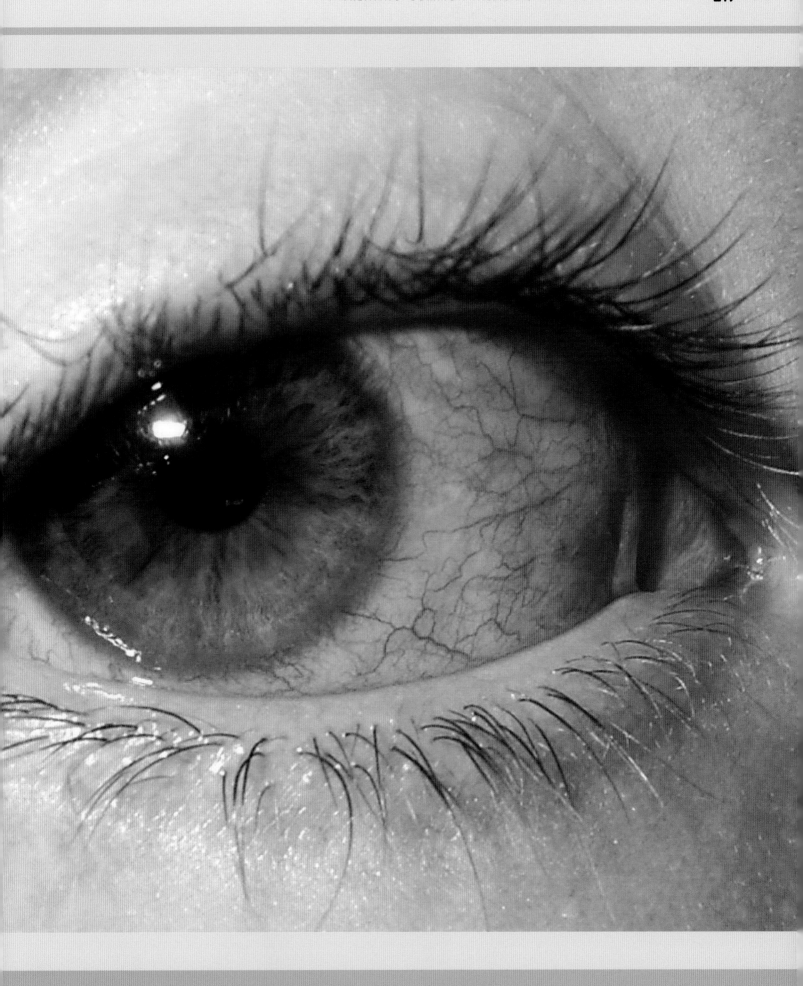

Flatulence (wind)

Flatulence, or wind, is caused by excessive gas in the intestines. The symptoms include bloating, abdominal cramps, unpleasant smelling emissions from the anus and belching. The causes of this condition may be a poor diet, incorrect combinations of food and not chewing food properly.

It is important to focus on the following reflex points when treating flatulence:

- the small and large intestines
- the rectum and anus
- the stomach
- the pancreas
- the duodenum
- the liver
- the gallbladder
- the solar plexus
- the adrenal glands
- the diaphragm
- the spine

Frozen shoulder

When a shoulder is 'frozen', it is stiff and ▶ painful, and the condition may worsen to the extent that normal arm movements become impossible (hence the term 'frozen'). The pain may radiate into the neck, down the arm and across the back and chest. A frozen shoulder may appear for no reason, but can also follow a minor injury to the shoulder.

It is important to focus on the following reflex points when treating a frozen shoulder:

- the affected shoulder
- the affected arm
- the neck
- the spine
- the solar plexus
- the adrenal glands

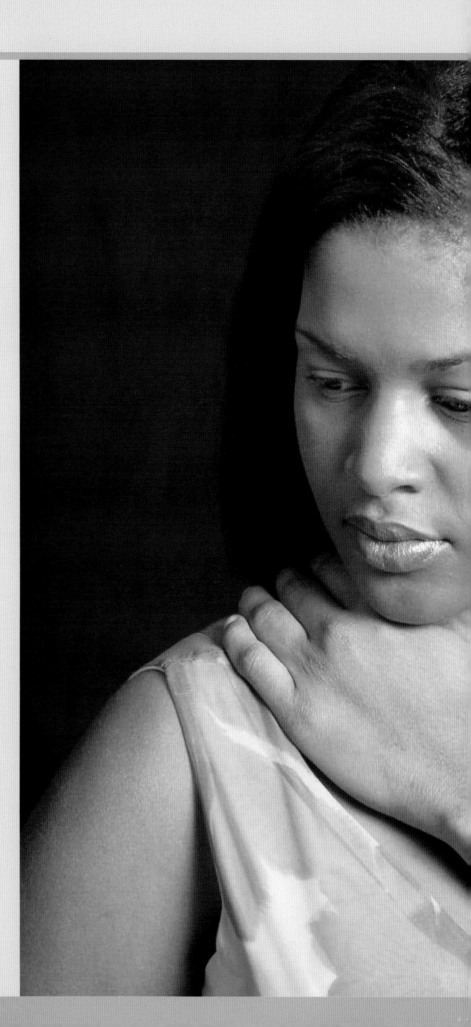

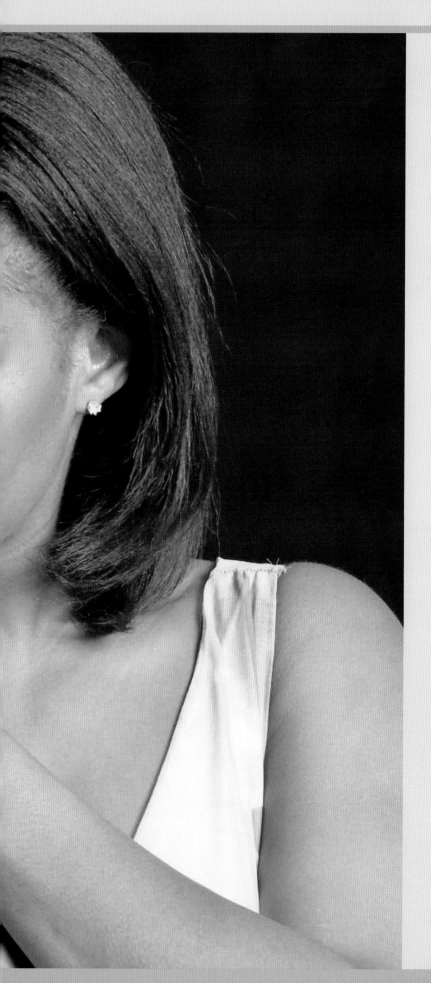

Gout

Gout is a common joint disease whereby uric acid crystals settle around the joints, and mostly around the big toe, which becomes red, hot, swollen and extremely tender. This disease is ten times more common in men than in women, and often has a family history. Heavy drinking and a poor diet can precipitate an attack.

It is important to focus on the following reflex points when treating gout:

- the corresponding thumb (because the big toe would be too tender to touch)
- the solar plexus
- the adrenal glands
- the kidneys and bladder
- the lymphatic system
- all areas of the digestive system
- the pituitary gland
- the thyroid gland
- the parathyroid glands

Haemorrhoids

Prolonged constipation, a diet that is low in fibre, a lack of exercise and not drinking enough water can all give rise to haemorrhoids, which are swollen veins in the lining of the anus. Haemorrhoids are also common during pregnancy and after childbirth. Symptoms of haemorrhoids include painful bowel movements, which may be accompanied by rectal bleeding.

It is important to focus on the following reflex points when treating haemorrhoids:

- the rectum and anus
- the small and large intestines
- the liver
- the gallbladder
- the stomach, pancreas and duodenum
- the solar plexus
- the diaphragm
- the adrenal glands
- the spleen

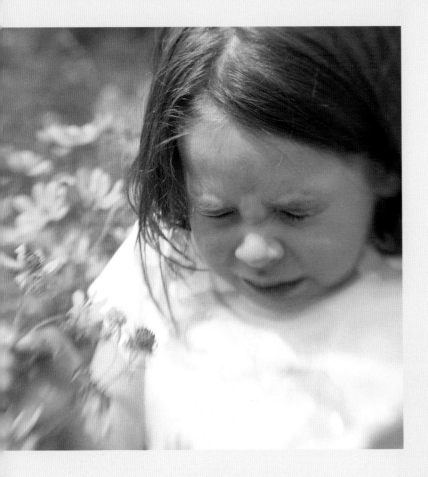

Headaches

▲ Most of us suffer from headaches from time to time, and there are a number of causes, including stress, sinus problems, hormonal imbalances, eye disorders, digestive disturbances, allergies and toxicity.

It is important to focus on the following reflex points when treating headaches:

- the head and brain
- the neck
- the sinuses
- all areas of the digestive system
- the solar plexus
- the adrenal glands
- the diaphragm
- the eyes
- the teeth
- the pituitary gland
- the reproductive organs
- the lymphatic system
- the kidneys and bladder

Hay fever

▲ Hay fever is an allergic reaction to pollens that causes sneezing, nasal congestion, a runny nose and watery, sore eyes. Sufferers are particularly affected when the pollen count is high during hot and windy weather.

It is important to focus on the following reflex points when treating hay fever:

- the sinuses
- the eyes
- the ears
- the throat
- the face
- the lungs
- the adrenal glands
- the solar plexus
- the thymus
- the neck
- all areas of the digestive system
- the lymphatic system
- the kidneys and bladder
- the pituitary gland

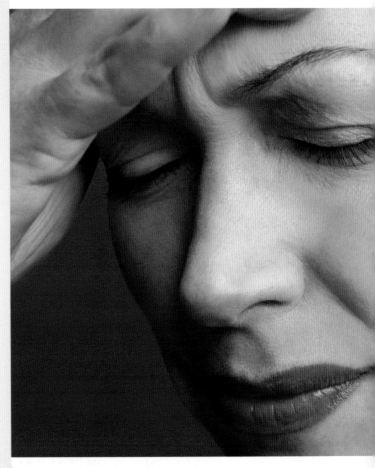

Heart problems

Common heart disorders include angina (see page 210), tachycardia (when the heart beats too fast), arrhythmia (an irregular heartbeat), bradycardia (when the heart beats too slowly) and high blood pressure. Following a healthy diet, not smoking, avoiding stress and taking regular exercise will help to prevent heart problems from developing.

It is important to focus on the following reflex points when treating heart problems:

- the heart (but see the caution)
- the left shoulder and arm
- the adrenal glands
- the pituitary gland
- the spine
- the lungs
- the solar plexus
- the diaphragm
- the kidneys and bladder
- the small and large intestines

Caution

Leave out the heart reflex in cases of severe heart problems or if a pacemaker has been fitted.

High or low blood pressure

▼ High blood pressure is a fairly common disorder whose incidence increases with age. Symptoms include headaches, visual disturbances, ringing in the ears, breathlessness and chest pains. Although low blood pressure is regarded as being far less serious, individuals who suffer from it are more prone to fainting and dizziness, as well as to experiencing fatigue and coldness.

It is important to focus on the following reflex points when treating high or low blood pressure:

- the solar plexus
- the adrenal glands
- the pituitary gland
- the thyroid gland·
- the parathyroid glands
- the kidneys and bladder
- the diaphragm
- the heart·
- the spine
- the lungs

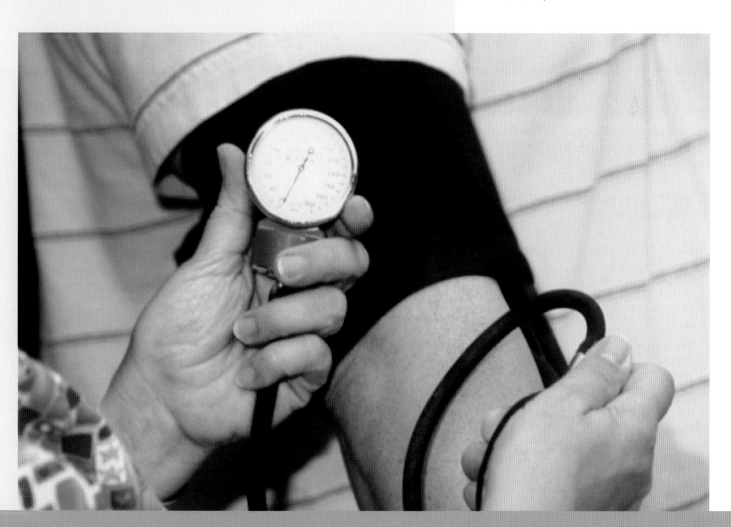

Impotence

Impotence is the most common male sexual disorder and affects most men at some point in their lives. Psychological factors, such as stress and tension, depression and lack of confidence, usually cause impotence, although physical disorders, such as diabetes and certain drugs, may also be implicated.

It is important to focus on the following reflex points when treating impotence:

- all reproductive organs
- the solar plexus
- the adrenal glands
- the diaphragm
- the pituitary gland
- the kidneys and bladder

Indigestion and heartburn

The main symptom of both indigestion and heartburn is a burning sensation behind the breastbone that may spread up the oesophagus to the back of the mouth. Stress and tension can induce heartburn, as can overeating, eating too quickly and not chewing food properly.

It is important to focus on the following reflex points when treating indigestion or heartburn:

- all areas of the digestive system, including the stomach, pancreas, duodenum, liver, gallbladder and large and small intestines
- the solar plexus
- the diaphragm
- the adrenal glands
- the chest
- the spine

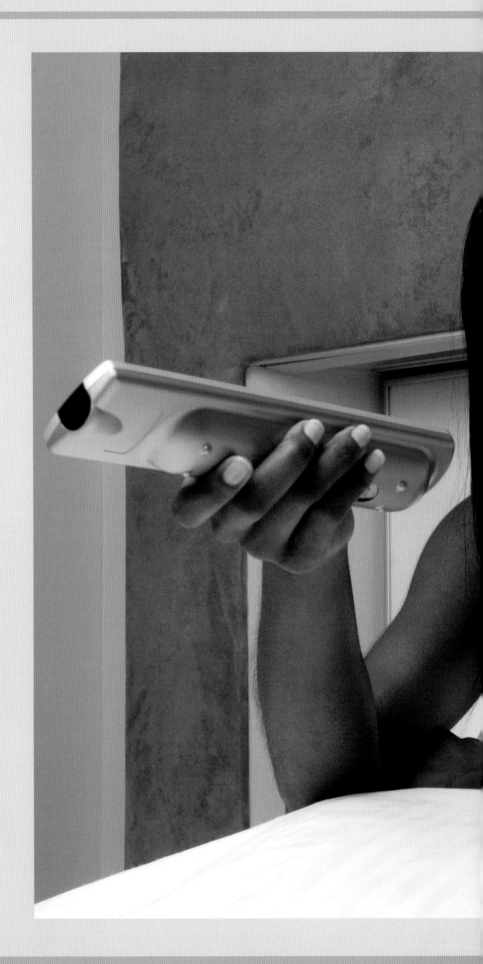

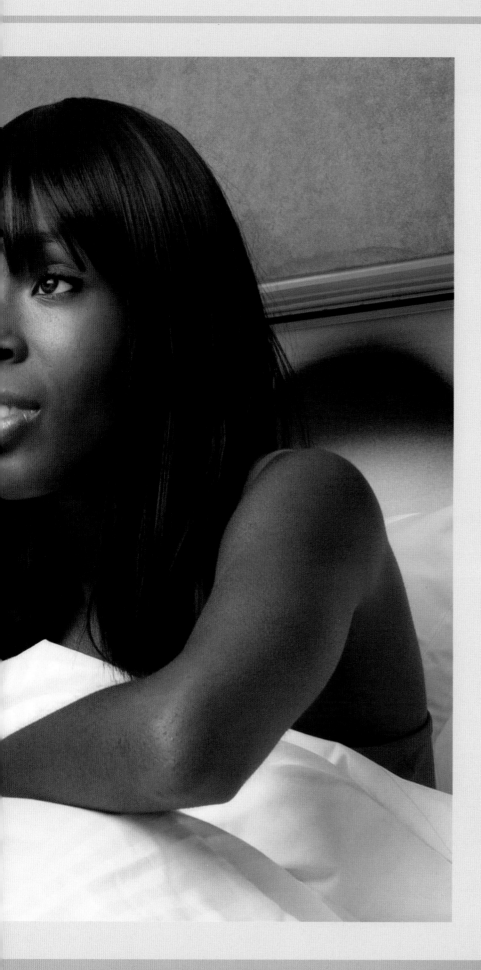

Infertility

Female and male infertility are common problems. Worry and tension can definitely decrease the chance of a woman becoming pregnant, as can such physical problems as disorders of the uterus, ovaries or fallopian tubes or a low sperm count. Ideally, both partners should be treated if a woman is having trouble conceiving.

It is important to focus on the following reflex points when treating infertility:

- the pituitary gland
- the ovaries or testes
- the uterus or prostate gland
- the fallopian tubes or vas deferens
- the thyroid and parathyroid glands
- the solar plexus
- the adrenal glands
- the spine

Insomnia

◀ When we are under a great deal of stress, most of us will find it difficult to go to sleep. Insomnia can result in daytime fatigue, irritability and an inability to concentrate and cope with day-to-day life.

It is important to focus on the following reflex points when treating insomnia:

- the solar plexus
- the head and brain
- the adrenal glands
- the pituitary gland
- the pineal gland
- the diaphragm
- the lungs
- the spine

Irritable bowel syndrome

Irritable bowel syndrome (IBS) is characterised by alternating constipation and diarrhoea, excessive flatulence, bloating, back pain, weakness and abdominal cramps, which may be severe. Stress is the main causative factor, although certain foods may also irritate the bowel.

It is important to focus on the following reflex points when treating IBS:

- all areas of the digestive system
- the solar plexus
- he adrenal glands
- the diaphragm
- the spine
- the lymphatic system
- the kidneys and bladder

Menopause

The menopause usually occurs some time between the ages of 45 and 55, and is normally a gradual process, with the changes associated with it taking place over a number of years. Women typically experience a whole range of physical and psychological conditions, including hot flushes, increased perspiration, night sweats, erratic menstruation, excessive bleeding, depression, insomnia, weight loss, irritability, vaginal dryness and loss of libido.

It is important to focus on the following reflex points when treating the symptoms of the menopause:

- the pituitary gland
- the uterus
- the breasts and chest
- the adrenal glands
- the hypothalamus
- the lymphatic system
- the kidneys and bladder
- the thyroid and parathyroid glands
- the ovaries
- the fallopian tubes
- the solar plexus
- the head and brain
- the liver
- the spine
- the heart

Liver and gallbladder conditions

Excessive consumption of alcohol, overindulgence in food, medications and stress all have an adverse effect on the liver and gallbladder.

It is important to focus on the following reflex points when treating conditions of the liver and gallbladder:

- the liver
- the gallbladder
- the small and large intestines
- the stomach
- the pancreas
- the duodenum
- the spine
- the solar plexus
- the adrenal glands
- the lymphatic system

Menstrual problems

▶ Menstrual problems are very common, and can take many forms, including an absence of periods (amenorrhoea), painful periods (dysmenorrhoea), profuse bleeding (menorrhagia), endometriosis, ovarian cysts and disorders of the fallopian tubes and uterus. Reflexology is an excellent way in which to regulate and normalise the menstrual cycle.

It is important to focus on the following reflex points when treating menstrual problems:

- the pituitary gland
- the thyroid and parathyroid glands
- the ovaries
- the uterus
- the fallopian tubes
- the breasts and chest
- the solar plexus
- the diaphragm
- the adrenal glands
- the head and brain
- the spine
- the kidneys and bladder
- the pancreas
- the small and large intestines

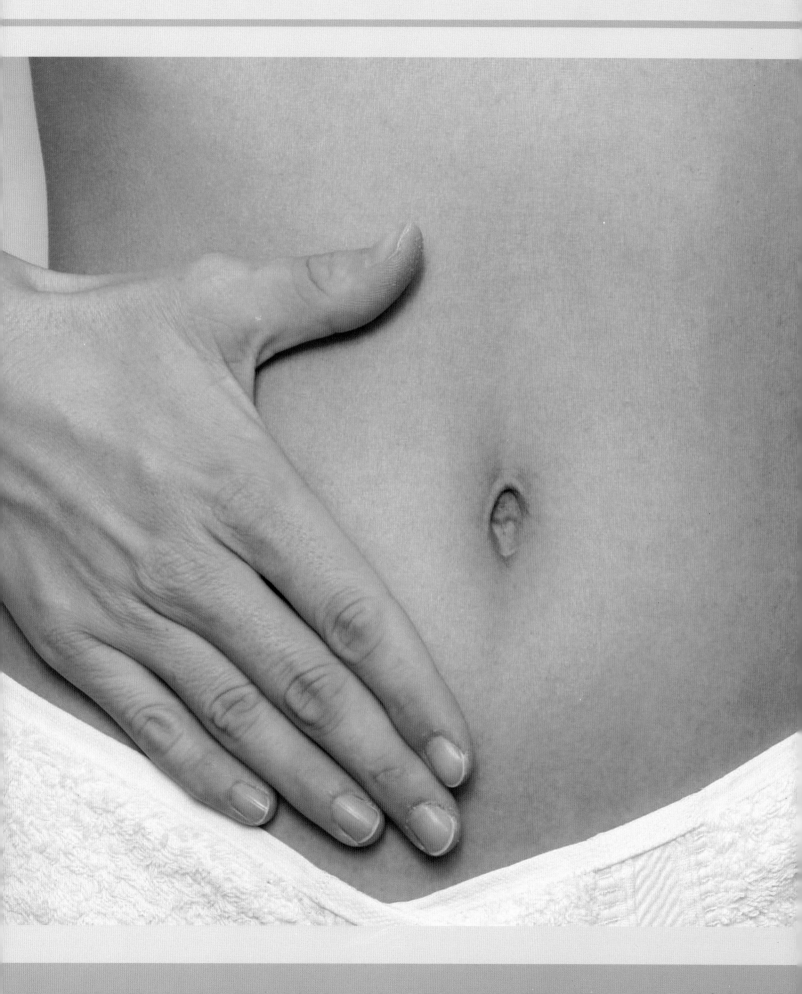

Migraines

▶ A migraine is an intensely painful headache that is usually confined to one side of the head and which is frequently accompanied by sickness. Prior to an attack, visual disturbances and extreme tiredness are very common. Susceptibility to migraines tends to run in families, and certain foods, particularly cheese, chocolate and red wine, can be triggers. Other contributory factors include stress, lack of sleep and erratic eating habits.

It is important to focus on the following reflex points when treating migraines:

- the head and brain
- the neck
- the adrenal glands
- the pituitary gland
- the lymphatic system
- the spine
- the solar plexus
- the diaphragm
- the eyes
- the kidneys and bladder
- all areas of the digestive system, especially the liver

Myalgic encephalomyelitis (ME)

Myalgic encephalomyelitis (ME), which is otherwise known as chronic fatigue syndrome or post viral syndrome, is a disorder of unknown cause. Its symptoms are very variable and include extreme tiredness, weakness, muscle pains, sleep disturbances, depression, loss of memory and panic attacks.

It is important to focus on the following reflex points when treating ME:

- the solar plexus
- the adrenal glands
- the lungs
- the lymphatic system
- the thyroid gland
- the spine
- the spleen
- the heart
- the diaphragm
- the head and brain
- the thymus
- the pituitary gland
- the tonsils
- the pancreas
- the liver
- the kidneys and bladder
- all digestive organs, including the ileocaecal valve

Caution

A shorter treatment than usual is advisable because ME sufferers are often in a very weakened state.

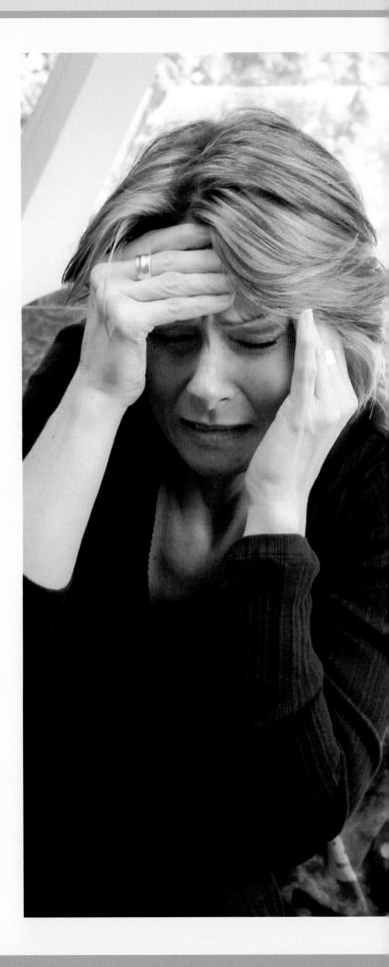

Osteoporosis

Osteoporosis most frequently occurs in women after the menopause, due to the loss of calcium, which results in a weakening of the bones that makes them more likely to fracture. Women may also develop a 'dowager's hump'.

It is important to focus on the following reflex points when treating osteoporosis:

- the pituitary gland
- the thyroid and parathyroid glands
- the spine
- the joints
- the adrenal glands
- the solar plexus
- the diaphragm·
- the ovaries
- the uterus
- the chest and ribs
- the lungs

Caution

In cases of osteoporosis, the pressure applied should be very light due to the fragility of the receiver's bones.

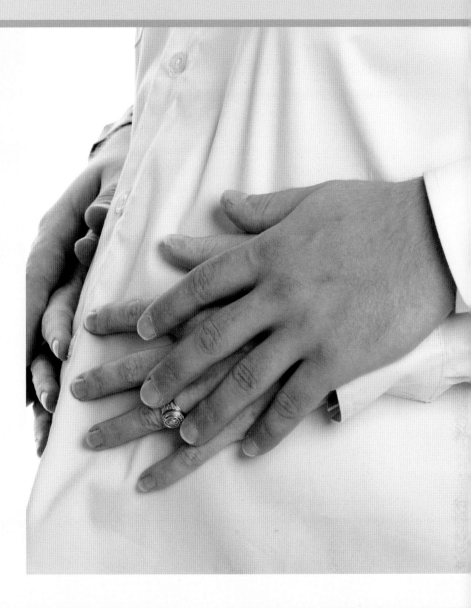

Pregnancy

Pregnancy is, of course, a completely natural state, not a disease! Common problems experienced during pregnancy include morning sickness, dizziness, backache, fluid retention, leg cramps, sore breasts, insomnia, haemorrhoids, varicose veins, tiredness and high blood pressure.

It is important to focus on the following reflex points when the receiver is pregnant:

- the pituitary gland
- the breasts
- the thyroid/parathyroid glands
- the solar plexus
- the adrenal glands
- the stomach
- the liver
- all digestive organs
- the spine
- the lungs
- the diaphragm
- the kidneys and bladder
- the reproductive areas (in the final stages of pregnancy only)

Caution

If the receiver is pregnant and has a history of miscarriage, reflexology is not recommended. Generally, however, reflexology can ensure a much easier and happier pregnancy.

Premenstrual tension (PMT)

▶ Women typically experience a wide range of symptoms – both physiological and psychological – prior to a period. The symptoms of premenstrual tension (PMT) include irritability and mood swings, depression, anxiety, poor concentration, breast tenderness, abdominal bloating, changes in bowel movements, fluid retention, sugar cravings, weight gain and skin problems.

It is important to focus on the following reflex points when treating PMT:

- the pituitary gland
- the ovaries
- the fallopian tubes
- the uterus
- the solar plexus
- the adrenal glands
- the diaphragm
- the thyroid and parathyroid glands
- the pancreas
- the head and brain
- the spine
- the lymphatic system
- the kidneys and bladder
- the small and large intestines
- the liver and gallbladder

Prostate problems

As men age, many of them experience enlargement of the prostate gland. The symptoms of this condition include increased frequency of urination, difficulty urinating and pain on urination. Prostate problems are particularly troublesome at night, and may lead to interrupted sleep.

It is important to focus on the following reflex points when treating prostate problems:

- the prostate gland
- the testes
- the vas deferens
- the kidneys and bladder
- the solar plexus
- the adrenal glands
- the diaphragm
- the lymphatic system
- the pituitary gland

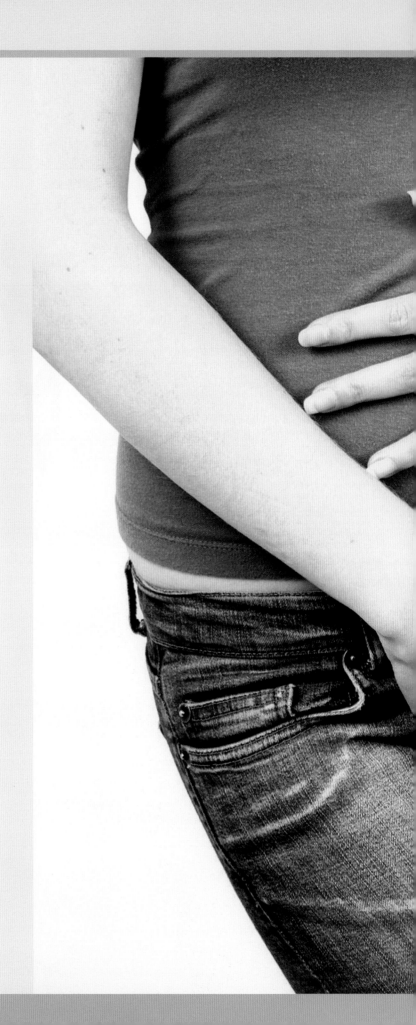

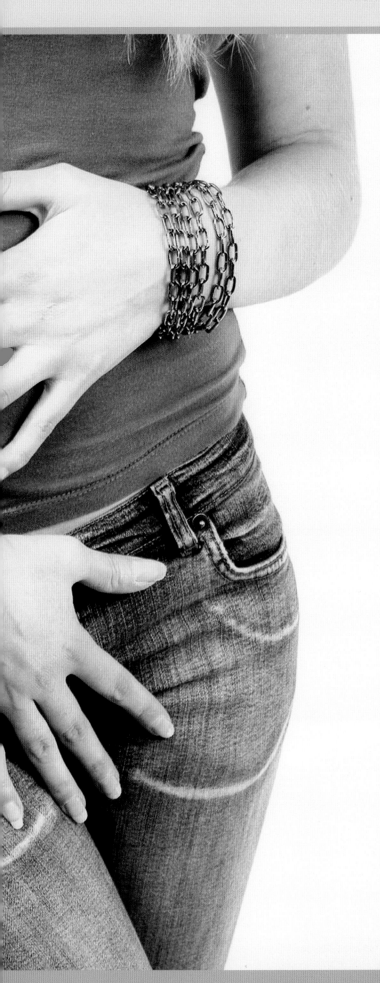

Psoriasis

Psoriasis is characterised by the formation of red patches, covered by scaly skin, on mostly the elbows, knees, palms of the hands, soles of the feet and scalp. Stress is a major cause of psoriasis, although it has a tendency to run in families.

It is important to focus on the following reflex points when treating psoriasis:

- all affected areas of the skin
- the solar plexus
- the adrenal glands
- the diaphragm
- the lungs
- all areas of the digestive system
- the pituitary gland
- the thyroid gland
- the kidneys and bladder

Sinusitis

Sinusitis is the inflammation of the membranes lining the sinuses. It is usually caused by infection, and occasionally by an infected tooth. Its symptoms include a throbbing facial pain, a feeling of fullness in the face, fever, headaches, tiredness and a loss of the sense of smell.

It is important to focus on the following reflex points when treating sinusitis:

- the sinuses
- the face
- the spine, especially the neck
- the eyes
- the ear
- the throat
- the teeth
- the head and brain
- the lymphatic system
- the adrenal glands
- the solar plexus
- the diaphragm
- the lungs
- the thymus
- the small and large intestines
- the kidneys and bladder

Stress and anxiety

▶ Stress is unavoidable, and we all experience it to varying degrees throughout our lives. It can affect all of the systems of the body, and such conditions as high blood pressure, problems with the digestive system and headaches are very common responses to stress.

Reflexology can be a powerful antidote to stress, and it is important to focus on the following reflex points when treating stress or anxiety:

- the solar plexus
- the diaphragm
- the adrenal glands
- the neck
- the head and brain
- the spine
- the lungs
- the heart
- the pituitary gland
- the kidneys and bladder

Tonsillitis

The tonsils are part of the body's defence against infection, and protect against respiratory infections. The symptoms of tonsillitis include fever, a sore throat, difficulty swallowing, swollen lymph nodes, earache and headaches.

It is important to focus on the following reflex points when treating tonsillitis:

- the throat
- the tonsils
- the lymphatic system
- the thymus
- the ears
- the head and brain
- the adrenal glands
- the solar plexus
- the diaphragm
- the lungs
- the neck

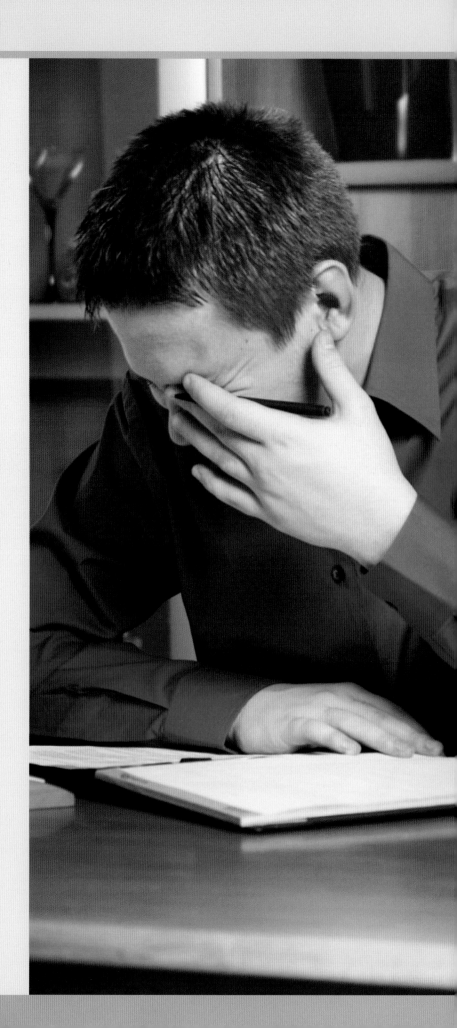

Varicose veins

Varicose veins are enlarged, swollen and twisted veins that are most commonly found in the legs. It is estimated that nearly half of all middle-aged adults suffer from this condition, whereby the valves in the veins become less effective. Long periods of standing, obesity, pregnancy, lifting heavy weights and genetic weakness of the veins can all lead to varicose veins. Heavy, aching sensations in the legs, pain and swelling are all symptoms that are typically experienced by sufferers.

It is important to focus on the following reflex points when treating varicose veins:

- the appropriate reflex points for the affected areas
- the heart
- the lungs
- the diaphragm
- the solar plexus
- the adrenal glands
- the spine
- the lymphatic system
- the kidneys and bladder
- all areas of the digestive system

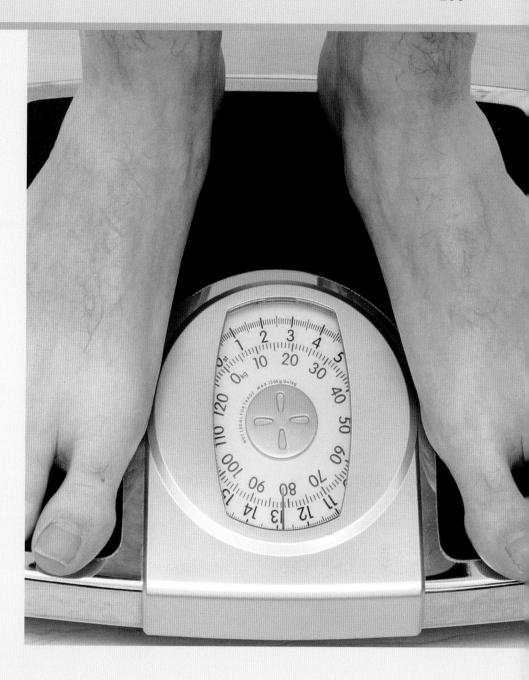

Weight problems

We are constantly being bombarded by magazine articles and books promising weight loss. Some individuals go through life trying all sorts of diets with little success, making them feel more and more miserable each time they fail. Instead of reaching for food when you feel bad about yourself, experience the joys of reflexology instead!

It is important to focus on the following reflex points when treating weight problems:

- the pituitary gland
- the head and brain
- the adrenal glands
- the stomach
- the duodenum
- the liver
- the kidneys and bladder

- the hypothalamus
- the solar plexus
- the thyroid
- the pancreas
- the small and large intestines
- the gallbladder
- the lymphatic system

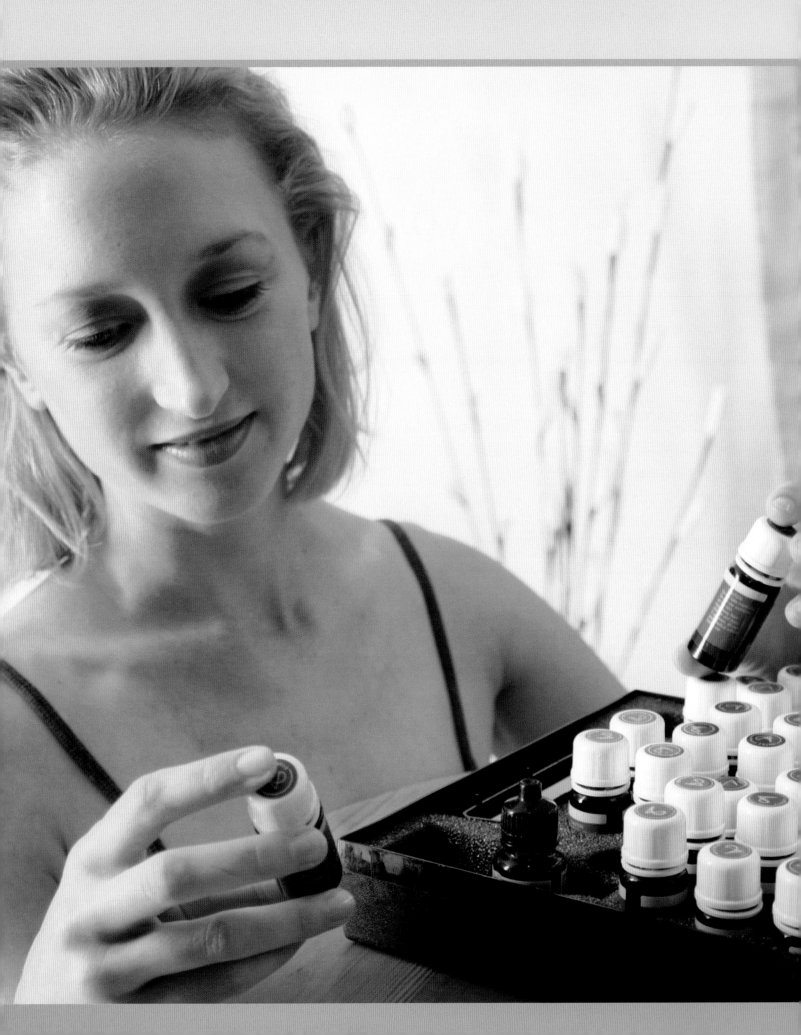

CHAPTER FOUR

Enhancing your treatments

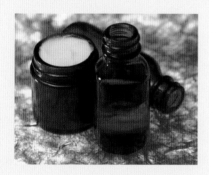 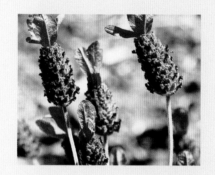 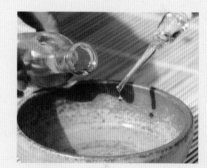

The use of healing aromatherapy oils at the end of a treatment is an excellent way to enhance and complement your reflexology. In this section you will learn how to prepare aromatherapy blends that are tailor-made for the individual.

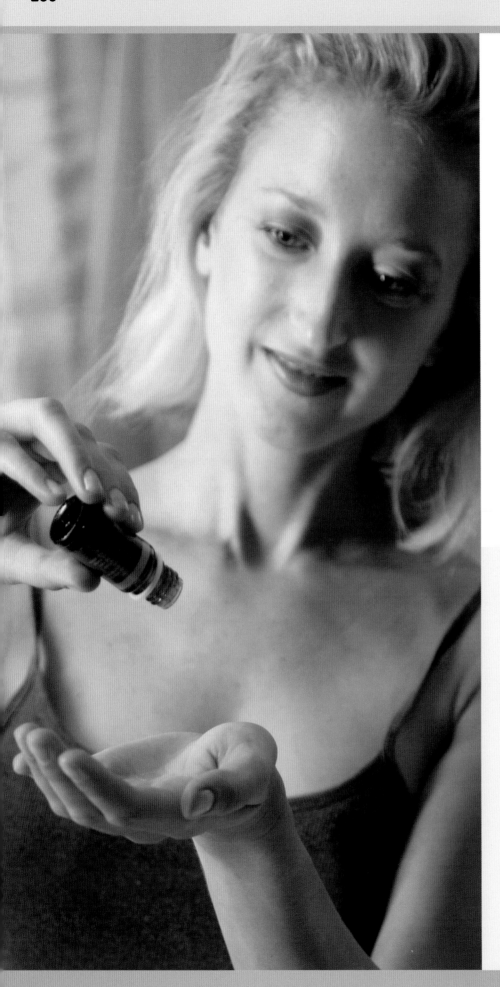

Enhancing your treatments

The healing effects of reflexology may be enhanced by the use of essential oils. Aromatherapy blends, tailor-made for the individual, can be massaged into the receiver's hands or feet at the end of a reflexology session, thereby complementing and reinforcing your treatment.

Do not, however, use aromatherapy oil or cream blends on the receiver's feet or hands during a treatment, otherwise your hands will slip and it will be difficult for you to feel and pinpoint the reflex points accurately.

Remember that essential oils may also be diffused into a room to create a healing atmosphere (see page 40). You could also add a few drops of an essential oil to a bowl of warm water in which you can then soak the receiver's feet or hands before the reflexology session begins.

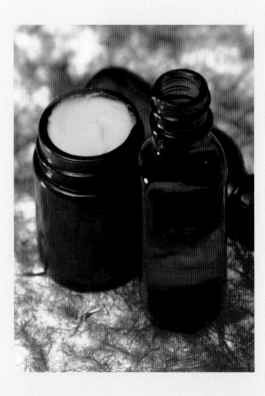

Preparing an oil blend

Essential oils should never be used undiluted on the hands or feet. They must be blended with a vegetable, nut or seed oil, and preferably with a carrier oil that is cold-pressed, unrefined and additive-free. Do not use a mineral oil (i.e., a commercial baby oil) as this will clog up the receiver's skin. Particularly suitable carrier oils include those made from sweet almonds, apricot kernels and peach kernels because these are light, and therefore easy to work with, and do not have a strong odour.

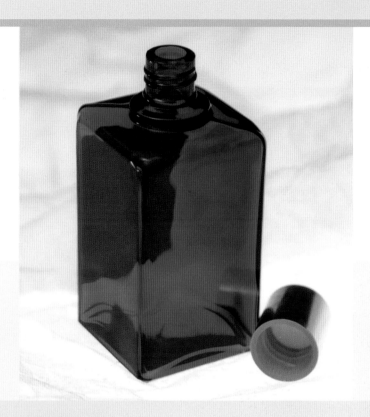

It is a good idea to make up 10ml (that is, 2 teaspoonfuls, for a teaspoon holds roughly 5ml) of an aromatherapy blend for use in your treatment. (Note that there should be some left over.) Just add 3 drops of essential oil to 10ml of your carrier oil.

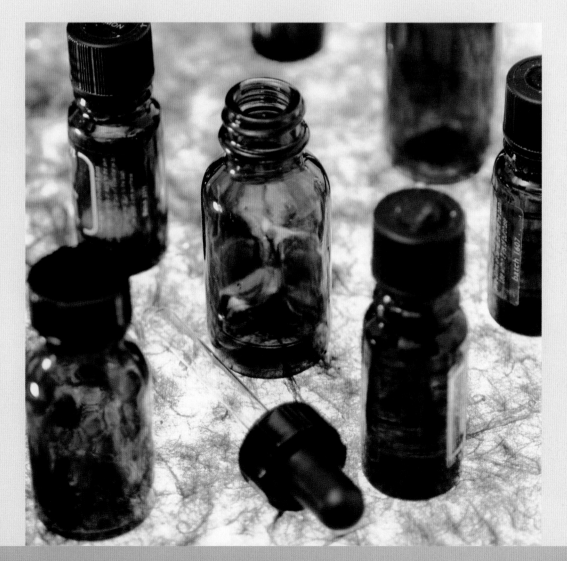

If you want to make up a larger quantity for the receiver to use between treatments, then store your blend in an amber-coloured glass bottle because essential oils are damaged by ultraviolet light. They are also adversely affected by extremes of temperature, and are volatile, too, which means that they evaporate rapidly. So do not place your treatment oils on a sunny windowsill and make sure that the tops of the bottles are tightly shut when the oils are not in use. If stored properly, pure essential oils will keep for several years, while a blended oil will remain usable for a few months.

Preparing a foot or hand cream

Creams are excellent for nurturing and protecting precious hands and feet. They are marvellous for healing cracked and chapped skin, and for relieving itching, redness and irritation, and also can help to reduce swelling in the hands and feet. They smell fantastic, too!

For best results, add your essential oils to a cream that is lanolin-free, non-mineral and preferably organic. You will need to store your creams in amber-coloured glass jars – jars that hold 30g (1oz) and 60g (2oz) are the most appropriate.

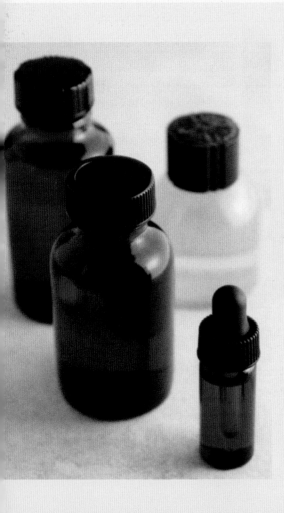

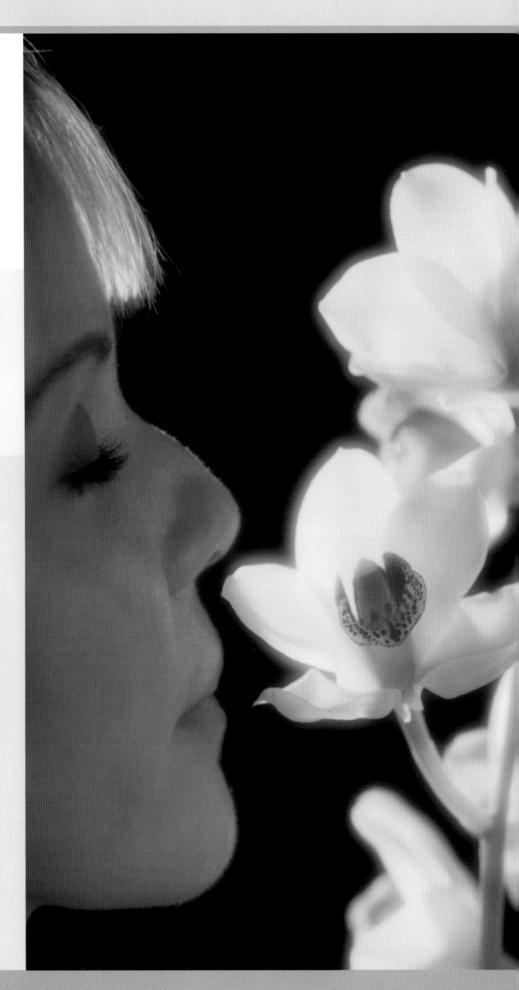

Recipes

Here are some recipes for oils and creams with which to treat dry or cracked, itchy, irritated or sensitive skin, or sweaty hands or feet. You'll also find some recipes for alleviating stress and tension and aches and pains, as well as one that revives and stimulates.

Using these aromatherapy blends during your final massage will add a wonderful finishing touch – an exquisite 'dessert'– to your hand and foot reflexology treatments.

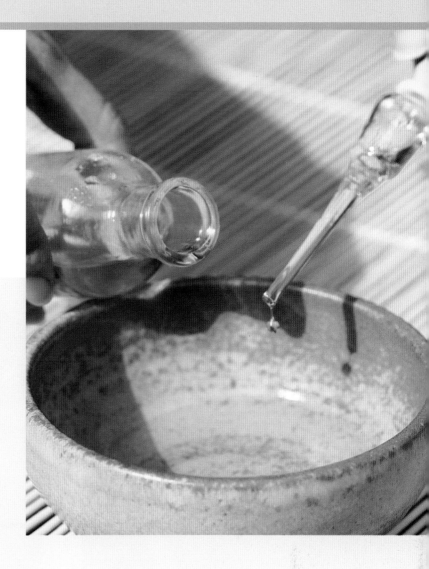

Formula for treating dry or cracked hands or feet

Aromatherapy oil blend
- 1 drop benzoin essential oil
- 1 drop myrrh essential oil
- 1 drop patchouli essential oil
in 10ml (2 teaspoons) carrier oil

Aromatherapy cream
- 2 drops benzoin essential oil
- 1 drop lavender essential oi
- 2 drops myrrh essential oil
- 2 drops sandalwood essential oil
in 30g (1oz) carrier cream

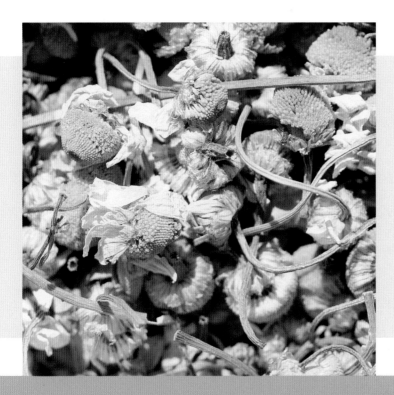

Formula for treating itchy, irritated or sensitive hands or feet

Aromatherapy oil blend
- 2 drops chamomile essential oil
- 1 drop lavender essential oil
in 10ml (2 teaspoons) carrier oil

Aromatherapy cream
- 2 drops chamomile essential oil
- 4 drops lavender essential oil
- 2 drops geranium essential oil
in 30g (1oz) carrier cream

Formula for treating sweaty hands or feet

Aromatherapy oil blend
- 1 drop cypress essential oil
- 1 drop lemon essential oil
- 1 drop peppermint essential oil

in 10ml (2 teaspoons) carrier oil

Aromatherapy cream
- 3 drops cypress essential oil
- 2 drops lemongrass essential oil
- 2 drops peppermint essential oil

in 30g (1oz) carrier cream

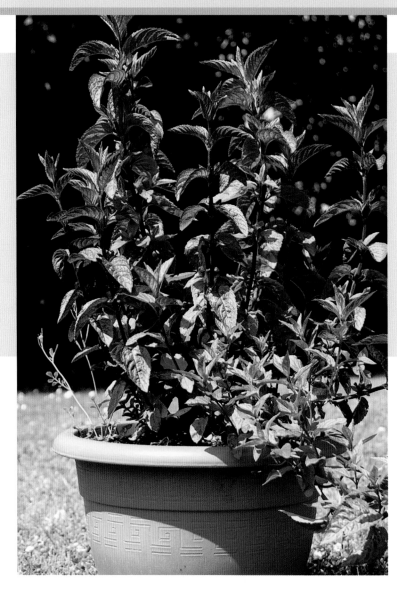

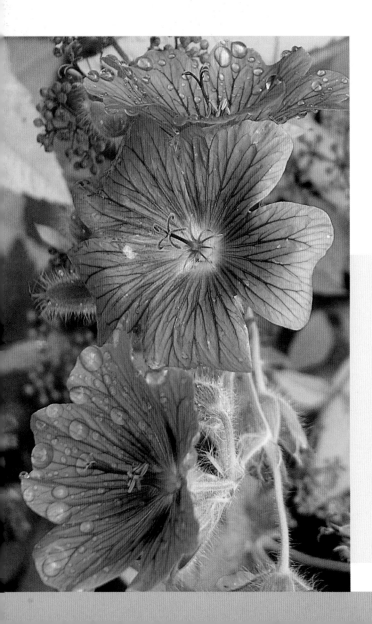

Formula for alleviating stress and tension

Aromatherapy oil blend
- 1 drop bergamot essential oil
- 1 drop frankincense essential oil
- 1 drop clary sage essential oil

in 10ml (2 teaspoons) carrier oil

Aromatherapy cream
- 2 drops geranium essential oil
- 3 drops lavender essential oil
- 2 drops bergamot essential oil

in 30g (1oz) carrier cream

Formula for alleviating aches and pains

Aromatherapy oil blend
- 1 drop chamomile essential oil
- 1 drop peppermint essential oil
- 1 drop lavender essential oil

in 10ml (2 teaspoons) carrier oil

Aromatherapy cream
- 1 drop frankincense essential oil
- 1 drop lavender essential oil
- 1 drop peppermint essential oil

in 30g (1oz) carrier cream

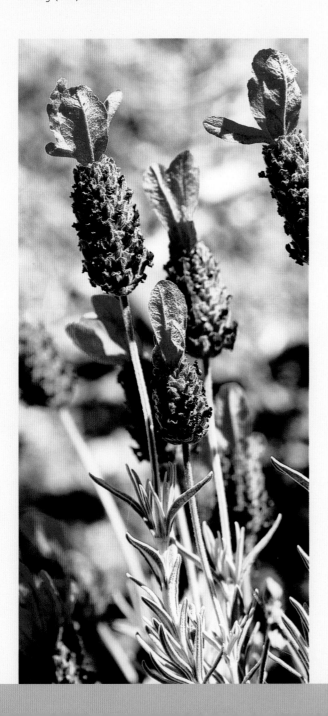

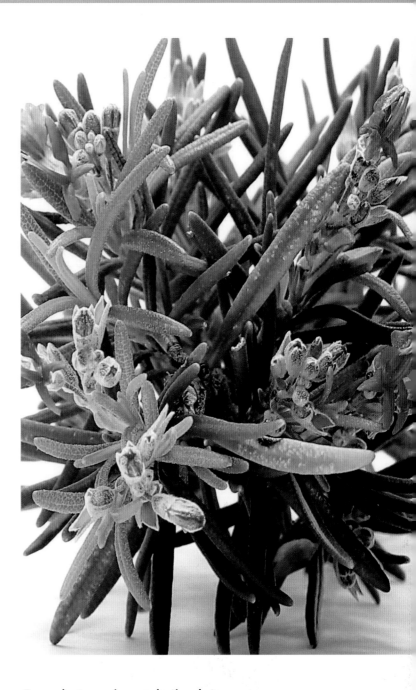

Formula to revive and stimulate

Aromatherapy oil blend
- 1 drop grapefruit essential oil
- 1 drop rosemary essential oil
- 1 drop bergamot essential oil

in 10ml (2 teaspoons) carrier oil

Aromatherapy cream
- 2 drops mandarin essential oil
- 3 drops rosemary essential oil
- 2 drops rosewood essential oil

in 30g (1oz) carrier cream

Charts

The following charts indicate the position of every reflex found on the feet and the hands. Study these charts to help you locate the points easily and accurately.

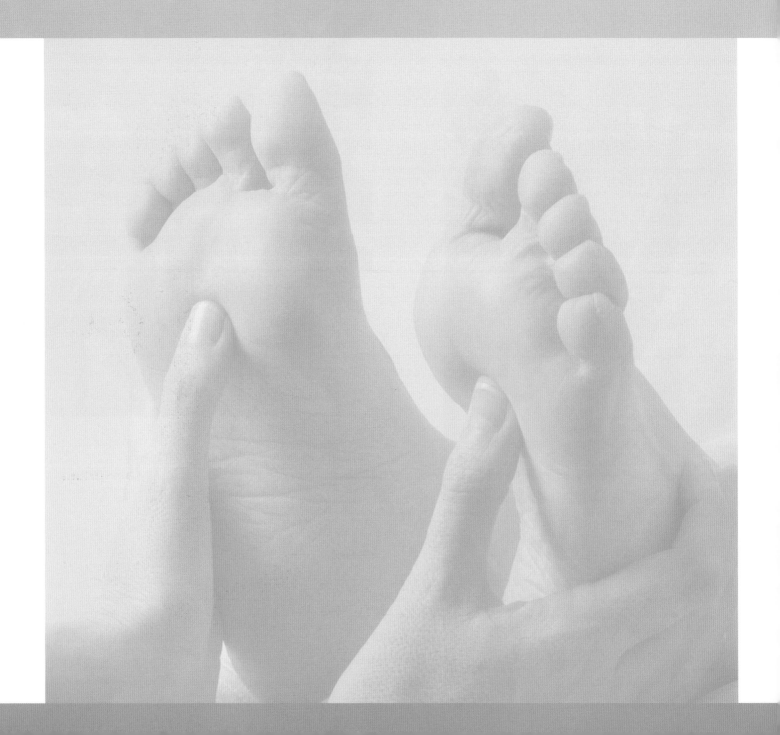

Medial and lateral sides of the foot

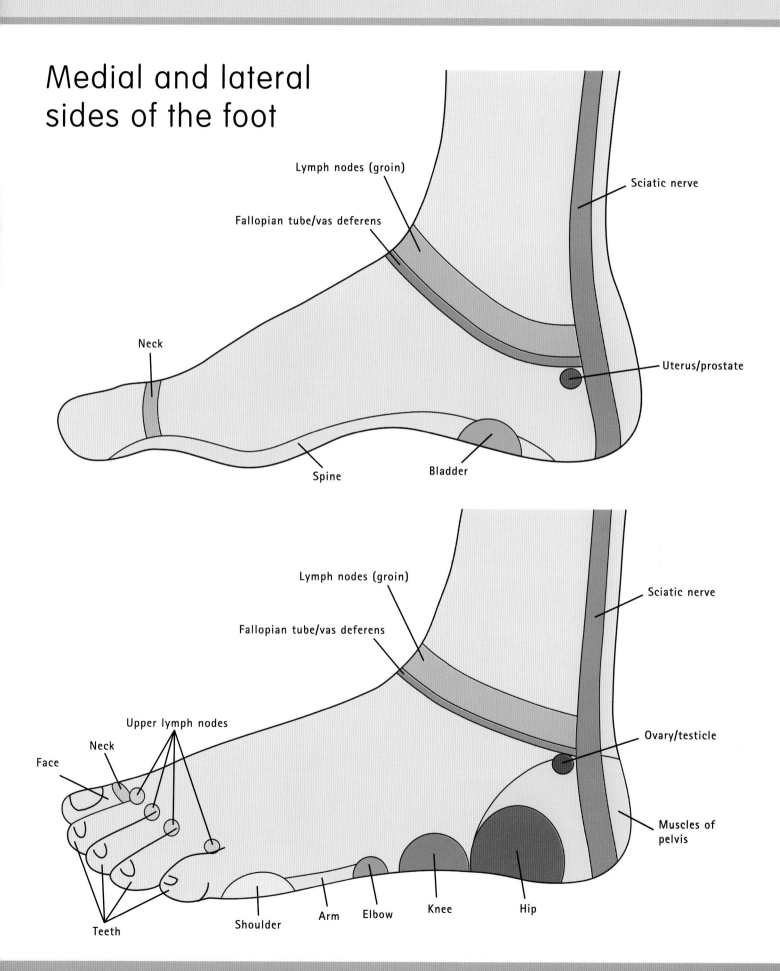

Lymph nodes (groin)

Sciatic nerve

Fallopian tube/vas deferens

Neck

Uterus/prostate

Spine

Bladder

Lymph nodes (groin)

Sciatic nerve

Fallopian tube/vas deferens

Upper lymph nodes

Neck

Face

Ovary/testicle

Muscles of pelvis

Teeth

Shoulder

Arm

Elbow

Knee

Hip

Sole of the right foot

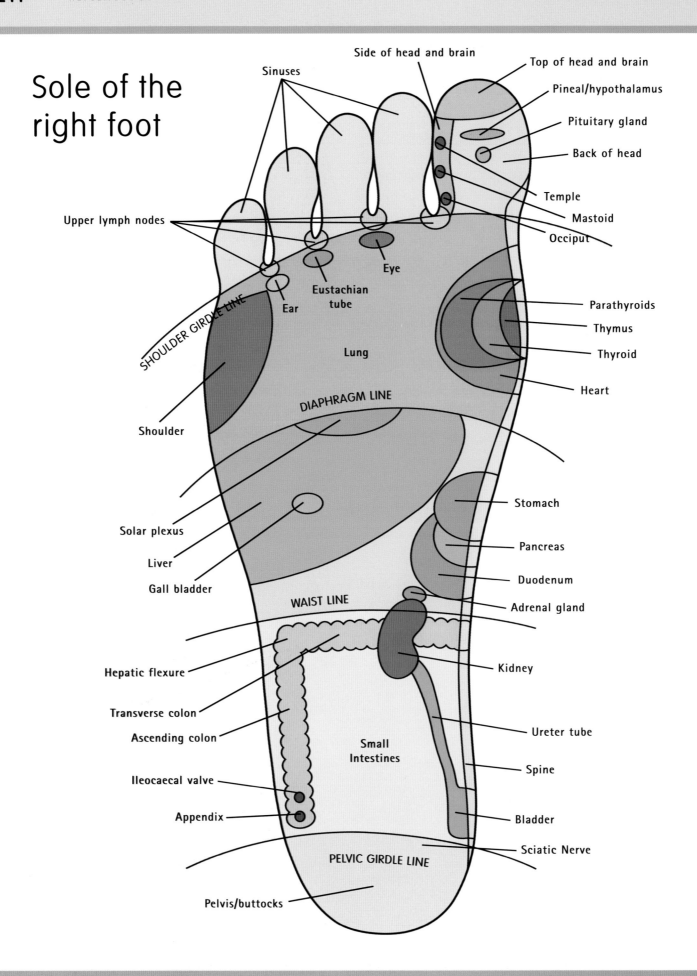

Sinuses

Side of head and brain

Top of head and brain

Pineal/hypothalamus

Pituitary gland

Back of head

Temple

Mastoid

Occiput

Upper lymph nodes

Eye

Eustachian tube

Ear

SHOULDER GIRDLE LINE

Parathyroids

Thymus

Thyroid

Heart

Lung

DIAPHRAGM LINE

Shoulder

Solar plexus

Liver

Gall bladder

Stomach

Pancreas

Duodenum

Adrenal gland

WAIST LINE

Hepatic flexure

Transverse colon

Ascending colon

Kidney

Ureter tube

Spine

Small Intestines

Ileocaecal valve

Appendix

Bladder

Sciatic Nerve

PELVIC GIRDLE LINE

Pelvis/buttocks

Sole of the left foot

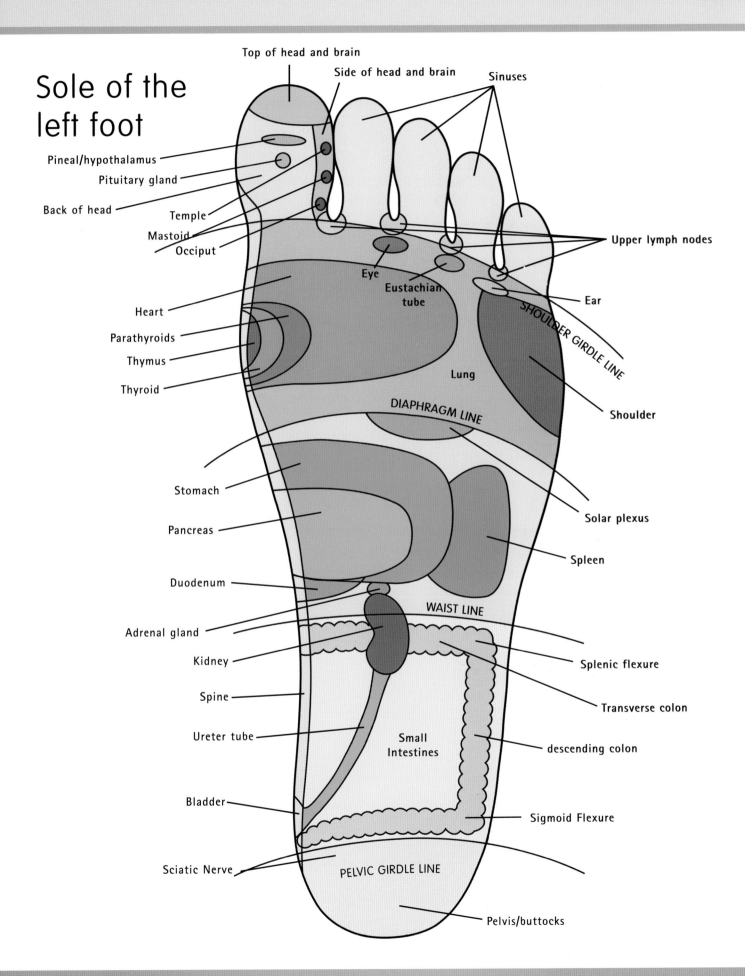

Top of head and brain
Side of head and brain
Sinuses
Pineal/hypothalamus
Pituitary gland
Back of head
Temple
Mastoid
Occiput
Eye
Eustachian tube
Upper lymph nodes
Heart
Parathyroids
Thymus
Thyroid
SHOULDER GIRDLE LINE
Ear
Lung
Shoulder
DIAPHRAGM LINE
Stomach
Pancreas
Solar plexus
Spleen
Duodenum
WAIST LINE
Adrenal gland
Kidney
Splenic flexure
Spine
Transverse colon
Ureter tube
Small Intestines
descending colon
Bladder
Sigmoid Flexure
Sciatic Nerve
PELVIC GIRDLE LINE
Pelvis/buttocks

Transverse zones of the feet

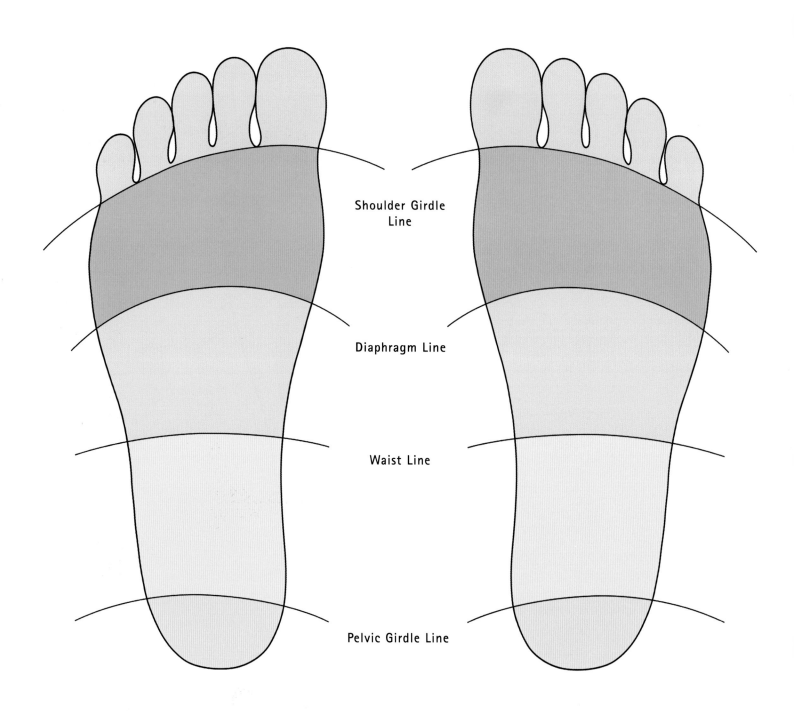

Shoulder Girdle Line

Diaphragm Line

Waist Line

Pelvic Girdle Line

Longitudinal zones of the feet

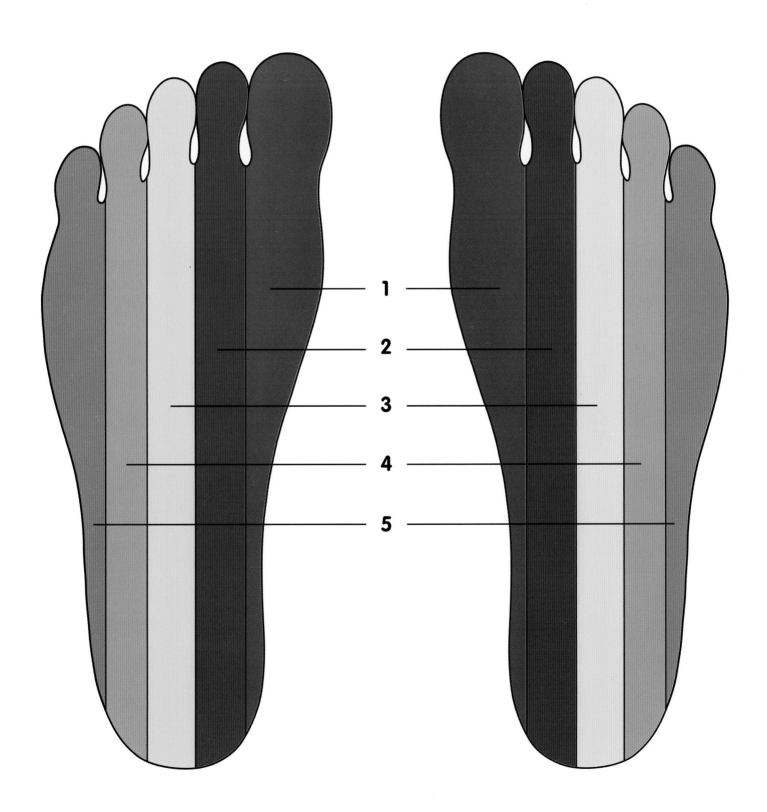

Palm of the right hand

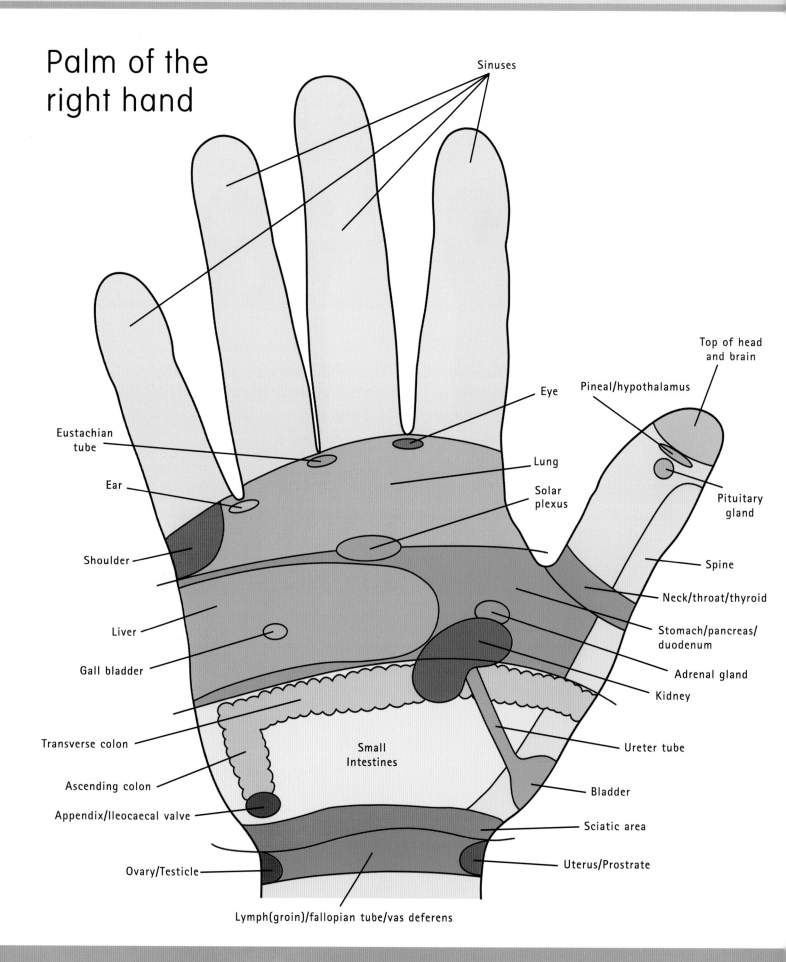

Sinuses

Eustachian tube

Ear

Shoulder

Liver

Gall bladder

Transverse colon

Ascending colon

Appendix/Ileocaecal valve

Ovary/Testicle

Eye

Lung

Solar plexus

Small Intestines

Lymph(groin)/fallopian tube/vas deferens

Top of head and brain

Pineal/hypothalamus

Pituitary gland

Spine

Neck/throat/thyroid

Stomach/pancreas/duodenum

Adrenal gland

Kidney

Ureter tube

Bladder

Sciatic area

Uterus/Prostrate

Palm of the left hand

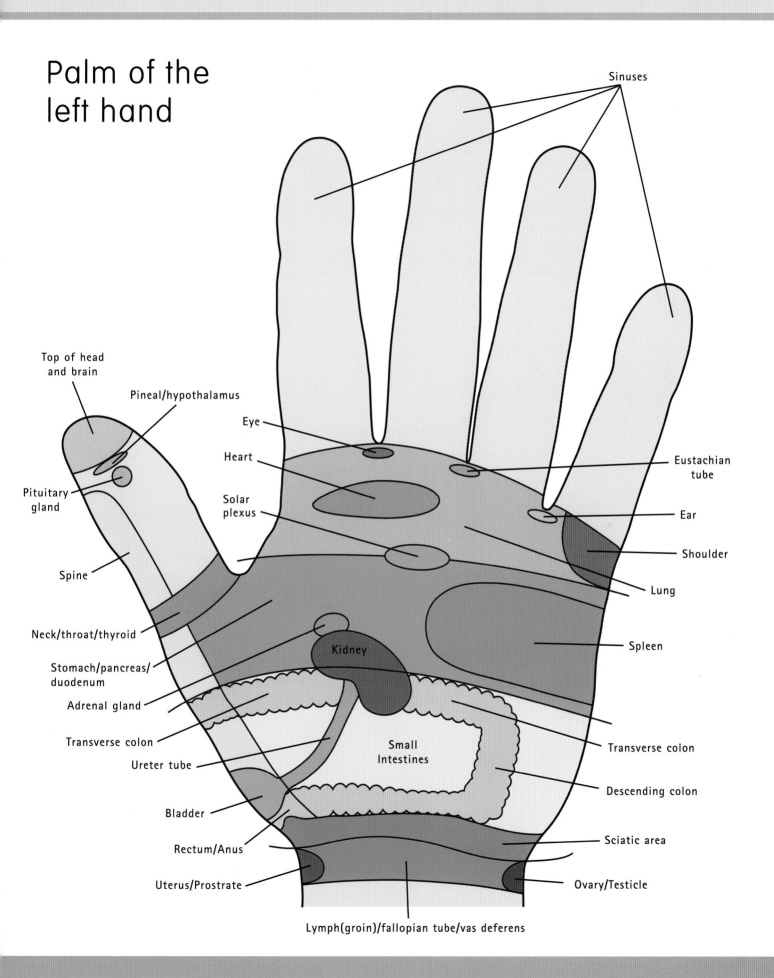

Sinuses

Top of head and brain

Pineal/hypothalamus

Eye

Heart

Solar plexus

Pituitary gland

Spine

Neck/throat/thyroid

Stomach/pancreas/duodenum

Adrenal gland

Transverse colon

Ureter tube

Bladder

Rectum/Anus

Uterus/Prostrate

Kidney

Small Intestines

Lymph(groin)/fallopian tube/vas deferens

Eustachian tube

Ear

Shoulder

Lung

Spleen

Transverse colon

Descending colon

Sciatic area

Ovary/Testicle

Transverse zones of the hands

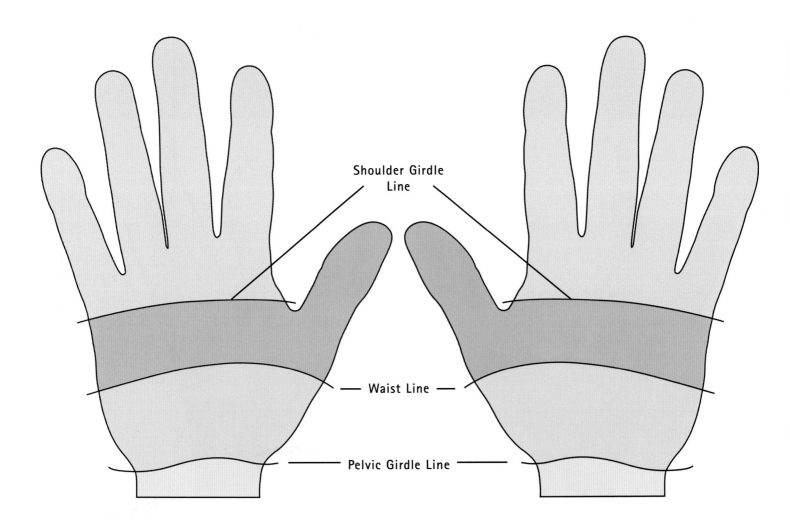

Shoulder Girdle Line

Waist Line

Pelvic Girdle Line

Longitudinal zones of the hands

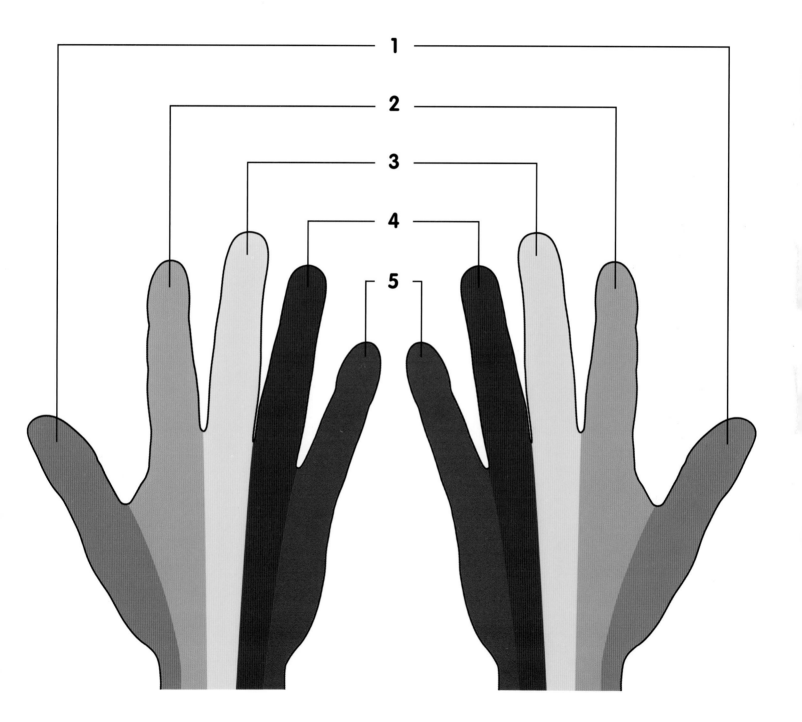

Index

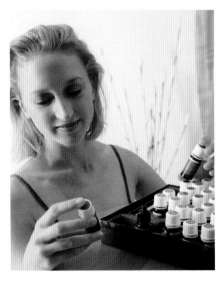

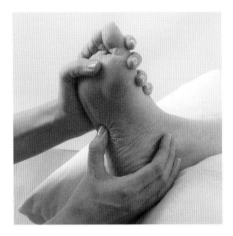

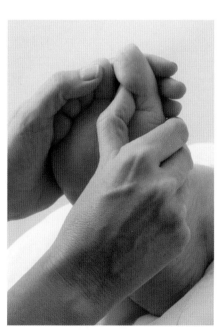

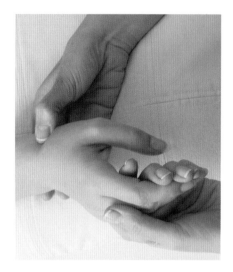

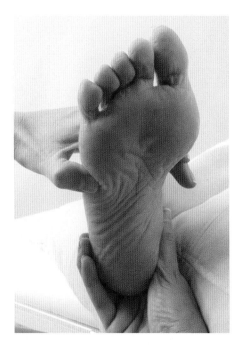

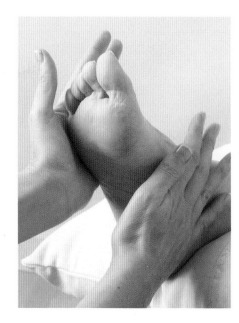

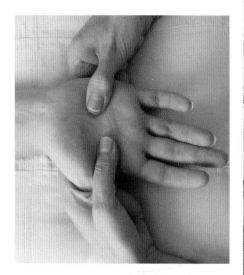